Bottom Line's HEALTHY HEART

The Breakthrough Program to Prevent, Halt and Even Reverse Heart Disease

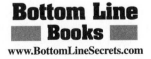

Bottom Line
Books
www.BottomLineSecrets.com

Michael Mogadam, M.D.

Bottom Line's Healthy Heart

The Breakthrough Program to Prevent, Halt and Even Reverse Heart Disease.
By Michael Mogadam, MD

Adaptation © 2009 by Boardroom® Inc.

ISBN 0-88723-517-4

10 9 8 7 6 5 4 3 2 1

Published by arrangement with Regnery Publishing, Inc.

Selected food ranking tables that appear on pages 188–232 are reprinted by arrangement with NAL Signet, a member of Penguin Group (USA) Inc. from *EATING FOR LIFE: One Simple Diet for Total Health* by Michael Mogadam, MD. Copyright © 2004, Michael Mogadam.

The information in this book has been carefully researched, and all efforts have been made to ensure accuracy as of the date published. Readers, particularly those with existing health problems and those who take prescription medications, are cautioned to consult with a health professional about specific recommendations for supplements and the appropriate dosages. The author and the publisher expressly disclaim responsibility for any adverse effects arising from the use or application of the information contained in this book.

Bottom Line Books® is a registered trademark of Boardroom Inc.
281 Tresser Blvd., Stamford CT 06901
www.BottomLineSecrets.com

Bottom Line Books® publishes the opinions of expert authorities in many fields. The use of this book is not a substitute for health or other professional services. Please consult a competent professional for answers to your specific questions.

Offers, prices, addresses, telephone numbers and Web sites listed in this book are accurate at the time of publication, but they are subject to frequent change.

Printed in the United States of America

TABLE OF CONTENTS

WHY THIS BOOK?

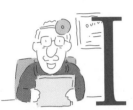I began this project because of a deep concern that for too long our healthcare system has been disease-oriented, and with a few exceptions has ignored prevention of a vast number of chronic diseases. We wait until people suffer heart attack, stroke, cancer, diabetes or any other ***preventable*** chronic disease, then we pounce on them with our expensive medical or surgical interventions, but we do very little or nothing to prevent these mostly preventable diseases. The consequence of this misdirected approach is that although we spend more per capita for our healthcare than any other country in the world, we are not a very healthy people! Look at table 1, and see what I mean.

Each year, more than one and a half million Americans suffer heart attacks, and many of them are in their 30s, 40s and 50s. Of the 500,000 who die from heart attacks each year, more than one-third won't even make it to a hospital; for them, all the sophisticated hospital based technology is worthless.

For more than three decades the medical community has promoted a flawed and outdated notion that elevated blood cholesterol is the principal cause of coronary artery disease, and that low-fat, low-cholesterol diets significantly lower blood cholesterol and therefore reduce the risk of heart attacks and strokes. Although an elevated blood cholesterol level is a major risk factor for coronary artery disease, so are 19 other major (and many minor) risk factors. Most of them are not affected by low-fat, low-cholesterol diets.

The sad state of misinformation prevails in the media and on internet sites concerning the causes of heart disease. When Vice President Dick Cheney suffered his fourth heart attack, newspapers across the country ran feature stories on the factors that contribute to coronary artery disease, and the "medical experts" on the television networks talked about the "major risk factors for heart attacks." Without exception, these reports parroted the conventional wisdom about coronary artery disease, citing only high cholesterol, high blood pressure, smoking and sedentary lifestyle as risk factors for heart attacks, with only a few mentioning diabetes as an added risk. None even hinted at the other 16 major coronary risk factors, some of which were relevant to Mr. Cheney's case.

Former President Bill Clinton had numerous coronary risk factors, most of which were either ignored or inadequately treated for years, until he nearly died before undergoing coronary artery bypass surgery. Only then, belatedly, his doctors began a more aggressive approach to

Table 1 **WILL THE "HEALTHY" AMERICAN PLEASE STAND UP! CHRONIC PREVENTABLE DISEASES IN AMERICANS**	
Preventable Diseases	**Millions**
• Weight Disorders	190
• Abnormal Blood Cholesterol	100
• Hypertension	95
• Coronary Artery Disease	60
• Osteoporosis	60
• Metabolic Syndrome*	50
• Diabetes and Prediabetes	45
• Alcoholism and other (Non-tobacco) Drug Addictions	30
• Peripheral Vascular Disease, Stroke/Dementa	10
• Cancers (Or Survivors) of Breast, Colon, Lung and Prostate	5
• Chronic Smoking-related Lung Diseases	5
• Chronic Liver Diseases (Hepatitis B and C; not counting fatty liver)	3
TOTAL	**653****

*Metabolic syndrome is a combination of three or more of the following: A sedentary lifestyle, abdominal obesity, cholesterol abnormalities and high blood pressure, with or without diabetes.

**Of course there are some overlaps!

Today, millions of Americans with major coronary risk factors are equally ignored or mismanaged. Recent data have shown that perhaps for the first time in generations, the baby boomers are less healthy and have far more chronic diseases than the previous generation. We live longer, but are not healthier. Fewer baby boomers smoke than their parents, but far more have weight issues, diabetes, high cholesterol, heart attacks and strokes. But this is not just an American tragedy; most developed and nearly all developing and underdeveloped countries have similar senseless models for their healthcare that ignore prevention and focus on treatment. Given this imbalanced and disease-oriented approach to healthcare, shouldn't we be more proactive in protecting and insulating ourselves against these preventable diseases?

Over the past decade a large number of studies have convincingly shown that coronary artery disease, diabetes, cancers of the breast, colon, lung or prostate, and a host of other chronic diseases are mostly preventable! (See table 2.) (US population is more than 300 million.) The good news is that prevention does not have to be convoluted, hard-to-follow, or require people to become dietary monks or elite athletes.

The risk reductions shown in table 2 are what we can achieve with the practical and easy-to-do dietary and lifestyle modifications I have presented in this book. Detection and correction of risk factors contributing to these preventable diseases will reduce the risk even more. What the risk factors are, how to detect, modify or effectively manage them are all detailed for you in these chapters. Do you need one special diet to control diabetes, another to lower cholesterol or blood pressure, and yet another to manage your weight? And one to reduce your cancer risk? Should your diet be low-fat, low-cholesterol? High-carb, low-fat, or low-fat high-carb? Should

control his multiple coronary risk factors. Women's cardiovascular health is still compromised by a pervasive gender bias, under-diagnosis and under-treatment, which former Director of the US National Health Institutes Bernadine Healy has called the "Yentl syndrome." She noted that, "The only way a woman can get a reasonable cardiovascular care is to be a man!" Gender inequality in cardiovascular care has improved, but ever so slightly.

Table 2
HEALTHY DIET AND LIFESTYLE
CONTRIBUTE TO:

- 91% reduction in type 2 DIABETES in women and 60% reduction in men[1]
- 83% reduction in the rate of CORONARY ARTERY DISEASE[2]
- 71% reduction in COLON CANCER[3]
- 65% reduction in ALL CAUSE DEATHS even in older persons[4]
- 60% reduction in METABOLIC SYNDROME[5]
- And, dramatic reductions in almost all other CHRONIC DISEASES![6]

1- Hu FB et al. N Eng J Med 2001; 345: 790–97
2- Stampfer MJ et al. N Eng J Med 2000; 343: 16–22
3- Platz EA et al. Cancer Causes Control 2000; 11: 579–8
4- Knoops KTB et al. JAMA 2004; 292: 1433–39
5- Esposito K et al. JAMA 2004; 292: 1440–46
6- Dansinger ML, Schaefer EJ. JAMA 2006; 295:94–5

---

it have high protein, but low calories? No meat, vegan? Do you have to starve yourself to be healthy? The simple answer is none of the above!

Bottom Line's Healthy Heart offers you a novel, all-in-one, state-of-the-art diet that will supplant all others. The plan here is an easy and enjoyable diet with a vast number of choices, limited only by your taste and culinary preferences. The diet helps people of all ages reduce their risk factors, promotes heart health and disease-free positive aging. The Twenty Risk Factor Diet, or TRF scoring system is fully explained, and I have provided the TRF ratings for everyday foods, grocery products and fast foods.

Almost every day I see men and women in my practice, many in their prime, who have undiagnosed or inadequately treated major coronary risk factors. According to the US Census Bureau, more than 93 million Americans are 45 years of age or older. At least one-half of this population has coronary artery disease in various stages;

almost everyone in this group has multiple identifiable coronary risk factors. We can dramatically reduce cardiovascular disabilities and deaths by hundreds of thousands by diagnosing and appropriately treating these treatable risk factors.

In the United States, the annual death toll from heart attacks, strokes and hardening of the arteries is over 920,000. This is equal to the next seven leading causes of death combined, including cancers, chronic lung diseases, AIDS and other infections, accidents, diabetes, suicides and homicides. Yet most of the cardiovascular diseases are preventable (and it is quite possible to predict with a reasonable degree of accuracy who is at high risk). As seen in table 3, coronary artery disease doesn't just happen when we reach 40 or 50 years of age; it begins at a young age, at times in infancy or childhood, and progresses slowly over the years before causing a fatal or nonfatal heart attack.

The goal is early intervention. I tell my patients that if they delay by one day, they are behind by one week; if they delay by one week, they are behind by one month; if they delay by a month; they are behind by a year! *Bottom Line's*

Table 3
PERCENT OF YOUNG AMERICANS
WITH EARLY OR ADVANCED
CORONARY ARTERY DISEASE

	White		African American	
Age	Male	Female	Male	Female
15–19	24	7	24	18
20–24	28	15	32	12
25–29	39	21	42	25
30–34	51	32	49	38

Based on autopsy data of 2,876 subjects who, died of non-cardiac causes.

Strong JP et al. JAMA 1999; 281: 727–35

Mc Mahan CA et al. Arch Intern Med 2005; 165: 883–90

Healthy Heart gives you the tools, and step-by-step directions, like the GPS in your car—your own GCP: *Global Cardiovascular Protection!*

For you, your family, your friends and anyone else you care to share your gained knowledge with, my wishes for happy and healthy hearts.

This is an epidemic that demands action, and this book provides you with a personal battle plan. *Bottom Line's Healthy Heart* means what it says—and shows you how to protect yourself, practically, from the most important coronary risk factors.

Bottom Line's Healthy Heart is a compelling all-in-one book that gives you the latest science—science your doctor might not even know. It will show you how to save your heart—and perhaps your life.

For convenience, I have included numerous easy-to-read tables and figures that illustrate what is being discussed in the text. You will find cross-references throughout the text to other sections of the book where more information can be found about the subject under discussion.

Also in the back is a useful glossary of scientific and medical terms.

—Michael Mogadam, M.D.

THE ABCs OF CORONARY ARTERY DISEASE

Blood Cholesterol

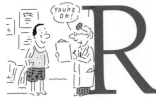

Right or wrong, the first item most people think about concerning heart attack or stroke is their blood cholesterol level. Although it is true that certain cholesterol particles circulating in the bloodstream have an essential role in the development of coronary artery disease, all cholesterol particles are not alike. Some are harmful and others carry significant benefits for the heart. So before we proceed with other issues, let's demystify and understand what it is we are talking about.

Cholesterol is a type of fat which is present only in animals. No plant or plant product contains cholesterol. Cholesterol is not a useless or harmful substance without any redeeming features. Nearly all animal and human cells have some cholesterol as a component of their cell wall or internal machinery. Without sufficient cholesterol, animal life could not exist. But as with blood sugar, calcium and sodium, it is the excessive levels of blood cholesterol that are harmful.

Cholesterol cannot dissolve in the bloodstream. To move from the intestine and liver into other tissues, cholesterol needs a vehicle. These vehicles are called "lipoproteins" (*lipo*, from the word lipid, means fat, so lipoprotein means plus proteins). The more protein and the less fat lipoproteins have, the heavier or "denser" they are. This is analogous to a lean steak being denser than a piece of steak with fatty streaks. On the basis of their protein content or density, lipoproteins fall into five major classes (Figure 1)…

1. Very low-density lipoproteins (VLDL)
2. Intermediate-density lipoproteins (IDL)
3. Low-density lipoproteins (LDL)
4. High-density lipoproteins (HDL)
5. Humans, primates and a few other animals have another lipoprotein called "lipoprotein(a)." But lipoprotein(a) is not measured in a routine cholesterol panel.

Triglycerides (tri=three connected fatty acids) are the predominant form of fat in the bloodstream, especially soon after consuming fatty meals. Triglycerides do not contain any cholesterol or protein; hence they are not lipoproteins. However, all lipoproteins, especially VLDL particles, carry some triglycerides in their core. With the exception of HDL (the "good" cholesterol), all other lipoproteins are coronary-unfriendly (the "bad" cholesterol).

The protein part of lipoproteins is called *apoprotein*. Apoproteins are essentially the "brain" or conductor of lipoproteins, and they are responsible

Figure 1
Lipoprotein Cholesterol Particles

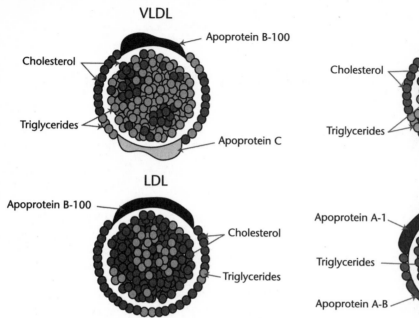

for the good or the bad deeds of these little fat globules. The three important apoproteins are A-1, which makes HDL cardio-protective, B-100, which is responsible for the misdeeds of LDL, and apoprotein E, which determines whether people's blood cholesterol goes up in response to fatty foods.

At present, the National Cholesterol Education Program (NCEP), which is composed of over 20 organizations including the American Heart Association, has set guidelines for blood levels of various lipoproteins and triglycerides (table 4). Unfortunately, these guidelines are confusing and often handcuff healthcare providers so that they become less active in the management of cholesterol disorders.

The NCEP guidelines were dated and practically useless when they were published in 2004. They should have a disclaimer stating, "These guidelines may be harmful to your health if followed as directed!" Look at figure 2

for a moment. Most of the heart attack victims have cholesterol levels that the NCEP calls "low risk" or "moderate risk" i.e., total cholesterol levels that range from 180 mg/dl to 240 mg/dl. How would you like to be dismissed casually

Figure 2
The Relation of Total Blood Cholestrol (mg/dl) to Risk of Heart Attack

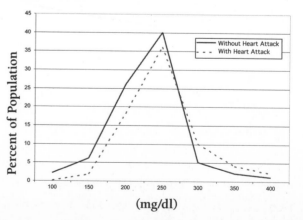

Table 4
NCEP ADULT TREATMENT PANEL GUIDELINES

Low Risk:	Less than 160 mg/dl	Over 190 mg/dl
0–1 risk factors		(160–189: drugs optional)
Moderate risk:	Less than 130 mg/dL	Over 160 mg/dL
2+ risk factors, and <10%		
10-year risk of CV events		
Moderately high risk:	Less than 130 mg/dL	Over 130 mg/dL
2+ risk factors and 10%-20%		
10-year risk of CV events		
Very high risk:	Less than 100 mg/dL	Over 100 mg/dL
CHD or CHD equivalents		(Less than 100: drugs optional)

CHD=Coronary heart disease

Grundy SM et al. Circulation 2004; 110:227–39

LDL-C=LDL-cholesterol   CV=Cardiovascular disease   CHD=coronary heart disease

Table 5
OPTIMAL BLOOD CHOLESTEROL
LEVELS FOR MEN, WOMEN AND
PEOPLE OF ALL AGES

Lipid Components	mg/dl
Total Cholesterol	Less than 180
LDL-cholesterol*	Less than 100
HDL-cholesterol:	
For Men	More than 45
For Women	More than 55
Vldl-cholesterol	Less than 25
Triglycerides	Less than 130
Non-HDL-cholesterol	Less than 130
Triglycerides/HDL Ratio	Less than 3

*LDL should be under 70 for those with cardiovascular diseases; diabetes; metabolic syndrome; chronic kidney disease; rhumatoid arthritis, lupus or AIDS and those with multiple major coronary risk factors.

Figure 3
Estimated Prevalence of Cardiovascular Disease (By Age and Sex)

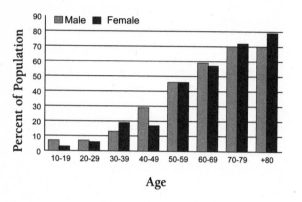

as having "moderate risk" cholesterol and be told "let's just watch it"? (Sometimes I wish I had the power to erase this sentence from healthcare providers' vocabulary!) What is it that you're supposed to watch for? Watch for a massive heart attack, a fatal or disabling stroke? Would you like to volunteer for this irrational watch and see program? Wouldn't you rather opt for a proactive intervention now to prevent such catastrophic cardiovascular events?

So what is an acceptable or "goal" cholesterol level? After reviewing several hundred recent studies dealing with the role of cholesterol abnormalities in cardiovascular diseases, I have developed a simplified and evidence-based alternative to NCEP guidelines. My guidelines are presented in table 5.

Anatomy of a Heart Attack: The "Coronary Quartet"

Heart attacks do not suddenly strike people when they reach their forties or fifties. In most cases the process begins in childhood and adolescence. Heart attacks are the end point or the last stage of the smoldering process I have called the "Coronary Quartet."

Stage One: Endothelial dysfunction

Unlike the skin, or the eye's cornea, which have multiple layers, the inner lining of arteries (the endothelium) is made up of a single layer of cells (the endothelial cells) like tiles on the kitchen floor, and damage can occur just like dirt and grime can accumulate on the kitchen tiles. Without dysfunction or damage to the endothelial cells, hardly anyone would develop heart attack, stroke or peripheral arterial closure. When these cells are damaged by the risk factors, they become leaky and allow white blood cells, platelets and LDL-cholesterol particles to pass into the artery's wall. The role of endothelial cells in protecting against coronary artery disease and heart attacks is so important that Dr. Robert Furchgott of the State University of New York in Brooklyn was awarded the Nobel Prize in Physiology and Medicine for his pioneering research in this area.

Stage Two: Oxidation of LDL-cholesterol

When we take a bite out of an apple and allow the apple to sit on the counter, it begins to turn brown within a short time. This is oxidation. A rusty nail is also the product of oxidation. In general, LDL-cholesterol particles are not harmful unless they are oxidized, either in the bloodstream or inside the wall of coronary or other arteries. When the endothelial lining of the arteries is damaged or dysfunctional, LDL particles trespass into a leaky arterial wall and become oxidized, especially if there are very few or no antioxidants present to defend these particles (figure 4). Oxidized LDL becomes the arsonist that sets the artery wall on fire, and then keeps fueling the flames.

Stage Three: Plaque formation

White blood cells in the artery walls consider oxidized LDL particles delicious morsels and gobble them up as fast as they can. When these white

Figure 4
Coronary Artery Disease Quartet

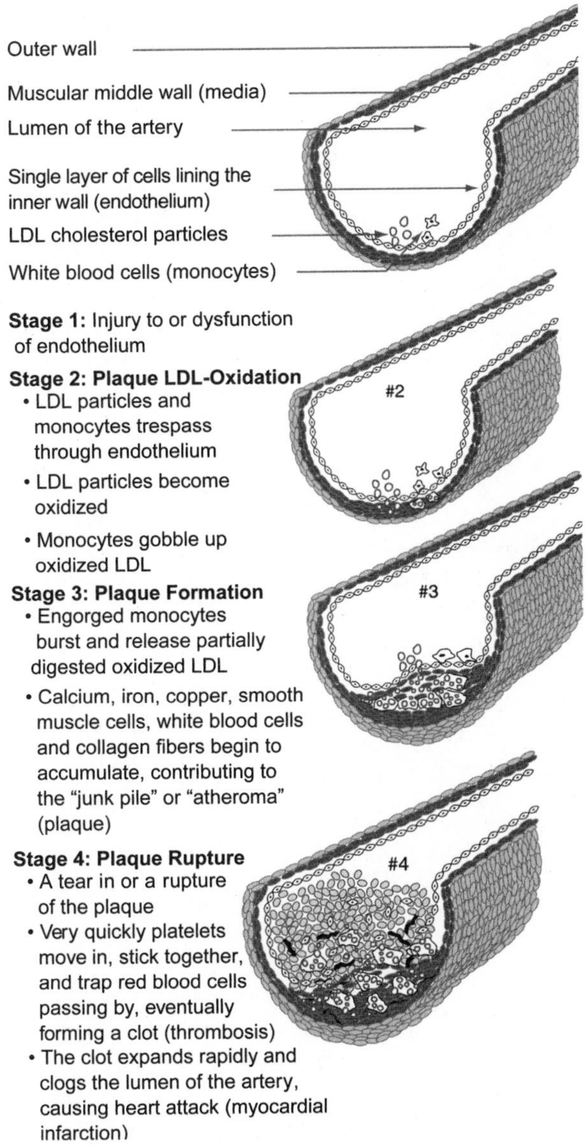

Outer wall

Muscular middle wall (media)

Lumen of the artery

Single layer of cells lining the
inner wall (endothelium)

LDL cholesterol particles

White blood cells (monocytes)

Stage 1: Injury to or dysfunction
of endothelium

Stage 2: Plaque LDL-Oxidation
• LDL particles and
  monocytes trespass
  through endothelium
• LDL particles become
  oxidized
• Monocytes gobble up
  oxidized LDL

Stage 3: Plaque Formation
• Engorged monocytes
  burst and release partially
  digested oxidized LDL
• Calcium, iron, copper, smooth
  muscle cells, white blood cells
  and collagen fibers begin to
  accumulate, contributing to
  the "junk pile" or "atheroma"
  (plaque)

Stage 4: Plaque Rupture
• A tear in or a rupture
  of the plaque
• Very quickly platelets
  move in, stick together,
  and trap red blood cells
  passing by, eventually
  forming a clot (thrombosis)
• The clot expands rapidly and
  clogs the lumen of the artery,
  causing heart attack (myocardial
  infarction)

blood cells have gorged on LDL particles, they burst at the seams or release partially digested LDL particles into the artery wall. These toxic by products cause biochemical turmoil within the wall of the artery. Slowly, smooth muscle cells and collagen fibers begin to move into the area of turmoil and entrap a number of substances from the circulating blood, including calcium, iron, copper, magnesium and fibrin. This "junk pile" thickens the arterial wall, and makes it bulge into the lumen of the artery. At this point, the junk pile is called a *plaque*, or a *coronary lesion*. When numerous coronary lesions are scattered throughout the arterial tree, the condition is called *atherosclerosis,* or *hardening of the arteries.*

The first three stages of a coronary quartet can be seen as early as childhood and adolescence. In fact, some autopsy data from infants who died of noncardiac causes have shown early changes in the first few weeks of life, suggesting that the process of heart disease can begin at any time. But it usually takes many years for the progression of the first three stages of the coronary quartet, and the process sometimes spans 30 to 50 years. It is this slow progression that lulls people into inaction until the catastrophic fourth stage.

Stage Four: Plaque Rupture

Tragically, for 500,000 Americans each year, the fourth stage is a fatal event. The goal is to prevent the progression of this deterioration long before its final stage. Fatty plaques are very fragile, unstable, and can crack or rupture easily. These "unstable plaques," or "vulnerable lesions," can rupture, and account for more than 80% of heart attacks (the other 20% are due to progressive clogging of the artery).

When a vulnerable plaque bursts, blood platelets quickly move in and clump together and form the core of a blood clot that gets larger and larger (within a few minutes to a few hours). This newly formed clot (or "thrombus") chokes off blood flow to the heart muscle. This is a heart attack or a "myocardial infarction." Depending on the size and the speed at which a coronary thrombosis expands, the individual may suffer a minor heart attack, or a massive and fatal one.

To prevent coronary artery disease and a subsequent heart attack, we must prevent the coronary quartet at the starting gate, or interrupt it as early as possible. Even among people with advanced coronary artery disease who have already suffered heart attacks, a future coronary event can be prevented by stopping the progression of the coronary quartet. Subsequent chapters will provide effective recommendations to achieve this goal by reducing major coronary risk factors and stabilizing existing coronary plaques.

Major Cardiovascular Risk Factors

Heart attacks and strokes—unlike diseases such as strep throat or specific injuries like a broken wrist—do not have a single identifiable cause. A variety of risk factors is almost always involved. I liken it to driving down a winding mountain road on a rainy night at 60 miles per hour—with bad brakes, worn tire treads, and streaking windshield wipers—while dozing off

Table 6
THE TWENTY MAJOR CARDIOVASCULAR RISK FACTORS

Risk Factor:	Relative Risk[1]	Risk Factor:	Relative Risk[1]
1-Diabetes (especially when poorly controlled)	5	11-Chronic inflammations, such as rheumatoid arthritis, lupus or infections (AIDS)	3
2-Abdominal obesity and metabolic syndrome	3	12-Hypertension	2
3-Sedentary lifestyle	3	13-High blood levels of lipoprotein(a) (over 65mg/dl[4])	2
4-Atherogenic ("Western") diet (especially high trans fats, low Omega-3 intake)	3	14-Family history of premature cardiovascular disease	2
5-Low levels of HDL-cholesterol (under 40 for men, 50 for women)	3	15-High blood levels of homocysteine over 15mol/l	2
6-Elevated LDL-cholesterol (over 100 mg/dl[2])	3	16-Negative affect or "HAD" syndrome (Hostility, Anger, Depression)	2
7-Elevated triglyceries, especially at high levels, more so in women	3	17-Hematocrit over 48% (or hemglobin over 17g/dl); anemia (Hg less than 11 g/dl)[5]	2
8-Age over 45 for men, over 55 for women[3]	3	18-Abnormal blood platelet function, or high fibrinogen levels over 300mg	2
9-Smoking	3	19-Chronic lung disease or obstructive sleep apnea[6]	2
10-Chronic kidney dysfuntion (more than 8 million Americans have CKD)	3	20-Low birth weight, under 5 lb	2

[1]For comparison, the relative risk of lung cancer in a heavy smoker vs. nonsmokers is 10.

[2]For those with cardiovascular disease; diabetes; chronic kidney dysfuntion; rheumatoid arthritis, lupus, and AIDS; or multiple major cardiovascular risk factor, optimal LDL should be under 70mg/dl

[3]Relative risk for men under 65 is 8 times and at under age 79 is 34 times higher than at under age 35.

[4]More so when associated with elevated LDL, eleveted fibrinogen or low levels of HDL

[#]Danik JS et al. JAMA 2007; 296: 1363-70

[5]Sabatine MS et al. Circulation 2005; 111: 2042-9

[6]Marin JM et al. Lancet 2005; 365: 1046-53

[6]Yaggi HK et al. N Eng J Med 2005; 353: 2034-41

behind the wheel. Numerous risk factors lead to a catastrophic accident. A single risk factor is, of course, less likely to result in an accident. Similarly, multiple interacting risk factors over the course of many years dramatically increase your risk of a heart attack or stroke.

In a few situations, the pace of coronary artery disease is greatly accelerated—especially after coronary angioplasty, with certain infections, including AIDS in people with rhumatoid arthritis or lupus, or after a heart transplantation. In these situations, the damage that usually takes 20 to 40 years can be compressed into months or a few short years. In each instance—whether the usual variety of coronary artery disease or the accelerated form—the more numerous and the more aggressive the risk factors are, the shorter the lag time to a fully developed coronary artery disease and heart attack.

How Many Risk Factors Are There for Cardiovascular Diseases?

For nearly 40 years medical thinking has focused on the four "traditional" risk factors: high cholesterol, high blood pressure, smoking and diabetes, and has ignored other equally important risk factors.

In a recent international study of 122,458 patients with coronary heart disease, one out of five patients did not have any of the traditional risk factors, and the majority of people who had one traditional risk factor also had one or more additional risk factors.

In fact, it is extremely unlikely for someone to develop coronary heart disease solely on the basis of a single traditional risk factor. The only exception is a severe familial disorder among adolescents and young people in whom blood cholesterol levels may be greater than 500 mg/dl. A large number of these young people

develop severe coronary artery disease in their teens and, on occasion, even earlier.

Coronary and cerebral artery disease and the subsequent heart attacks and strokes are nearly always "multifactorial;" they are the consequences of the damaging impact of multiple risk factors over many years, often beginning at an early age. A narrow focus on one or two risk factors, while leaving many "foxes in the chicken coop," is a major reason why nearly one million Americans die each year of cardiovascular diseases.

"MINOR" CARDIOVASCULAR RISK FACTORS

- Certain genetic defects of enzymes involved in metabolism of fat and cholesterol

- Chronically elevated white blood cell count, high levels of blood iron (hemochromatosis)

- Alcoholism, gout, underactive thyroid, migraines, chronic periodontitis or sinusitis

- Not taking afternoon nap (working, not chronically ill or sedentary persons)

- Long-term use of immune suppressing drugs such as steroids or cyclosporine, and some antiviral drugs

- Certain occupations (for example air traffic controllers, firemen, police, clergy and coal miners)

- Air pollution, soft water, including most bottled waters that are low in magnesium and calcium

- Certain backgrounds, African-Americans, Middle Easterners, Eastern Europeans, Indians and Pakistanis

There are also a large number of *risk markers* such as elevated blood levels of C-reactive protein, rapid heart rate at rest and social factors, such as being single, divorced or widowed, lack of justice at work or poverty, that are associated with higher risk for cardiovascular events but are not risk factors for cardiovascular disease.

As seen in table 6, there are 20 major cardiovascular risk factors that contribute to more than 95% of all heart attacks, strokes and peripheral vascular disease. However, there is also a large, expanding list of minor, or less common, risk factors. These minor risk factors add to the burden of pre-existing major risk factors. In addition, there is a growing list of "markers" that are actually warning signals for ongoing, active cardiovascular disease. These markers are similar to smoke coming out of a burning building; the smoke is a sign of the fire but not the cause of it.

Don't assume that because you don't smoke, and have normal blood pressure or level of LDL-cholesterol that you are unlikely to suffer a heart attack or stroke. I wish that were true. The fact is that the vast majority (95%) of adults in the US, Northern and Eastern Europe, Australia, the Middle East and other parts of the world have one of the 20 major coronary risk factors.

Every major cardiovascular risk factor counts and we cannot "cherry pick" one or two for intervention and ignore the others. Would it help much if you only replace the battery in your stalled car but ignore the spark plugs, water pump, the empty gas tank and flat tires? We need a basket of interventions to correct every risk factor or as many risk factors as we can.

The impact of a certain coronary risk factor is not the same for each person. The response of an individual to high levels of homocysteine or LDL-cholesterol, high blood pressure or smoking may be greater or less than that of another person. But having several risk factors significantly increases the risk of coronary artery disease and eventually a heart attack in almost every person. In subsequent chapters, I will demystify all the major coronary risk factors, and provide you with a state-of-the-art road map that will enable you to deal with any risk factors you may have.

Minor Cardiovascular Risk Factors

Many of the minor risk factors are chronic diseases or socioeconomic factors. In most cases, their negative impact on coronary arteries is indirect and is due to their association with, and contribution to, a variety of major risk factors. For example, an underactive thyroid gland can not only raise the LDL-cholesterol by 30 to 50%, it can also cause hypertension which will then increase the risk of coronary artery disease.

Chronic infections, such as periodontitis or sinusitis, contribute to the release of certain inflammatory compounds that add to the turmoil within the artery plaques. So we must make every effort to treat and eradicate such chronic infections. Air pollution in most large American cities and Europe (and even greater in developing parts of the world) has steadily increased. Recent studies reported in the *New England Journal of Medicine* have shown that long-term exposure to fine particulate air pollution increases the risk of cardiovascular events by more than 70% compared to people who are not exposed to heavy air pollution.

Socioeconomic factors contribute to poor access to, or lack of, medical care and to undertreatment of major risk factors such as hypertension, abnormal blood cholesterol levels, diabetes and stress or negative affect. Excessive drinking, smoking, lack of exercise, poor nutrition and low intake of antioxidants may also be contributing factors. It is highly unlikely that poverty, overcrowding or a given occupation—by themselves and independent of the 20 major risk factors—have a direct and robust impact on coronary arteries.

Estrogen deficiency in young, post-menopausal women (but not in women past their late 60s) is a relatively easy risk factor to remedy for those who are motivated. Balding, early graying and short stature are markers for a genetic predisposition to low HDL-cholesterol, abdominal obesity, elevated blood cholesterol and triglycerides. They are not associated with a stand-alone, genetic abnormality which can independently harm coronary arteries.

Certain blood types (such as Lewis a-negative or b-negative) can increase the risk of coronary artery disease, but the underlying mechanisms are not well defined. Presumably in these blood types, the risk of clot formation inside the coronary artery is somewhat increased. A combination of low-dose aspirin (81 milligrams per day) and three to four seafood meals a week is often sufficient to counteract the negative impact of these blood types, provided there are no other associated major risk factors.

What you should do

The contribution of minor risk factors to coronary artery disease may be relatively small. Their presence should heighten your awareness and your doctor's effort to look for and correct any coexisting major risk factors. Although you should try to correct as many of these minor risk factors as you can, your main focus should still be on major risk factors.

What you must do is ask you doctor to see whether you have any of the minor risk factors. And if you do have any minor risk factors, ask your doctor to test you for the major risk factors and to treat you for all your risk factors. Of course if you live in a large polluted city or have a highly stressful job, your doctor won't be able to do much about those risk factors. In that case, focus on controlling any associated major risk factors that you may have. ❦

2

THE TWENTY MAJOR RISK FACTORS

Risk Factor #1
Diabetes

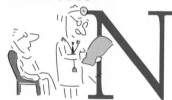 early 21 million Americans have diabetes, yet one in three—about six million people —do not know it. Another 20 million American children and adults have insulin resistance or pre-diabetes, according to the US Centers for

Disease Control and Prevention. In fact, some experts predict that one-third of all Americans born in 2000 will eventually develop diabetes.

Recent data show that within the next 20 years, the number of diabetics in the US, Western Europe and Australia will double, while in China, India, Pakistan, Indonesia and even in the very poor country of Bangladesh, it will triple.

We know that *diabetes is mostly a preventable disease, but do very little to prevent it!* Just as tragically, in my view, there is *"clinical inertia"*— the failure of healthcare providers to initiate and follow a vigorous treatment plan to prevent serious, multi-organ disease caused by poor diabetes control. This phenomenon has been reported in the *Annals of Internal Medicine.* So it is enormously important for the public to take a proactive role in preventing diabetes, and for those who already have diabetes, to be aggressive in managing their disease.

What is diabetes?

Diabetes is a disease in which the body is either unable to produce any insulin, a hormone needed to convert sugar, starches and other food into energy needed for daily life (type 1 diabetes), *or it produces insufficient amounts* (type 2) of needed insulin. Type 1 diabetes is caused by destruction of insulin-producing glands of the pancreas

---

WHO'S AT RISK?

According to the San Antonio Heart Study, the rate of diabetes has skyrocketed within the past decade—tripling among white Americans and doubling among those of Hispanic origin. Although type 2 diabetes has traditionally been a disease afflicting those in middle age and older, researchers reported a 76% increase in diabetes rates among men and women in their 30s compared to the previous decade.

The demographic breakdown of American adults who develop diabetes, pre-diabetes or insulin resistance...

- 1 in 7 whites
- 1 in 4 African-Americans
- 1 in 2 Native Americans
- 1 in 5 Hispanic-Americans

EXPLAINING INSULIN RESISTANCE

Insulin resistance means that the body's muscle, fat and liver cells do not respond properly to insulin. So the pancreas tries to produce and release increasing amounts of insulin, trying to overcome the body's resistance. Eventually the pancreas cannot keep up with the body's need for insulin. As a result, excess glucose builds up in the bloodstream.

Here's an example to illustrate the process: If someone has a sore throat caused by "Strep" germs, it can usually be treated with a seven-day course of a low-dose antibiotic. But if the strep germs are antibiotic-resistant, the low dose antibiotic will be ineffective. What do we do? We double or triple the dose of that antibiotic to overcome the germ's antibiotic resistance.

What causes insulin resistance? A sedentary lifestyle is a major contributor to type 2 diabetes, because non-exercising muscles become insulin resistant. Dietary miscues, especially refined sweets and starches, trans fatty acids and high-calorie diets, also contribute heavily to type 2 diabetes. More than 50% of adults with insulin resistance become diabetic within five to seven years. Conversely, many studies have shown that practical dietary and lifestyle modifications can reduce the risk of developing diabetes by 90% in women and by 60% in men.

The bottom line: Type 2 diabetes is merely an advanced form of insulin resistance. It is a preventable disease.

FACTORS IN INSULIN RESISTANCE

People with insulin resistance tend to have...

- A family history of diabetes
- Sedentary lifestyle
- Obesity, especially with excess intra-abdominal (belly) fat
- Low HDL- (good) cholesterol levels
- High levels of triglycerides, another fat in the blood
- A diet rich in sweets, starches and highly-caloric, greasy or deep-fried foods and with little or no seafood, fruit and vegetables
- Aging
- History of gestational diabetes
- Birth weight less than 5 lb or more than 9 lb.

In its early phase, sometimes referred to as *pre-diabetes*, the disease often remains unrecognized for several years, mostly because healthcare providers and the public rely on dated and obsolete "fasting blood sugar" level testing. During this time, the pancreas keeps pumping insulin into the bloodstream and keeps the fasting blood glucose (sugar) "normal," but the ruinous multi-organ damage already has started. As this process continues, eventually the pancreas falls behind and cannot catch up with demands placed upon it, especially when frequent sweet or starchy food and snacks are consumed. The exhaustion or inability of the pancreas to keep up has two simultaneous consequences, both serious: on the one hand, the blood sugar (glucose) level stays high, which is very toxic to nearly every organ, and on the other, blood levels of insulin are also high, which have their own toxic side effects.

Thus type 2 diabetes is an insulin resistance disease resulting in simultaneously high levels of both blood glucose (hyperglycemia) and insulin (hyperinsulinemia). Nearly all serious and life threatening complications of diabetes are directly the result of this combination.

by viral infections and immunological disorders. Type 1 diabetes, which accounts for 7%–10% of all cases, usually starts at an early age; hence it has been referred to as "juvenile" diabetes. In contrast, in type 2 diabetes, pancreatic glands are preserved, and are actually working the very hard to keep pace with the body's ever-increasing demands. The culprit here is the body's poor response and *resistance to insulin*, not its absence.

Every effort must be directed at correcting them, especially hyperglycemia!

Type 2 diabetes used to be called "maturity onset" diabetes since usually it occurred in people after age 40. Until the mid-1990s, Type 2 diabetes was unheard of among children and adolescents; today an estimated 650,000 people have type 2 diabetes in the US alone, and the numbers are rapidly climbing. Over 90% of all diabetes cases are type 2 and the age of onset has become alarmingly younger and younger.

Fat cells in the abdomen, around the intestine, kidneys and liver are distinctly different from fat cells elsewhere. These intra-abdominal fat cells produce many compounds that increase the body's resistance to insulin. One important compound is resistin, which, as the name suggests, increases insulin resistance. Even worse, abdominal fat cells cut back or stop producing a substance called adiponectin, a "good guy" that reduces insulin resistance. This explains why the "tummy tuck" does not significantly impact the risk of diabetes or other cardiovascular risk factors. These procedures remove fat from under the skin but not from inside the abdomen.

Is diabetes really an epidemic?

- According to the US Department of Agriculture, in the past 25 years Americans have increased their total caloric intake by more than 500 calories a day. And they have become even more sedentary so that about 65% of the US adult population is either overweight (30%) or obese (35%)! The switch from liquid oils to solid fats such as margarine, shortening and cooking fat with high concentrations of trans fat; repeatedly heated fats; high fructose corn sweeteners and sugars in our food and snacks have further contributed to this modern-day epidemic. This dietary practice is also at the core of worldwide diabetes epidemics.

- The US Centers for Disease Control and Prevention found a worrisome 76% rise in diabetes among men and women in their 30s over the past decade. In addition to the culprits listed above, long-term consumption of trans fatty acids (common in deep-fried foods from the mushrooming fast food industry) starting in childhood is a contributing factor.

- Today an estimated 21 million Americans have type 1 and type 2 diabetes, a number that may exceed 30 million by the year 2030. Another 20 million Americans have pre-diabetes (insulin resistance) or undiagnosed diabetes, and will eventually join those with established diabetes.

- More than 60% of Pima Indians in the United States, compared to less than two percent of Apache Indians in Chile, develop type 2 diabetes or insulin resistance by the time they reach the age of 40. This vastly different number is primarily due to the Pima's sedentary lifestyle, diet and high rate of alcoholism, all risk factors.

- Recent data from the United States, Europe, Asia and South America have shown that low birth weight (less than five pounds) doubles the risk of type 2 diabetes. Similarly, the risk of type 2 diabetes is significantly increased among individuals whose mothers had gestational diabetes.

- More than one-third of children of a diabetic parent (especially the father) will develop type 2 diabetes. The percentage may exceed 50% for obese and sedentary offspring.

- *Study:* In a six-year follow-up of 8,633 nondiabetic men between the ages of 30 and 79, those who were the least physically fit had more than a 300% higher risk of developing type 2 diabetes.

What causes type 2 diabetes?

A diet that promotes obesity is the biggest risk factor, because the more fatty tissue, the more resistant cells become. High calorie foods rich in sugar, high fructose corn sweeteners, refined starches, deep-fried foods and snacks loaded with trans fatty acids prompt overall weight gain and abdominal obesity. Such an unhealthy diet is made worse when it also includes little fruit, vegetables, fish and monounsaturated fats, such as olive oil.

Age, too, plays a role: Type 2 risk increases as we get older, especially after age 45. Often, that's because people tend to exercise less, lose muscle mass and become more insulin resistant. Also, any genetic predisposition to diabetes will appear as we get older.

How can you find out if you have insulin resistance or diabetes?

The diagnosis of insulin resistance and diabetes is not complicated; it requires an up-to-date understanding of what constitutes normal and abnormal blood sugar levels.

When the fasting blood glucose level is more than 100 mg/dl on two separate occasions, it may suggest either insulin resistance or diabetes. However, other factors can impact these

---

METABOLIC SYNDROME

A combination of factors that leads to insulin resistance—and increased risk of heart disease—can also lead to Metabolic Syndrome, defined by the National Cholesterol Education Program as the presence of any three of the following conditions…

- A waist measurement of more than 40 inches for men and more than 35 inches for women
- High triglycerides (150 mg/dl or higher)
- Low levels of HDL (below 40 mg/dl for men and below 50 mg/dl for women)
- High blood pressure (130/85 mm Hg or higher)
- High fasting blood glucose levels (110 mg/dl or higher)

---

readings—diet, weight, alcohol consumption, acute illness or taking medications such as diuretics, niacin or cortisone-like drugs. Since measurement of blood insulin levels is somewhat more cumbersome than blood glucose levels, we usually rely on glucose measurement for the diagnosis and management of diabetes.

A large number of recent studies have clearly established that currently accepted "normal" blood glucose levels, set in 2003 by the International Expert Committee on the Diagnosis and Classification of Diabetes and the American Diabetes Association, need downward adjustment. Although we have made such adjustments for blood cholesterol levels, we have been slow to correct our dated diabetes guidelines. The current guidelines suggest that the upper limit of normal for *fasting blood glucose* level is 100 mg/dl, and two fasting blood glucose readings greater than 126 mg/dl one or two weeks apart, is indicative of diabetes. To add to the confusion, blood glucose levels of 100–110 are referred to as *"impaired fasting glucose"* and levels of 111–125 are classified as *"impaired glucose tolerance."*

One major drawback of this mixed bag of classifications is that it has contributed to a dismissive and lackadaisical attitude of healthcare providers in recognizing and properly managing insulin resistance and pre-diabetes before serious multi-organ damage has occurred.

A recent 12-year study of 13,163 men between 24 and 40 years of age strongly suggests that with current guidelines we are inappropriately assuring a vast number of people that their blood sugar is normal, when in fact it is not. This well-conducted study from Israel followed up these otherwise healthy adults for 11 years. It showed that the risk of diabetes in those whose fasting blood glucose levels were 91–99 mg/dl was nearly three times higher than in those with fasting blood glucose levels of less than 90 mg/dl. In fact, among those with fasting blood glucose levels of 91–99 mg/dl who also had even slightly elevated blood triglyceride levels of over 150 mg/dl, the risk of developing diabetes during the follow-up period was more than eight times higher than in those with fasting blood glucose of lower than 81 and triglycerides of lower than 150. In other words, the lower the fasting blood glucose level, the lower the risk of future diabetes.

For many years, I have advocated that a *normal fasting blood glucose level for men, women and people of all ages should be lower than 90 and certainly not more than 100.*

What about people whose fasting blood glucose levels are over 90 mg/dl?

We can't classify someone as insulin resistant or diabetic based on a single fasting blood glucose level of over 90 mg/dl. When fasting blood glucose level is over 90 mg/dl (on two separate occasions), especially if there is abdominal obesity, elevated blood triglycerides over 150 mg/dl, a sedentary lifestyle, or a family history of diabetes, a challenge test is needed. A two-hour glucose tolerance test (two-hour GTT) is the best available means to determine whether the higher blood glucose levels are accurate, due to insulin resistance, or reflect the presence of diabetes.

A two-hour GTT is the counterpart of a stress electrocardiogram in someone whose baseline ECG is either "normal" or "not diagnostic."

HEMOGLOBIN A1c AS A TEST FOR UNCONTROLLED INSULIN RESISTANCE AND DIABETES

As the blood glucose level increases, some glucose will seep into various cells throughout the body. The uninvited entry of glucose into cells or compounds (such as LDL-cholesterol or HDL-cholesterol) is called *glycation*. In persons with elevated blood glucose levels, glycation of red blood cells occurs continuously and is proportionate to the ambient blood glucose level. Glucose is readily bound to one of the pigments in the red blood cells called *hemoglobin A1c* (or HgA1c).

Since red blood cells live for about three to four months, measuring the glycated Hb A1c (or glycohemoglobin) gives us a reasonably accurate mirror into previous three to four months. A person with normal blood glucose levels over that period would have no more than 5% to 5.5% HgA1c, whereas in diabetics with inadequate control the levels are much higher. The current "desirable" or "goal" for HgA1c is also set too high by the American Diabetes Association at 7%. This allows many diabetics to be exposed to the ravages of high blood glucose while thinking that their disease is under control. To reduce the risk of cardiovascular events, neuropathy, chronic kidney disease or retinal damage and blindness, we should aim for HgA1c under 6% and preferably below 5.5%.

INTERPRETING RESULTS OF A TWO-HOUR GLUCOSE TOLERANCE TEST*			
Glucose status	Fasting blood Glucose	One hour post challenge	Two hour post challenge
Normal	Under 90 mg/dl	Under 160 mg/dl	Under 125 mg/dl
Insulin resistance	91–125 mg/dl	161–180 mg/dl	126–140
Type 2 diabetes	Over 125 mg/dl	Over 180 mg/dl	Over 140 mg/dl

*At present, guidelines set by the American Diabetes Association for diagnosis of diabetes are set at 20 mg/dl higher for both 1- and 2-hour post-challenge samples. These threshold levels are too high and miss a large number of cases with early diabetes. They should be adjusted in the near future.

The treadmill exercise test measures whether the heart muscle can get enough blood and oxygen in response to exercise challenge. Similarly, the GTT can determine whether the body responds adequately to a sugar (glucose) load by producing sufficient amounts of insulin.

For the 2-hour GTT, a fasting blood sample is obtained, and the person then drinks a glass of water containing 75 grams of glucose. Additional blood samples are drawn one and two hours later. The chart on the previous page provides a guide for interpreting the results of 2-hour GTT. So if your fasting blood glucose (sugar) level is more than 90 mg/dl or especially if it's more than 100 mg/dl, don't assume that your blood sugar level is "normal." Ask your healthcare provider to order a repeat test after an eight-hour fasting. If it is still elevated, you should have a two-hour glucose tolerance test.

The Diabetes-Heart Disease Link

More than 80% of diabetics eventually die of cardiovascular complications. Once diabetes is diagnosed, nearly all patients have developed coronary plaques. This is why diabetes is called "coronary artery disease equivalent." In lay terms, having diabetes means having diabetes plus coronary artery disease. It explains why diabetes is the most serious and the strongest risk factor for coronary artery disease, heart attack and stroke.

There are several ways diabetes increases the risk of a heart attack…

First, elevated blood glucose directly damages the lining of coronary arteries.

Higher blood insulin levels are also toxic to the arteries of the heart, brain, eyes, kidneys and other organs. So someone with inadequately or poorly controlled diabetes risks double jeopardy —higher blood levels of both glucose and insulin.

People with inadequately controlled diabetes have a heavy "oxidant load" with too many internal oxidants, and not enough antioxidants to deal with them. The high oxidant load is one of the most important reasons for many cardiovascular complications of diabetes.

Blood glucose also binds with LDL proteins and quickly oxidizes them and causes clumping of the LDL particles in the artery walls. In non-diabetic adults, less than two percent the bloodstream. That percentage can increase up to 10% in people with diabetes. High concentration of oxidized LDL is a potent toxin for endothelial cells in the entire arterial system (including the arteries of the brain, eyes, kidneys and lower extremities) and contributes to various complications of diabetes.

Diabetics also have higher triglycerides and lower HDL levels, both of which make a bad situation even worse. An additional concern with HDL-cholesterol in diabetics is that it can become glycated and lose its potency as an antioxidant and a transporter of cholesterol from the arteries to the liver. Under these circumstances, even "normal" levels of HDL may be inadequate and unable to provide any protection for the heart, especially in the presence of other major coronary risk factors.

The Diabetes-Stroke Link

At an American Stroke Association's International Conference, researchers from Canada reported that new-onset diabetics have double the rate of stroke in the first five years after diagnosis.

Another study from the US showed that African-Americans with diabetes had a seven- to nine-fold higher risk of stroke before the age of 45 compared to those without diabetes. Among the white diabetic population, the risk of stroke before the age of 55 was six to 17-fold higher than in non-diabetics. Similarly, the risk of fatal or non-fatal heart attacks is three to five times higher among diabetics, more so when their disease is poorly controlled.

Since many diabetics have additional major coronary risk factors, an aggressive intervention to treat all of these risk factors is essential. Regrettably, very few persons with diabetes have adequately controlled diabetes, LDL-cholesterol, HDL-cholesterol, triglycerides, blood pressure or other co-existing coronary risk factors.

Diabetes, especially when it is inadequately controlled, is at least twice as likely as an elevated blood cholesterol level in causing various cardiovascular complications. Because diabetes, whether type 1 or 2, can affect practically every organ and cause devastating complications, it must be treated vigorously. Unfortunately, diabetes requires frequent—and, for type 1 diabetics, daily attention. Most complications resulting from diabetes are preventable. The problem is that they are not prevented.

Often patients do not comply with the recommended diet and lifestyle changes and anti-diabetes drugs. This may be compounded by "clinical inertia" and the passive attitude of some healthcare providers.

Diabetes and Other Serious Complications

Diabetics have a much higher risk for infections, in part due to reduced ability of their white blood cells to fight off infections. Recent data have shown that in diabetics who undergo surgical procedures, adequate blood sugar control during their hospital stay dramatically reduces post-operative infection rates, and lowers it to the level of non-diabetic people.

Several recent studies have shown that retinal (eye) damage occurs in nearly 60% of

---

EXERCISE GOALS FOR PEOPLE WITH TYPE 2 DIABETES

Based on evidence accumulated in the past 15 years and published in *Diabetes Care,* there are specific recommendations prepared for the American Diabetes Association.

If you are overweight by 30 pounds or less and/or have been diagnosed as pre-diabetic:
At the very least, strive to get 150 minutes per week of moderate exercise, such as brisk walking. More intense exercise, such as running, bicycling or swimming, are even better and likely to result in faster weight loss.

If your goal is to improve blood glucose levels because you have been diagnosed as pre-diabetic or if you already have type 2 diabetes:
The recommendation is the same 150 minutes per week, but you need to kick up the intensity—enough so that your heart rate during exercise is at 50–70% of its maximum level. That's a minimum of fast-paced walking.

As a general guideline, you can determine your maximum heart rate by subtracting your age from 220, and then multiplying that number by .50 to .70. That means a 40-year-old has a predicted maximum heart rate of 180, and the target range during exercise would be 90 to 126 beats per minute.

If you're more than 30 pounds overweight and/or already have type 2 diabetes:
Work toward at least one hour each day of moderate to vigorous exercise. In addition to regular aerobic exercise, resistance training two-to-three times a week is recommended. Ideally, this resistance training should involve all major muscle groups. Work toward three sets of eight to 10 repetitions of each exercise.

diabetics, which without prompt attention can cause irreversible blindness. In fact, diabetes is the second most common cause of adult blindness in the US—the most common cause is macular degeneration.

Diabetes also increases the risk of colorectal and pancreatic cancers by more than twofold. Recent studies have shown that the risk of colorectal cancer in type 2 diabetics who require insulin is threefold higher than non-diabetics. This is an important reason for type 2 diabetics to have periodic screening colonoscopy.

Kidney damage is present in a large number of diabetics, and along with cardiovascular complications accounts for more than 90% of deaths in diabetics.

The damage to various peripheral nerves (neuropathy) can cause severe disabling pain in the feet and legs. Moreover, poor blood circulation to the legs, if not managed properly, may result in gangrene and eventual amputation.

Progressively worsening impotence due to neuropathy of pelvic nerves and hardening of the penile arteries is also common, and may be one of the early manifestations of diabetes among men.

What you should do

• **Get active.**

A sedentary lifestyle aggravates insulin resistance and diabetes. Regular exercise is crucial in preventing and managing diabetes, and it offer numerous benefits. In addition to burning excess fat, exercise improves the body's use of insulin, lowering blood sugar levels and blood pressure levels, and improving cardiovascular health.

Since 70% of the body's insulin resistance is in the muscles, regular exercise, at least four to five times a week for 30 to 40 minutes each is essential to lower insulin resistance. The more intense the exercise, the better your insulin response will be.

THE IMPACT OF EXERCISE ON INSULIN RESISTANCE

Since the primary cause of type 2 diabetes is insulin resistance, you must make every effort to lower your insulin resistance and thereby your blood glucose level. Seventy percent of insulin resistance is in the muscles and the remainder is in the liver, brain and other organs. Regular vigorous exercise will significantly reduce insulin resistance and improve the muscle's processing of glucose. In contrast, the muscles in sedentary people become less efficient in burning glucose; hence they tend to show more insulin resistance. Regular exercise provides a vast number of other benefits. Thus it is absolutely essential for everyone with insulin resistance and diabetes to engage in regular exercise, at least four to five times a week.

What you should eat

The main focus of diabetes management is to reduce blood sugar and prevent glycation of LDL-cholesterol and vascular damage. A dietary program based on the Twenty Risk Factor diet explained in Chapter 4 and with a TRF score of 30 is ideal for nearly all diabetics.

Carbohydrates and starches, such as white bread, bagels, pasta, rice and potato, aggravate diabetes and are undesirable for diabetics of all ages. Studies show that long-term, frequent consumption of dark fruits and vegetables reduces the risk of diabetes by 30%. Small amounts of table sugar or honey, however, are not harmful if you eaten only on occasion.

• **Eat plenty of seafood.**

Seafood with dark (pink or red flesh) have heart-healthy omega-3 polyunsaturated fat.

• **Reduce vegetable oils and fats.**

Vegetable oils, especially stick margarine and shortenings, increase oxidation of LDL particles. That's dangerous for anyone—it leads to more plaque accumulating on arterial walls—but it's especially bad for diabetics.

Replacing vegetable oils and fats with olive oil (a fruit oil) will not only reduce the oxidation of LDL-cholesterol, but will also improve insulin resistance.

- **Eat dark, not white.**

In two recent studies a diet rich in dark produce and whole grains (usually also dark) was shown to help lower the risk of diabetes by more than 30%.

- **Seek medication.**

Diabetics with elevated triglycerides or cholesterol disorders require a far more intensive intervention than nondiabetics with these conditions. Even in diabetics with minimal cholesterol elevation, cholesterol-lowering measures can reduce the very high risk of coronary events by 30%.

Since nearly one in five people with cardiovascular disease also has diabetes or insulin resistance, aggressive cholesterol-lowering in this group may require a multipronged attack. Because of the increased rate of oxidation of almost every tissue in diabetics, you should not rely solely on vitamin E or vitamin C to deal with the large oxidant load. Moreover, not all oxidants are necessarily neutralized by vitamin C or vitamin E (it would have made everyone's life a lot easier if they were!). For this reason, all diabetics should enrich their diet with many servings of dark green, leafy vegetables and deeply colored fruits such as berries, plums, nectarines, peaches and figs. Drinking one or two glasses of a mixed vegetable juice such as V-8 is also a reasonable alternative to colas or other drinks with meals.

Diabetes is not only the most potent risk factor for cardiovascular diseases, it is also a serious disease that impacts and impairs nearly every organ. It requires aggressive long-term intervention. In the early years of the disease, insulin resistance and diabetes are not painful and have no particular warning signs or symptoms. Healthcare providers are often casual when blood glucose levels are elevated and practice a wait and see approach with a disease that needs intervention from day one.

Be proactive to save your life

If your blood glucose is under 126 mg/dl, it's a good bet that you'll be told "you don't have sugar diabetes." However, if your fasting blood glucose level is more than 100 mg/dl on at least two occasions, ask for a more accurate two-hour glucose tolerance test. Make sure the data on page 14 is used to interpret your results.

This more accurate testing can allow you to take action that could save your life. Recent studies show that early intervention may help you prevent nearly all complications, and dramatically reduce your risk of heart attack, stroke or death from cardiovascular disease.

Improved and sustained blood glucose control also reduces the risk of serious and irreversible damage to the retina, blindness, kidney failure, peripheral vascular disease requiring amputations, painful neuropathy and various digestive disorders.

- **What about alcohol?**

Many studies suggest that a small amount of alcohol with dinner may reduce insulin resistance; it also raises "good" HDL-cholesterol levels and lowers the risk of a heart attack by about 30%. So if you have no objection to alcoholic beverages, a drink or two each night with dinner might be helpful. But don't overdo it—alcohol is high in calories and more than the recommended amount can impede diabetes control.

As alcohol is metabolized, it is initially converted to acetaldehyde, which stimulates the production and accumulation of fatty acids in the liver. Long-term excessive alcohol use can cause severe fat accumulation in the liver cells—a serious complication that may progress to cirrhosis of the liver.

• **Coffee or tea?**

Several large studies from the US and Europe have shown that coffee consumption is associated with a significant protective effect against type 2 diabetes.

- A study from Finland, where the population has the highest coffee consumption in the world, followed more than 14,000 men and women for 12 years. The study showed that frequent daily coffee intake was associated with a lower risk of developing type 2 diabetes. For men with the highest coffee consumption, the risk of diabetes was reduced by 55% and for women, the risk was reduced by 80%. However, this study and other coffee studies did not separate the impact of regular versus decaffeinated coffee.

- The Iowa Women's Study examined the impact of regular versus decaffeinated coffee, tea and other caffeinated beverages such as soda pop among over 28,000 post menopausal women. After adjusting for diet and lifestyle factors, regular coffee, tea and caffeinated beverages had no significant protective effect. However, consuming more than four cups of decaffeinated coffee reduced the risk of type 2 diabetes by more than 30%.

• **Does decaffeinated coffee reduce the risk of diabetes?**

Coffee beans are a rich source of many minerals and antioxidants that can potentially protect the insulin producing glands inside the pancreas from oxidation. And they improve the muscle's and liver's response to insulin. Also, coffee beans contain substances which help to reduce carbohydrate absorption, so less sugar is released in the bloodstream. Since tea and other caffeinated beverages have shown no protective effect, it is unlikely that caffeine has any beneficial impact and it may even increase the risk of diabetes. In heavy coffee drinkers, the high intake of chlorogenic acid and other ingredients has a more dominant impact and explains the lower rates of diabetes in very heavy coffee drinkers, and the lower rates of diabetes in the very heavy coffee drinkers in the Finnish study and other studies.

The impact of vitamins and minerals on insulin resistance and diabetes

One of the most important reasons for multi-organ damage in diabetes is the high concentration of oxidants in the bloodstream and in nearly every organ. This abundant "oxidant load" is further fueled by hyperglycemia (high blood glucose level).

Since there are many oxidants some specific to certain organs, a dose of vitamin C or E cannot offer a cure-all remedy. The majority of oxidants produced in diabetes are resistant to vitamins C and E, even at 1,000 times higher than usual doses. This is more reason to reduce the oxidant load in the first place by intensive treatment of hyperglycemia and by eating as many servings of different dark fruits and vegetables as possible. The operative word here is different (because fruits and vegetables have different antioxidants)!

Dark fruits and vegetables have many other cardiovascular and non-cardiovascular benefits. Except for a few high glycemic items (dates, potatoes and sweet potatoes), fruits and vegetables reduce insulin requirements and improve insulin resistance and diabetes. Plus, they generally do not pack many carbohydrates, fat or calories.

• **Take vitamins**

As a supplement to several servings of *different* fruits and vegetables daily, taking one or two multivitamins with minerals (without iron, since iron is actually an oxidant) each day is preferable to taking vitamin C or E separately.

- *Chromium*, in doses of 400 to 1,000 micrograms per day, reduces insulin resistance. Specifically, this trace mineral can

VARIETY OF PRODUCE IS MOST PRODUCTIVE

Although dark-skinned produce is the clear choice for preventing and managing diabetes, there is no magic food. That's because no single nutrient prevents the high "oxidant load" that causes multi-organ damage in diabetics.

Eat as many servings of *different* dark fruits and vegetables as possible. Antioxidants are in varying amounts in different types of produce. Unfortunately, no single nutrient—say, vitamin C or E—will offer a cure-all to battle the dangerous oxidant load.

Studies show that the vast majority of oxidants produced in diabetes, especially when it's poorly controlled, are resistant to vitamins C and E, even at doses 1,000 times above the Recommended Daily Allowance.

But this much is clear: In data pooled from eight separate studies involving more than 257,000 people and published in *The Lancet,* eating five or more servings of fruits and vegetables a day reduced the risk of stroke by more than 25%.

stimulate muscle and liver cells to produce insulin receptors, enhancing insulin entry into various tissues. However, for diabetics who require insulin, chromium supplements are unlikely to have any significant impact. Note that vitamin C in doses above 200 milligrams can interfere with chromium absorption, so they shouldn't be taken together.

- *Magnesium*, in doses of 200 to 400 milligrams daily, may be a safe way to improve insulin resistance. Recent studies suggest that people with high magnesium intake may reduce their risk of metabolic syndrome by 30%.

- *Selenium* is another trace mineral that acts as a potent antioxidant. The recommended dose is 200 to 400 micrograms a day. In addition to its diabetes benefit, it's been found to help reduce the risk of colorectal and prostate cancers. (*Folic acid*, one of the B vitamins, at 1 to 2 milligrams a day, may also reduce the risk of colorectal cancer—a risk that is significantly higher in diabetics than the general population.)

Diabetes is a serious disease with a high risk of serious or fatal cardiovascular complications. Thus treating diabetes should never be a do-it-yourself approach. Since the requirements of each person with diabetes may vary from one day to the next, treatment should always be individualized under the supervision of a physician. Whether the choice is insulin or oral anti-diabetes drugs, diabetics always need a variety of interventions to prevent cardiovascular, neurological, kidney, eye and other serious complications.

Blood glucose monitoring

I have stressed that the negative multi-organ impact of diabetes is a consequence of high blood glucose and high (but ineffective) insulin levels. Although many healthcare providers assure their patients that sporadic or intermittent rise in blood glucose levels are "ok," this is a dated and unsupportable attitude that serves the public poorly. Blood glucose fluctuations, especially after meals, trigger the release of far more oxidants than sustained elevation of blood glucose, and contribute to a greater multi-organ damage.

Diabetes and co-existing coronary risk factors

Among all 20 major coronary risk factors, diabetes is the most dangerous, increasing the risk of heart attack, stroke or peripheral vascular disease by four- to five-fold. Unfortunately, diabetes is rarely a stand-alone disease, and almost always it is accompanied by two or more major coronary risk factors. Most often diabetics have elevated triglycerides, low levels of cardio-protective HDL-cholesterol, and even when their LDL-cholesterol levels are normal, a high percentage of them are the small, "atherogenic" LDL particles. This triad or combination of three abnormalities is referred to as the *atherogenic lipid profile,* and contributes to the high risk of cardiovascular events in diabetics.

The risk of various cardiovascular diseases, such as coronary artery disease, peripheral vascular disease and heart failure, among diabetic women is twice as high as in diabetic men. But a pervasive gender bias has contributed to a dismissive approach in management of

diabetes among women. To dramatically reduce the risk of cardiovascular events in men and women, it is absolutely essential to intensively correct the atherogenic triad. Moreover, the threshold for many of these risk factors among diabetics is much lower. For example, in the absence of diabetes or other coronary risk factors, the desirable or "goal" LDL-cholesterol is less than 100 mg/dl. However, among diabetics, the LDL-cholesterol should be lowered to under 70 mg/dl. Similarly, the threshold for an acceptable blood pressure must be set at less than 120/80 mmHg. Everyone with diabetes should be tested, at least annually, to rule out the existence of other coronary risk factors, but more frequent testing is required to make sure co-existing ones are adequately controlled.

WHEN TO TEST BLOOD GLUCOSE

Conventional wisdom on when to monitor blood glucose levels is anything but wise. The American Diabetes Association recommends that patients with type 1 diabetes check their blood glucose levels three to four times a day—before meals—but it does not advise diabetics to test post-meal levels. This is a gross error!

Even more puzzling: The ADA makes no specific monitoring recommendations for type 2 diabetics, who represent 90 percent of those with the disease.

Reality: Blood glucose fluctuations after meals trigger the release of more oxidants, which cause multi-organ damage in diabetics. So in addition to checking fasting blood glucose two to three times a week, blood sugar levels should be periodically checked two hours after dinner to ensure there are no extreme peaks. If there are, speak to your doctor about appropriate action.

Accurate blood glucose self-monitoring devices are available at nearly all drug stores in the US (and are reimbursable by most health insurers).

Risk Factor #2
Abdominal Obesity and Metabolic Syndrome

Weight mismanagement is a disease that affects two out of three adults and one out of six children or adolescents in the US. The numbers are even higher among Native Americans, Hispanics and African-Americans. But this is no longer a disease limited to Americans or populations of developed countries. It is a global epidemic that cuts across all continents. Weight mismanagement has many forms and many negative health consequences.

A critical feature of weight mismanagement is where and how the fat is distributed, rather than the actual weight. An obesity pattern with body fat distribution around the waist and inside the abdomen (potbelly or beer belly) is distinctly different from one which involves the chest, arms or hips. This is because fat cells inside the abdomen act quite differently from fat cells everywhere else, even though they may look like regular fat cells.

WHAT YOU SHOULD DO IF YOU HAVE INSULIN RESISTANCE OR DIABETES

Reduce abdominal obesity

Diet: Follow the Twenty Risk Factor Diet, and keep your score at least 20 per day initially and not more than 30/day

Regular exercises four to five days a week, and for more than 30–40 minutes each time

Control blood glucose level aggressively. Self-monitor your blood glucose frequently, both before and at least two hours after dinner

Control LDL-cholesterol to less than 70 mg/dl, **often requires cholesterol-lowering drugs**

Control HDL-cholesterol to below 45 mg/dl for men and below 55 mg/dl for women

Control triglycerides to less than 150/dl

Control blood pressure to under 120/80, **frequently requires anti-hypertension drugs**

Control homocysteine to under 10 mmol/l, **requires high-dose vitamin B-12 and folic acid**

Low-dose aspirin, 81 mg/day (to reduce the risk of heart attack and stroke by 30%)

Insulin-sensitizers such as metformin, pioglitazone (Actos)

Kidney-protective drugs such as ACE-inhibitors, commonly used for hypertension

Oral anti-diabetes drugs or insulin when necessary for strict blood glucose management

Multivitamins with minerals without iron, two tablets per day

Chromium, 400–600 microgram/day, magnesium, 200–400 mg/day, selenium, 200 mcg/day

Permitted but not necessary: Alcohol, a glass or two with dinner; tea (black or green); preferably decaffeinated coffee, 2–4 cups/day; caffeine-free, sugar-free sodas one to three per day

---

Weight mismanagement can be measured in several ways...

1. *Weight on the basis of height:* Although this tool has been used for over 50 years, it is an inaccurate way of judging the presence or extent of abdominal obesity.

2. *Waist to hip ratio:* This ratio is obtained by measuring the circumference of the natural waistline and the widest part of the hips. The waist measurement is divided by the hip measurement to obtain the waist/hip ratio. Desirable waist/hip ratios are less than 0.90 for men and less than 0.75 for women.

   However, there is always a range for all biological markers like waist circumference. For the purpose of defining abdominal obesity the threshold is set at 35 inches (88 cm) for women and 41 inches (102 cm) for men. But these numbers are quite arbitrary. For people who are tall and muscular or "big-boned," the threshold is higher by as much as two to four inches (five to 10 cm), whereas for people from the Far East or for short people the threshold is 34 inches (85 cm) for women and 38 inches (96 cm) for men.

3. *Body Mass Index (BMI):* BMI is presently the most popular means of expressing body weight, and has a wide international acceptance.

   You can determine your BMI by dividing your body weight in kilograms by the square of your height in meters. The table on page 23 provides a wide range of BMIs based on body weight in pounds and height in inches. Optimal BMI for men should be less than twenty-five, and for women,

22

BODY MASS INDEX (BMI) BASED ON WEIGHT AND HEIGHT

Weight (lbs)	5'0"	5'1"	5'2"	5'3"	5'4"	5'5"	5'6"	5'7"	5'8"	5'9"	5'10"	5'11"	6'0"	6'1"	6'2"
130	25	25	24	23	22	22	21	20	20	19	19	18	18	17	17
135	26	26	25	24	23	22	22	21	21	20	19	19	18	18	17
140	27	26	26	25	24	23	23	22	21	21	20	20	19	18	18
145	28	27	27	26	25	24	23	23	22	21	21	20	20	19	19
150	29	28	27	27	26	25	24	23	23	22	22	21	20	20	19
155	30	29	28	27	26	26	25	24	24	23	22	22	21	20	20
160	31	30	29	28	27	27	26	25	24	24	23	22	22	21	21
165	32	31	30	29	28	27	27	26	25	24	24	23	22	22	21
170	33	32	31	30	29	28	27	27	26	25	24	24	23	22	22
175	34	33	32	31	30	29	28	27	27	26	25	24	24	23	22
180	35	34	33	32	31	30	29	28	27	27	26	25	24	24	23
185	36	35	34	33	32	31	30	29	28	27	27	26	25	24	24
190	37	36	35	34	33	32	31	30	29	28	27	26	26	25	24
195	38	37	36	35	33	32	31	31	30	29	28	27	26	26	25
200	39	38	37	36	34	33	32	31	30	30	29	28	27	26	26
205	40	39	37	36	35	34	33	32	31	30	29	28	28	27	26
210	41	40	38	37	36	35	34	33	32	31	30	29	29	28	27
215	42	41	39	38	37	36	35	34	33	32	31	30	29	28	28
220	43	42	40	39	38	37	36	34	33	33	32	31	30	29	28
225	44	43	41	40	39	37	36	35	34	33	32	31	31	30	29
230	45	43	42	41	39	38	37	36	35	34	33	32	31	30	30
235	46	44	43	42	40	39	38	37	36	35	34	33	32	31	30
240	47	45	44	43	41	40	39	38	36	36	34	33	33	32	31
245	48	46	45	43	42	41	40	38	37	36	35	34	33	32	31
250	49	47	46	44	43	42	40	39	38	37	36	35	34	33	32

To calculate any Body Mass Index not listed above:
1. Multiply weight (in pounds) by 700
2. Square height in inches (H x H)
3. Divide #1 by #2

less than twenty-four. Although BMI is a more accurate way of determining obesity, waist/hip ratio is the best tool for assessing abdominal obesity.

Although intra-abdominal fat cells (not the fat under the skin, but the fat inside the abdomen and around various organs) may look like other fat cells, they are distinctly different. These cells are microscopic chemical factories that produce a host of chemical compounds and fatty acids directly carried by intra-abdominal vessels into the liver. The response to these uninvited and unfriendly compounds is summarized on the following page. The fatty acids released from intra-abdominal fat cells stimulate the liver to produce more triglycerides and release them into the bloodstream, which raises the blood levels of triglycerides. Some excess triglycerides produced by the liver are stored in the lever cell, contributing to development of an enlarged fatty liver.

Elevated blood triglycerides have two problems; they lower the blood levels of the good HDL-cholesterol and convert many LDL-cholesterol particles into smaller, more harmful ones. This combination creates a hostile, coronary-unfriendly environment and can increase the risk of coronary artery disease or heart attack by five- to tenfold. Fatty liver is a potentially harmful condition that should not be ignored. The surge of triglycerides into the bloodstream forces the less harmful large LDL particles to exchange some of their cholesterol for triglycerides and become smaller and more atherogenic. At the same time, the HDL-cholesterol levels fall, contributing to the *atherogenic lipid profile* similar to that occurring in diabetics. All of these collectively raise the risk of heart attack, stroke and other cardiovascular events.

Alcohol intake of more than one or two drinks per day also stimulates the production and storage of more triglycerides inside liver cells, making the fat burden of liver cells even worse. Some of the triglycerides trapped inside liver cells are oxidized, and set in motion a cascade of inflammatory reactions and scarring that may cause destruction and death of liver cells. As this liver inflammation and scarring or *fatty hepatitis* continues, many liver cells that are still struggling to stay alive are surrounded and choked by scar tissue. At this late stage the liver is a dysfunctional, scarred and hardened organ. This is referred to as *cirrhosis of the liver*, which is mostly irreversible. This condition is further aggravated by high-carbohydrate, high calorie diets, and especially trans fatty acids.

We have already begun to see a large number of people in their 40s and 50s with liver failure caused by fatty cirrhosis. Experts predict that by 2015, there may be an epidemic of liver failures due to this new type of cirrhosis.

The American Cancer Society researchers reported its findings of a fourteen-year study of over one million adults in the United States (457,785 men and 588,369 women).

The results: Among nonsmokers, the body mass indexes associated with the lowest death rates (from all causes) were 23.5 to 25 for men, and from 22 to 23.5 for women. High BMI (greater than 30) among white men and women increased their all-cause mortality by 2.5-fold and 2-fold, respectively. Although the impact of obesity among African-Americans was less pronounced, this difference is partly due to other risk factors that result in deaths before the impact of obesity becomes fully apparent.

For a similar reason, obesity seems to affect older persons (more than seventy years of age) less than it does their younger counterparts. Still, because these groups have a higher overall risk of mortality from cardiovascular events and cancers, their obesity should be taken even more seriously.

WHAT DO INTRA-ABDOMINAL FAT CELLS DO?

- **Produce** fatty acids that go to the liver and stimulate over-production of triglycerides
- **Raise** blood triglycerides
- **Lower** HDL-cholesterol level
- **Make** LDL-cholesterol particles smaller so they more easily cross into artery's wall
- **Increase** oxidation of small LDL-cholesterol and make them more atherogenic*
- **Force the liver** cells to store some of the excess triglycerides and cause fatty liver
- **Increase** insulin resistance within liver cells
- **Produce** a compound called resistin that increases insulin resistance in the muscles
- **Reduce** production of the compound adiponectin that reduces insulin resistance
- **Contribute** to metabolic syndrome, insulin resistance and type 2 diabetes
- **Make** the arteries stiffer; therefore raising the blood pressure
- **Increase** the risk of heart attack, stroke and peripheral vascular disease
- **Produce** estrogen-like compounds that increase the risk of breast and prostate cancers
- **Increase the risk of colon cancer** by 50% due to low adiponectin levels**

*Weinbrenner T et al, Am j Clin Nutr 2006;83: 30–5
**Wei Ek et al. J Natl cancer inst 2005;97: 1688–94

Unfortunately, except for liver transplantation, often a $200,000 expense, there is no other treatment option on the horizon for this disease. We already have a painful shortage of donor organs, especially livers, and thousands of Americans die each year while waiting for liver transplantation.

The complications of abdominal obesity are shown in the table above.

Metabolic syndrome: Why is it so important?

Metabolic syndrome is a collection of *any three* of these disorders in a person…

- Abdominal obesity: Waistline over 40 inches (102 cm) for men, and over 35 inches (88 cm) for women
- Sedentary lifestyle
- Elevated fasting blood glucose over 100 mg/dl
- High blood pressure over 120/80 mmHg
- Elevated triglycerides more than 150 mg/dl
- Low levels of HDL-cholesterol less than 40 for men and less than 50 for women

More than 50% of adults with abdominal obesity have metabolic syndrome, but abdominal obesity is not a necessary component of metabolic syndrome. This collection of metabolic disorders significantly increases the risk of cardiovascular disease, diabetes, fatty liver and various cancers. Elevated triglycerides and low levels of cardio-protective HDL-cholesterol are the best predictors of future cardiovascular events, whereas elevated fasting blood glucose is the strongest marker for development of type 2 diabetes, increasing the risk by sevenfold.

Among adults with metabolic syndrome the risk of a heart attack increases by more than fivefold. If they are also diabetic or their LDL-cholesterol particles are predominantly small, the risk rises 10-fold.

In the Framingham Offspring Study, when one component of metabolic syndrome was type 2 diabetes, the 10-year risk of stroke was increased by nearly 3½ times compared to those who did not have diabetes.

In a recent study of 6,038 Americans, a waist circumference of more than 35 inches (88 centimeters) was associated with a significantly higher risk of having high blood pressure, elevated triglycerides, low levels of good HDL-cholesterol, or elevated fasting blood glucose levels. In fact, for "overweight" persons (body mass index of 25 to 30), abdominal girth over 35 inches (88cm) for women and over 38 inches (95cm) for men is far more relevant to cardiovascular risk factors than total weight based on height or body mass index.

Obesity and metabolic syndrome in children and adolescents

Obesity is now the fastest growing non-infectious epidemic among children and adolescents in the US and most of the rest of the world. More alarming is the fact that 50% of obese children and adolescents have metabolic syndrome, prematurely mimicking their adult counterparts. Unfortunately, these youngsters are at a significantly elevated risk for developing premature cardiovascular events and diabetes.

Study: In a recent 30-year follow-up study of 917 children and adolescents (five to 19 years of age), the risk of experiencing a cardiovascular event was 8.5 times higher in those who had the pediatric version of metabolic syndrome compared to those without the metabolic syndrome.

Study: In another study of 1,175 girls, those who had abdominal obesity at age 18, had a sixfold higher risk of metabolic syndrome compared with those who did not have abdominal obesity at 18. These studies and many other studies strongly affirm that obesity and metabolic syndrome in children and adolescents are serious and life-threatening disorders that need aggressive intervention.

Until a few years ago, type 2 diabetes was unheard of among children and adolescents. In fact, most pediatric textbooks did not even bother to include it. Type 2 diabetes was considered the maturity-onset diabetes affecting men and women past their 40s and 50s. Today, more than 650,000 children and adolescents in the US have type 2 diabetes, nearly all associated with or as a complication of obesity and metabolic syndrome. This unfolding tragedy is just the tip of the iceberg; by 2010 the number may exceed one million! It is now nearly a worldwide epidemic.

Metabolic syndrome and obesity in children and adolescents are harbingers of not only type 2 diabetes, but many premature cardiovascular complications that will begin to unfold as they grow older.

Childhood and adolescent obesity, like its adult version, is a disease with many contributing factors. One major factor in childhood obesity is parents who allow children to eat what they want rather than what they need.

Have you noticed what children eat? They get an abundance of trans fatty acids from margarines, shortenings and fats that are invariably present in cakes, candies, cookies, donuts, pastries, pies and deep-fried foods like french fries or chicken nuggets. They also eat greasy and high calorie processed cheeses, pizzas and cheeseburgers with fatty garnishes their little bodies do not need and cannot use. And what about snacks? Most snacks are loaded with high glycemic carbohydrates such as sugar, high fructose corn sweeteners and of course, the omnipresent (but hidden) trans fats, which increases their risk of obesity and metabolic syndrome. This tragedy is often made worse by the parents' own eating habits or weight mismanagement. In approximately one out of five cases, there is also a family history of type 2 diabetes or maternal gestational diabetes.

An equally important and almost universal contributing factor to the worldwide epidemic of obesity and metabolic syndrome in children and adolescents (very much like the adults) is a sedentary lifestyle that creates a vicious cycle. Unfortunately, many youngsters are ignored by healthcare providers who lack time, knowledge or the interest in managing children and adolescents with obesity and metabolic syndrome.

In early 2007, the Institute of Medicine sent Congress detailed recommendations for replacing many food and snack items in vending machines and from school lunch menus. However, they are not likely to be acted upon anytime soon. Only a few schools—less than one percent—have begun to make some small changes to cut down on fat, sugar and total calories in their lunch menus.

Why are parents and school boards so silent? Perhaps it will require legislation or a directive from the Department of Education or Health and Human Services to require schools to offer healthful menus. So responsibility lies with the parents. Remember, *we* are responsible for our own children's well-being; *we* must act responsibly.

"Overweight": A tempest in a teapot!

For decades, public health institutions, medical establishments, insurance companies, the media and the public have described millions of healthy people as overweight, implying a metabolic disorder or disease. The overweight classification is based on a more than half century-old weight and height table developed by an insurance company. Recently, we have tweaked the BMI index to define "overweight" as a BMI of 25–30.

At present, we stigmatize 35% of US adults by labeling them "overweight," creating millions of "instant patients!" Surely, not everyone who happens to be 10 or 20 lbs. heavier than an arbitrary number is diseased or carries a significant risk for future disease. One unfortunate consequence of this "overweight" stigma is that several billion dollars is wasted every year on useless weight loss aids, supplements or diets. In a way, we have made this huge population a renewable source for commercial exploitation!

There is no valid scientific evidence that in the absence of abdominal obesity, insulin resistance, metabolic syndrome or diabetes, being 10, 20 or even 30 pounds overweight has any significant negative health impact, especially among older persons. Does it make any sense to classify everyone who has one or two drinks with dinner as a "moderate alcoholic"? Imagine the social, emotional, and healthcare cost associated with such labeling! What we should strive for is fitness and firmness, not thinness!

I believe that it's time to liberate an estimated 40 million otherwise healthy Americans who are stigmatized by a bogus disease.

The argument has been made that obesity starts out as excess weight; hence the need to focus on the overweight population. However, millions of "overweight" people stay healthy and never approach or cross the obesity line. Obesity is not an inevitable result from overweight status; obesity is the consequence of long-term weight mismanagement *at all levels*, starting with *normal* weight.

A recent study of 320,252 adults enrolled in a California health maintenance organization showed that being overweight (BMI 25 to 30) increased the risk of chronic kidney failure by about 70% compared to 500% excess risk for severely obese persons. However, when the researchers looked at presence of diabetes and hypertension, the increased risk of chronic kidney failure for overweight persons almost disappeared, but still remained quite strong for severely obese persons. The problem is not excess weight; the problem is the co-existence of risk factors that should be dealt, regardless of the person's weight.

I recommend screening all "overweight" and obese persons of all ages for various coronary risk factors, insulin resistance, metabolic syndrome and diabetes. If any risk factors are found, they should be corrected, and weight management can significantly improve this effort. The high risk individuals with multiple risk factors or an existing disease are the ones to focus on and not the healthy "overweight" people.

Considering the enormous healthcare costs, we should spend our limited resources on high risk people or who have a narrow window of opportunity to prevent disability or death. I urge healthcare providers to stop promoting the diet industry by re-enforcing the false notion that every "overweight" person must go on a diet to lose weight.

The diet industry thrives by promoting thinness, convincing millions of people that they are overweight and need the "guaranteed to make you lose weight" products. Thus, we have diet drinks, diet foods, diet snacks, diet gums, diet beers and diet wines, diet books, diet cooks, diet gimmicks, diet gurus and diet everything else!

The desire for a particular body image or body part such as nose, face, breasts or figure, is an esthetic issue, not a health-related one. People can choose to lose weight for esthetic reasons, but I candidly discourage the notion that esthetic weight loss in healthy "overweight" persons has any significant health benefit. Liposuction can remove fat from thighs, hips and abdominal wall (not from intra-abdominal fat), but it does not improve cholesterol levels, insulin resistance or other cardiovascular concerns.

On the other hand, losing weight through dietary and lifestyle modifications presented here will help you lose intra-abdominal fat and other fat. It also dramatically reduces your risk of insulin resistance, metabolic syndrome, diabetes, cardiovascular events and various cancers.

Another concern about abdominal obesity: the risk of stroke is also significantly higher among both men and women. A recent study of 28,000 US male health professionals between the ages of 40 and 75 showed that the risk of stroke was 2.3 times greater in those with the highest waist/hip ratio (greater than 0.97) than in those in the lowest category (less than 0.89).

Another study, a long-term follow-up of more than 116,000 female nurses in the US showed almost identical results—the risk of stroke among women with marked abdominal obesity was 2.4 times greater than among those with a waist-to-hip ratio less than 0.8.

What you should do

In 2007, the US Centers for Disease Control and Prevention (CDC) released a sobering assessment of our nation's poor diet and lifestyle. Only 12.4% of men and 16.6% of women (or one out of seven adults) engage in moderate intense exercise for at least 30 minutes five days a week, and eat at least five servings of fruits, and vegetables, a day.

But if the CDC had focused on those who eat a healthful diet—as presented here—the number would be less than five percent (or one in 20) of American adults. The healthful diet includes plenty of seafood, healthful nuts (almonds, hazelnuts, pistachios and walnuts) and olive oil, and contains very little or no trans fats, high glycemic carbs or calorie-stuffed foods and snacks. So here are some practical steps for successful weight management...

1. *You must reduce your total calories from both fat and, even more importantly, carbohydrates.* This is essential! Use my Twenty Risk Factor (Chapter 4) system of scoring foods and snacks. It's a convenient way to avoid unnecessary fat in your diet. Start by limiting yourself to a TRF score of less than 20, until you achieve your goal. Then your score should be below 30, preferably below 25 for long-term weight maintenance.

The argument that "calories are calories no matter where they come from" is sensible, but not entirely true. For example, out of every 100 calories from proteins, the body burns 20 calories to facilitate the absorption process, leaving only 80 calories for use. In contrast, out of each 100 fat calories, the body spends only two calories absorbing the fat, leaving 98 calories for use. With carbohydrates, the body spends eight out of 100 for the work of the intestine during absorption, leaving 92 calories for use. Gram for gram, fat has 250% more calories than carbohydrates or proteins. Thus all fat-containing foods are more energy dense (pack in more calories) than those without fat or with very low fat.

Although it is easy to avoid visible fat, reducing hidden fat requires more vigilance because it is often disguised and hard to identify. For example, in many fast food restaurants, salad dressings added to a garden salad can supply as many calories as one serving of a roast beef sandwich and french fries. The salad dressing may have 50 percent more fat. The chart below provides examples of hidden fats in some common foods.

All carbohydrates, simple or complex, can contribute to obesity. Since carbohydrates provide about 60% of daily calories, cutting their intake by half (even without a significant fat reduction) can promote weight loss. Ideally, a balanced approach of reducing

HOW MUCH FAT IS IN YOUR FOOD?
PERCENTAGE OF CALORIES FROM FAT

Food	%	Food	%
Beans	4	Tenderloin Beef, Lean	41
Most Shellfish	5	Dark Chicken (without skin)	42
Breast of Turkey (without skin)	7	Breast of Chicken (with skin)	44
Most White Meat Fish*	10	Ground Turkey	45
Salmon, Tuna or Mackerel*	14–18	Whole Milk	50
1 Percent Milk	17	Extra Lean Hamburger	53
Breast of Chicken or Turkey (without skin)	17	Dark Chicken (with skin)	56
Dark Turkey (without skin)	23	Turkey or Chicken Hot Dogs	70
Top Round Beef, Lean	29	Most Processed Cheeses	75
2 Percent Milk	36	Beef Hot Dogs	80
		Potato or Corn Chips	80

*Depending on the type of fish and its fat content, the percentage of calories from fat may vary somewhat.

both carbohydrates and fat intake, and increasing exercise is more effective and can be followed indefinitely. This combination can prevent the yo-yo syndrome or "weight cycling" that occurs in more than 90% of dieters.

The five carbohydrate culprits are bread, pasta, rice, potato and all sweets (including cakes, cookies, pies, pastries, chocolate, donuts and ice cream).

All foods with high fat content (except those prepared with olive oil, canola oil or hazelnut oil) have TRF scores exceeding +10, and many exceed +15 to +20. So when in doubt, always use the TRF scores.

For the purpose of weight management, calories from olive oil or other monounsaturates are not different from butter or margarine. Reduce the amount of all fats and oils, as well as all carbohydrates, simple or complex.

Good choices include many kinds of seafood, provided it's not deep-fried; lean cuts of meat; fruits such as berries, plums, nectarines, fresh peaches; dark vegetables and leafy green leafy vegetables, broccoli, beans and herbs. Consider this—habitual consumption of chili pepper (which contains capsaicin) actually reduces insulin resistance and deceases food-stimulates rise in blood sugar. High glycemic foods (sweets, starches, sugared cereals), *not* total carbohydrate intake, increase the risk of fatty liver by twofold.

2. *Exercise and weight management:* Weight mismanagement and abdominal obesity result from an imbalance between calories consumed and calories burned. This simple fact is clear but, amazingly, many people, including healthcare providers, can't see it!

An obese person may have 20 to 30 billion fat cells. When we lose weight, we lose fat, muscle and water. When we gain weight, we reverse the process. However, the number of fat cells remains unchanged. They are enlarged or made smaller with weight gain or loss. But for many obese people, once the fat cells have grown by more than 70%, they will begin to reproduce and increase the total number of fat cells. The reverse does not happen, no matter how much weight is lost.

There is a fierce competition among fat cells, especially intra-abdominal, for every unused calorie. Among people who are sedentary, abdominal fat cells seem to beat out other less biologically active fat cells in the race to capture the unused calories and convert them into stored fat. Unfortunately, when we lose weight, skeletal fat cells tend to downsize more than intra-abdominal ones. This uneven downsizing partly explains why it is harder to lose that big tummy.

Many people with weight problems say that they don't really eat excessively. In fact a number of studies support their claim, and show that the total caloric intake of some obese persons may even be lower than normal weight persons. Many studies have shown that people with weight problems often underestimate their total caloric intake, often by a wide margin, especially their calories from fats and snacks. It's an understandable mistake—many people don't have the tools to estimate their calorie consumption exactly.

An obese person and a slim person, walking together, may not burn the same amount of energy. If the slim person burns 100 calories by fast-walking for one mile, the obese person may burn only 50 to 70 calories. This explains why overweight people have a hard time losing weight and keeping it off. The additional burden of a "slow metabolism" puts millions of people at a distinct disadvantage. To lose weight they will have to cut their total energy intake further, and increase their exercise level by 30% to 50%.

When people with obesity lose weight, approximately 60% of the weight loss is from fat, 30% from muscles, and 10% is water. When they regain weight, they reverse these. Regular exercise, unless it is very intensive, cannot and does not produce weight loss without calorie restriction. Very few obese people can or should exercise intensely. Many should also be wary of rewarding themselves with a snack after exercising. Exercise does help with your dietary effort, prevent weight regain and firm up the muscles that may have become weak.

Weight management for children and adolescents

Obesity and metabolic syndrome in the pediatric age group is similar to that of adults but the cardiovascular complications and diabetes will affect them when they are in their 20s and 30s. The treatment approach is similar to adults but requires tweaking and compromise to get them to comply.

The belief that, "if they don't eat it at home they'd eat it at school or at friends' homes," is true, to some extent. Children need consistency and firmness, not inflexibility or parental dictatorship. I believe that with firm but loving consistency they can be taught healthy habits, and not to "cheat" behind your back.

Remember the adage that "children eat what their parents eat"? Parents need to look at what and how much they eat, drink and weigh. We can't lecture our children about good nutrition if we have a similar problem. Very often the child's weight issue is a family problem. In fact, our own short-term risk of developing cardiovascular or diabetic events is far greater than our children's. You can't convert an adolescent who

is a pizza, hamburger and potato chip "junkie," or an adolescent who is a sweet snacker into a fish eater overnight.

Start setting goals on a weekly or monthly basis to change your children's dietary practices to reach the Twenty Risk Factor Diet (Chapter 4) score of less than 30 points of a day. Give them dietetic candies or sugar-free and fat-free ice cream as treats. Few American teenagers are going to get excited about three to four seafood meals a week. So, go gradually by serving it at home once a week, and after several weeks, make it twice a week.

Just as important, dramatically cut back on all high glycemic foods and snacks, such as sugar, high fructose corn sweeteners, frosted or glazed cereals, bread, pasta, potato and rice and all sweets. Since one gram of fat (any fat) has approximately 10 calories versus four calories for proteins or carbohydrates, it is essential to reduce all greasy, fried or cheese-loaded foods from their diet.

In 2006, major American beverage bottlers and distributors (with former President Clinton's help) agreed to stop supplying elementary and middle schools with sodas or sweetened fruit juices by 2008. They further agreed to supply high schools with only diet sodas and unsweetened juices, all in an attempt to reduce total daily calories. Although this was presented as the first step toward reducing obesity in children, in my view, it is only a tiny step with doubtful benefits. What do these children eat and drink before and after school?

The benefit is brief, if they return to the sugary drinks after school. Replacing regular sodas with sugar-free soda may reduce 120–240 calories. Moreover, soft drinks and all sodas, regular or dietetic, contain phosphoric acid, which may wash calcium out of the bones and eliminate it through the kidneys. Long-term and frequent consumption of sodas may contribute to osteoporosis.

To me, a more rational plan would have been complete elimination of soda from schools coupled with a dramatic change in school cafeterias to healthful food choices. If parents do not commit to limit high glycemic foods and snacks, replacing regular soda with sugar-free soda is highly unlikely to have a significant long-term benefit.

Teaching and coaching children to eat properly requires patience. An interested and knowledgeable pediatrician can be immensely helpful, especially since children frequently tend to listen to an outsider. Importantly, the pediatrician can check for other components of metabolic syndrome and provide helpful guidance.

Stress the need for regular exercise

For successful weight management, encourage youngsters to have regular, vigorous exercise. Regular walking, biking, basketball, swimming, skateboarding, roller-skating and other activities (but not bowling, spectator sports or computer games), *must* be a component of any weight management in this age group.

They may resist and complain, but eventually they'll get over it. A parent's frustration may make the child more likely to push for a return to an unhealthy diet. Children may be more likely to adapt than their parents.

Anti-obesity drugs

Weight management is never an all-or-nothing issue. Even a five percent to 10% weight loss in three to six months can significantly improve insulin resistance and help improve components of metabolic syndrome. For a 200-pound person, a 10- to 20-pound weight loss (5% to 10%) is sufficient to see the initial benefits.

Although diet, lifestyle and behavioral modifications can help achieve modest goals, some people need help to jump-start weight management. And, some people do lose and regain their weight.

For those people, especially if they have metabolic syndrome, abdominal or generalized obesity, the use of an anti-obesity drug with demonstrated long-term safety and efficacy would have a great appeal. Regrettably, we do not have such a drug! The few FDA-approved anti-obesity drugs and others currently in the investigational phase have been primarily used for a relatively short time (from a few months to two years). Fen-phen was taken off the market a few years after a controversy related to possible heart valve injury. That lesson should be remembered when we recommend or take any anti-obesity drug entering the bloodstream.

Prescription drugs

One recent drug, sibutramine, marketed in the United States under the trade name Meridia, has been shown to be relatively safe on a short-term basis. Unlike fenfluramine and dexfenfluramine, which could potentially cause heart valve lesions after long-term use (over six months) or result in vascular damage in the lungs, sibutramine does not seem to have these potential effects.

One concern with sibutramine is that it may raise blood pressure. Other relatively mild side effects include headaches, insomnia and constipation. However, as with any new drug, we can't assume that these are the only side effects. Only long-term studies with a large number of individuals can provide adequate information regarding both safety and efficacy.

Sibutramine (like other anti-obesity drugs) does not work by itself and without dietary and lifestyle modifications. It's not a miracle drug that sheds weight overnight. Sibutramine is a prescription drug and should be taken under close medical supervision. It is also expensive and often not reimbursed by many health insurers.

Orlistat, marketed as Xenical, is another prescription drug promoted for weight loss and weight management. In early 2007, a lower dose of Orlistat was approved by the USFDA as an over-the-counter weight-loss aid. Orlistat blocks the function of an intestinal enzyme—lipase—necessary for the breakdown and absorption of dietary fats. When the action of lipase is blocked, a good part of dietary fat passes through the intestine unabsorbed (which may cause loose bowel movements or even diarrhea).

In a recent European study of 688 obese adults, participants were placed on low-calorie diets and Orlistat, 120 milligrams three times per day. After one year, the Orlistat group lost 10% of their body weight, compared with six percent for those not taking it. However, as soon as they stopped taking Orlistat they experienced a rebound, regaining nearly all their weight in a short time. So, you have to ask the question: Is it worth taking a drug three times a day for one year to lose only four percent of body weight (10% for the drug, minus six percent for the placebo)? For a 200-pound person, four percent is approximately eight pounds after one year. This is hardly a breakthrough or even a modest improvement in obesity treatment.

This raises a question about the over-the-counter version. Undoubtedly such lower doses will prove even less effective. It's my view that the FDA's approval of this drug for over-the counter sale was a mistake.

Acarbose is also a prescription drug (marketed as Precose) that partially blocks the breakdown of sugar and some starches so that it slows the absorption of sugar into the bloodstream and reduces the insulin surge. In theory it might help reduce the risk of abdominal obesity and perhaps be of some value in weight management. However, there are not enough data to recommend acarbose for this reason.

Self-directed obesity management is not easy. The urge and desire to eat can never be simply turned off. A US government survey estimates that 5%—nearly 10 million adults—are now extremely obese. In 2007, the Rand Corporation, a nonprofit think tank, reported that the prevalence of extreme obesity (or "morbid obesity," body mass index of more than 40) increased by 33% between the years 2000 and 2005. Would we have been silent if a food borne illness, or other serious disease had increased by one-third in five years?

Rimonabant is an investigational drug that may be approved by the USFDA. It has been shown in several studies to cause 10–15 pound weight loss, when taken on a daily basis for a year. However, more than one-third of the subjects discontinued it because of side effects including nausea, depression and anxiety. As with sibutramine, I find it hard to justify the use of this drug every day for one year to lose 10–15 pounds, then regain it when the drug is stopped.

The absence of an effective and safe long-term anti-obesity drug (like blood pressure-lowering or cholesterol-lowering drugs) reinforces my original argument: Weight mismanagement results from an imbalance between calorie intake and calorie output; calorie reduction is always the primary way to loss weight.

Obesity and metabolic syndrome are often associated with insulin resistance or diabetes, low levels of the good HDL-cholesterol, elevated levels of triglycerides and extremely harmful small LDL-cholesterol particles, hypertension and other coronary risk factors. Weight loss alone will not control or normalize all these abnormalities. To minimize your risk of a cardiovascular

> Almost every overweight person has tried one or more "diets" and has failed. For this population of the extremely obese, a surgical approach is a viable option.

event, you must address each and every one of these co-existing coronary risk factors. Successful weight management will improve all your risk factors and may reduce the need for drugs to control them.

Surgical management of obesity

Surgical treatments for severe obesity are not new; they have been performed for nearly 40 years. Technical and safety aspects of obesity surgery, referred to as bariatric surgery, have dramatically improved. Until recently most healthcare insurers, including Medicare and Medicaid, did not cover the cost of bariatric surgery. In 2006, however, the Centers for Medicare and Medicaid Services announced that they will provide national coverage for obesity surgery, prompting a number of healthcare insurers to do likewise.

To qualify for coverage, candidates must have...

1. A body mass index of greater than 35 (severe to extreme obesity)

2. At least one medical complication of obesity such as hypertension, heart disease, stroke, severe fatty liver, diabetes, breast, colon or prostate cancers (which are more common among obese persons)

3. Failed medical treatments

4. The procedure performed at a Center of Excellence for bariatric surgery by experienced surgeons, who have expertise in pre- and post-operative management of these cases. This requirement is mandated to minimize poor outcomes that are more common with less experienced surgeons.

To qualify as a Center of Excellence for bariatric surgery, each affiliated surgeon must have done at least 125 cases and performed 50 or more such surgeries per year to maintain his/her skills. This important requirement encourages people to pick qualified, experienced surgeons.

There are several types of surgeries. "Adjustable gastric banding," done with laparoscopic technique (requiring a few small incisions, no resection of any part of the stomach, and a very short hospital stay) has gained worldwide popularity, especially in Europe and South America. In the US, gastric bypass surgery is the preferred method, but the adjustable gastric banding is now available throughout the country.

Before you decide to go the surgical route, you must understand that these procedures do not offer an easy and lifetime "cure." There are many rules and dietary restrictions that you should follow to achieve the desired goal and avoid significant complications. This is why you need a Center of Excellence with a team of knowledgeable people who can educate and support you, both before and after surgery.

Over-the-counter drugs, herbs and supplements

Taking 200 mcg of chromium two times per day may somewhat improve the body's response to insulin, especially among people with abdominal obesity, whether diabetes is present or not. Chromium is not likely to help without following diet and lifestyle modifications.

Several over-the-counter appetite suppressants use phenylpropanolamine as the active ingredient. At manufacturers' recommended doses, these products are relatively safe but they are not effective unless combined with both diet and exercise. Rare major side effects include stroke, heart attack and severe irregularities of heart rhythm, which can be fatal. Minor side effects include nervousness, sleep disturbance, elevated blood pressure, dizziness, headache and nausea.

Various herbs, ginseng, DHEA, melatonin and many other supplements have no appreciable weight loss effect unless accompanied by the two pillars of weight management: eating less and exercising more.

Abdominal and generalized obesity is a chronic disease that takes years to develop, and therefore requires sustained long-term treatment. As with any other chronic disease, if treatment stops, the condition recurs. If it were easy to treat, no one would be overweight. To repeat— no matter what approach you choose, it must include the two pillars—reduce energy intake (calories) and increase energy output (exercise).

Risk Factor #3
Sedentary Lifestyle

Over the last decade, a wealth of information has reaffirmed what everyone intuitively knows— vigorous physical exercise has numerous health benefits. Unfortunately, less than 25% of the US population does any kind of exercise. Even more alarming is the fact that less than eight percent of men and less than five percent of women engage in regular, moderate to intense exercises three or more times a week. This is the case in most other developed countries.

Sedentary lifestyle is one of the worst example of a self-inflicted disease. You may argue that smoking, excessive drinking, obesity, metabolic syndrome or diabetes may have some genetic predisposition or addictive component. Not so for being sedentary!

According to the US Centers for Disease Control and Prevention, sedentary lifestyle accounts for more than 250,000 deaths each year. That's more than the total deaths from breast, colon and prostate cancers.

Why exercise?

Regular exercise dramatically reduces the risk of cardiovascular events, diabetes, abdominal obesity and several cancers, including breast, ovarian, prostate and colon.

Study: An eight-year study of 3,120 healthy women showed that physical fitness (as assessed by treadmill testing) dramatically affected cardiovascular health. The age-adjusted death rate from cardiovascular disease among the most fit women in the study was eight in 10,000 persons each year, as compared to 74 among the least fit women —a more than 900% difference.

Exercisers also live longer. According to a study of 5,000 people published in the *Archives of Internal Medicine*, people who walk or do other moderate exercise for at least 30 minutes a day, five times a week, live up to four years longer than their sedentary counterparts—largely because they put off developing heart disease.

Increased body weight, especially in the obese range (BMI over 30), is associated with elevated blood levels of a number of inflammatory compounds released by intra-abdominal fat cells. For example, one of these compounds,

In the US Nurses' Study, scientists monitored more than 84,000 women for eight years. Women who exercised regularly (even brisk walking) had a 54% lower combined risk of heart attack and stroke than their sedentary counterparts.

A recent, 25-year study from Sweden showed that men who exercised on a regular basis were 70% less likely to die from cardiovascular disease than were sedentary persons. In another 22-year follow-up study of 2,014 middle-aged Norwegian men, the risk of dying from cardiovascular disease among those who exercised regularly was 53% lower than that of nonexercising men.

Finnish researchers studied the relationship of leisure-time physical activities and death from all causes in 16,000 male and female Finnish twins, followed up for about 17 years. Among the twin pairs who were healthy at the beginning of the study, the relative risk of death from causes other than accidents, violence or suicide was 34% less for occasional exercisers and 56% less for regular exercisers. This study confirms that longevity is not necessarily genetically predetermined, and that lifestyle is a paramount factor to living healthier.

C-reactive protein (CRP) is a marker for ongoing inflammation within the wall of the arteries or joints. Obese persons are 10 times more likely to have high CRP levels than normal weight persons. However, physically active obese persons are less likely to have high CRP levels than inactive ones. Similarly, physically active obese persons are less likely to have significant cholesterol abnormalities than their sedentary counterparts. In other words, regular physical activities/exercises can improve cardiovascular risk factors, and reduce the intensity of inflammatory processes within coronary plaques.

For men and women with preexisting coronary artery disease, regular exercise is just as important as any heart medication. Exercise helps to open up side channels (collaterals) in the coronary artery, which improves blood circulation to the heart muscle. Regular physical activities also increase the production of an enormously important compound called nitric oxide within the wall of the arteries. Nitric oxide (a distant cousin of nitroglycerin that is used by heart patients to relieve angina) plays a significant role in dilating coronary and cerebral arteries in times of need so that the heart and the brain will be able to receive adequate blood flow and oxygen supplies. Studies have consistently shown that regular exercise decreases death rates from coronary artery disease among these individuals by 30% to 50%.

A recent long-term study (46 years) from the Framingham study, revealed that regular physical activities increased healthy life expectancy by 3.5 years, compared with sedentary people or non-exercisers. Many people confuse thinness or

HEALTH BENEFITS OF REGULAR EXERCISE

CARDIOVASCULAR BENEFITS
DECREASES:

Risk of heart attack by 50%

Risk of stroke by more than 35%

Risk of peripheral vascular disease by more than 30%

The "bad" LDL-cholesterol by 10%–15%

Triglycerides by 20%–30%

Abdominal obesity

Metabolic syndrome

Risk of diabetes by 60% in men and by 90% in women

Blood pressure

Blood fibrinogen, a potent clotting factor
Insulin resistance
Number of small, harmful LDL particles
Total body oxidant load and inflammatory compounds

INCREASES:
The "good" HDL-cholesterol by 10%–20%
Arterial wall nitric oxide, a potent vasodilator
Blood levels of TPA, a potent clot buster, by more than 20%

ANTI-CANCER BENEFITS
DECREASES:
Risk of breast cancer by 20%
Risk of colon cancer by 50%
Risk of prostate cancer by 30%
Risk of lung, ovary, pancreas and uterus cancers by 10% to 20%

OTHER BENEFITS
DECREASES:
Risk of premature aging
Weight regain after weight loss
Risk of depression and anxiety disorders
Risk of various infections
Muscle wasting and weakness
Osteoarthritis
Osteoporosis
Chronic fatigue syndrome, sleep disorders
Fibromyalgia
Risk of cognitive decline and of dementia
Constipation and irritable bowel

INCREASES:
Stamina
Well-being
Libido and sexual functions
Self-esteem
Muscle tone
Lean body mass
Healthy life expectancy by more than 3.5 years
Immune system

leanness with health. They are *not* the same. This has been demonstrated in a recent eight-year study of 21,925 men between the ages of 30 and 80. Physically unfit, lean men had a much higher risk of cardiovascular-related death than did men who were fit but obese. In other words, what counts is fitness, not leanness.

The vulnerable weekend athlete and the occasional exerciser

Almost everyone—young or old, fit or unfit—can and should exercise. As the late Arthur Fiedler, conductor of the Boston Pops, once said, "He who rests, rots!" Unfortunately, occasional bursts of exercise are not only useless, but may actually be harmful. Weekend athletes have more aches and pains, pulled muscles, shinsplints, fascitis of the feet and heel problems than regular exercisers.

Researchers recently compared the impact of exercise on the oxidation of LDL-cholesterol in two groups of college students. In students who were not long-term exercisers, oxidation of LDL-cholesterol actually increased after occasional exercise sessions. In contrast, among track team members who had been regular exercisers for more than two years, LDL oxidation was reduced considerably. Why this 180-degree difference in response? During all physical activities the body produces many oxidants (free radicals). The body's ability to procure antioxidants and cope with the oxidants increases in regular exercisers but not in occasional or weekend exercisers.

The benefits of exercise and a healthy lifestyle cannot be banked for long-term benefits. In reality, the benefits of exercise are limited to days or weeks. Exercise—like eating, sleeping and good hygiene—is necessary for good health and requires repetition. "What have you done for me lately?" is the body's response to the assertion, "I used to be very athletic."

Can exercise be harmful?

Although the risk of an exercise-induced heart attack is very low, each year one out of 2,500 men over 40 suffers a heart attack while exercising. Overall, it is estimated that anywhere between four percent and 20% of all heart attacks occur after a bout of moderate to heavy exertion, especially among the least-fit individuals. This explains why the most important aspect of any exercise program is to avoid sudden, strenuous exertion, especially for unfit or nonexercising individuals.

For example, the risk of a heart attack after a bout of strenuous physical activity, such as shoveling snow, for a 50-year-old, sedentary, "out of shape" man is more than 10,000% greater than it is for a regularly exercising and well-conditioned man of the same age. For the unfit, it is a lot smarter and safer to pay the local teenager to clear the driveway than to risk a massive heart attack.

The annual incidence of exercise-related deaths in the United States is approximately one death per 100,000 young male athletes and one per 700,000 young female athletes. For middle-aged men, the risk is one per 18,000. Viewed from another perspective, the risk per total hours of exercising, it is even more miniscule: For men between the ages of 20 and 39, the risk is one per four million hours of exercise; between 40 and 49, it is one per 1.3 million hours; and between 60 and 69, the risk is one per 900,000 hours. For women, the risk at all ages is even lower than for men.

The intensity and duration of exercise must be tailored to each person's overall health and fitness level and should increase only gradually. Exercise regimens should take into account physical ability, age, gender, presence and severity of cardiovascular disease or other medical problems, the environment (e.g., hot and humid versus indoors and air-conditioned), time of day (there is more risk of an exercise-induced heart attack in the early morning), tiredness and physical or medical limitations.

What is reasonable for a 25-year-old man is not necessarily applicable to a 55-year-old. Of course, the level of physical activity for a 55-year-old healthy person is not applicable to a 55-year-old with preexisting coronary artery disease, diabetes, high blood pressure, or other risk factors. Men older than 40 and women older than 50 with any major coronary risk factor should have an exercise stress test (or exercise echocardiogram—an ultrasound version of the exercise stress test) before the start of an intensive exercise program.

What you should do

You should look at regular exercise the same way that you look at eating or sleeping—as a necessary part of your life. There are 1,440 minutes in a day, so set aside 40 or 50 of those minutes for exercise. For most sedentary people, the greatest reduction in overall mortality occurs when they move to the next level of physical activity, or to 40% of their maximum capacity. The common belief that people should exercise at 60% to 70% of their maximum capacity is true for conditioned and fit persons, especially those under 60.

What kind of exercise should you do?

Exercise does not need to be strenuous, or of very long duration, especially early in your program, or for people over 40. For older people, or people who have coronary risk factors, and people with knee, or hip problems, it should be less intense. The consequence of rigorous exercise for a physically unfit person may be a skeletal injury (muscles, ligaments, joints) which may sideline them for weeks or months.

Choose an exercise that you like—and that you want to do repeatedly. Not everyone likes tennis, racquetball, jogging, etc. Some people prefer fast walking; others may enjoy exercise along with other people at a gym or club; others may enjoy using exercise equipment at home. No matter what your preference, start exercising now...

How much exercise?

For most people, exercising for 35–45 minutes, including a few minutes to warm-up and cool down, four to five times a week may be adequate. I use a simple formula to estimate the benefit of exercise: Benefit = Duration × Intensity. So you'll be better off doing 30–35 minutes of fast walking compared with three hours of shopping at a mall (and it will be less expensive!)

What kind of equipment?

The first rule is repeat-likability. Always try the equipment for a week or two before you buy it. And never buy a cheap exercise machine; they clink and rattle and will fall apart. A good piece of equipment should last 10 years. Don't take the advice of friends, family or salespeople who may have different abilities and limitations than you.

In an 18-year study of 69,693 women (The Nurses' Health study), the absolute risk of sudden cardiac death during exercise was one per 36 million hours of exercise. Even for people who have previously suffered heart attacks, in a supervised program the risk of exercise-related death is extremely low—at one per 784,000 hours. And the risks vary among different types of exercises: for instance, the risk of a sudden cardiac death is nearly seven times higher for jogging (associated with profuse sweating, magnesium loss and dehydration) than for other forms of exercise.

And don't buy anything that's not suitable for you especially if you have certain foot, knee, hip or back problems.

Generally, an elliptical exerciser is more suitable for people with arthritis of the lower extremities, or leg, foot or back problems. An elliptical is more effective equipment for those with weight problems; it can help you burn 20% more calories than treadmills, and 30%–50% more than stationary bikes or rowing machines.

Before you buy an exercise machine, test various machines several times to choose one that is right for your temperament, needs and, most importantly, your long-term use.

For people with foot, knee or hip problems, you may find treadmills uncomfortable or painful. Instead choose the elliptical exercisers that eliminate the pounding of your feet on a hard surface (it works like gliding bike pedals; you start slowly).

What's the measure?

For years, exercise physiologists have used the heart rate as the standard indicator of exercise intensity. For people without heart disease, exercise should be intense enough to increase the heart rate to between 60% and 80% of the maximum heart rate. (Maximum heart rate is calculated as 220 minus a person's age. For example, the maximum heart rate for a fifty-five-year-old person is 220-55=165, and the desirable, exercise-induced rate is 60% to 80% of that, which is between 100 and 132 beats per minute.)

Caution: People with coronary artery disease and people with coronary risk factors should have an exercise electrocardiogram or echocardiogram before doing vigorous exercise.

Exercise has to be sustained for 30 or more minutes (plus a warm-up and cool-down of five to 10 minutes each). Activities that are not rigorous or sustained enough to be of much value include window shopping, swimming two laps and sunbathing, house chores, gardening, painting, mowing, golf, leisure walking (except perhaps for the elderly, those with severe cardiovascular diseases, or people with physical disabilities).

Brisk, long walks, jogging, rowing, ballroom dancing, elliptical exercise, biking, lap swimming, aerobic or aquatic exercises, handball, racquetball and bodybuilding are all reasonable choices. Older persons should incorporate gentle resistance training exercises into their routine. Two recent studies suggest that for older persons breaking the exercise time into two 15- to 20-minute periods is as heart healthy as one sustained period of exercise. You need to find the time, and the discipline to follow this approach.

Avoid mid-day workouts outdoors

When is exercise unhealthy? When it's done in a polluted environment. After analyzing six years of data on 1.2 million people, researchers found that long-term exposure to air pollution—specifically from car exhaust and coal-fired power plants—poses a greater risk of death from heart disease than from respiratory ailments. The reason is because air pollution provokes inflammation and accelerates atherosclerosis. Since air and ozone pollution tends to peak between noon and 4 pm, it may be wise to limit outdoor workouts during those hours—especially if you are running or walking near traffic-filled streets.

The most intensive exercises have more heart-healthy benefits, but any degree of activity—whether sustained or interrupted—does burn calories that would otherwise be converted into fat.

We burn about 60% of our calories from our basic metabolism. Another 10% is used to process what we eat and 30% are burned during daily activity including exercise. Remember that all activities help burn calories—climbing stairs and using your brain for reading, working, playing a musical instrument.

Risk Factor #4
Diet

Many studies over the past decade have shown that diet and lifestyle have an enormously important role in our health and disease. Since the mid-18th century when the average lifespan in the US and Europe was about 47 years, we have increased our longevity by about 80% to 78–80 years. We have achieved this not because our genetic pool has changed; that would take one to two million years, and it is highly unlikely that we will be around that long!

The increase in our lifespan is attributable to better sanitary conditions, vaccinations, dramatic changes in medicine and surgery and a vast number of "lifesaving drugs." Yet, we are not a very healthy people.

The longer lifespan has increased our exposure to risk factors for chronic diseases and carcinogens for 30 additional years. We add to the risk with our diet and lifestyle practices. Consequently, the risk of acquiring some diseases is greater as we age. Although the risk of various chronic diseases in an older person is 1,000 times more than in someone 20–25 years of age, aging is not the cause, but aging is *associated* with these chronic diseases.

The evidence is overwhelming that dietary abuses and sedentary living contribute to most of these age-associated diseases. The reverse is equally convincing—prudent diet and lifestyle practices over the years will dramatically reduce the risk of these age-associated diseases.

Most cardiovascular and lung diseases, obesity, diabetes and cancers of the breast, colorectal, lung and prostate can be prevented by diet and lifestyle modifications. I will recommend them in this book.

As I will show in the later chapters, most American diets are loaded with unhealthy ingredients, including...

- Fat (both visible and hidden) and which is often saturated, trans fats or partially hydrogenated fat
- High glycemic index carbohydrates (sugar, fructose, corn sweeteners, starches)
- Calories—on average 300–500 more daily calories than you need
- Salt (two or three times the daily requirement).

The typical diet also lacks important healthy ingredients, such as...

- Vitamin D—inadequate intake of this vitamin contributes to high rates of colon, prostate, pancreas and kidney cancers as well as osteoporosis
- Antioxidants and anticarcinogens from dark fruits and vegetables
- Seafood—low consumption of seafood results in little intake of seafood omega-3 fat which reduces the risk of heart attack by 40% and the risk of sudden death by heart attack by 70%
- Monounsaturated fat from olive oils which have a 3,000-year history of safety and healthfulness
- Adequate dietary fiber, which helps to avoid constipation, diverticulosis and irritable bowel disease.

Plus, instead of one or two glasses of wine with dinner (which reduces the risk of coronary artery disease), we drink beer or cocktails—a process that has contributed to more heart attacks and strokes and to more than 20 million alcoholics in the US.

So what should I eat?

The Twenty Risk Factor Diet explained in this book offers you many choices for healthy, enjoyable eating. It is the product of many years of extensive research, and has drawn from over 3,000 scientific and peer-reviewed studies published in medical and other scientific journals in the past 10 years.

Remember, *food is not the enemy*, unless we make it so. To take advantage of the vast benefits of a variety of available foods, we must have clear ideas why we should eat certain foods and reduce or avoid others. The TRF scoring system provides you with the most precise and scientific tool to choose your foods among endless varieties, limited only by your preferences and culinary inventiveness. Always use the TRF scoring system and try to keep your TRF scores below 30 each day.

Risk Factor #5
Low Levels of
HDL-Cholesterol

For decades we have promoted the notion that the "bad" LDL-cholesterol is the main culprit in heart attacks and strokes. A low level of the "good" HDL-cholesterol is an even greater culprit than elevated LDL, especially among women. Using the normal values for HDL-cholesterol from Table TK, at least 50% of men and 70% of women with coronary artery disease have low levels of HDL-cholesterol.

In a recent study of 8,200 men and women with documented coronary artery disease, 30% had total cholesterol levels below the current "normal" level of 200 mg/dl. Among this group, 52% had HDL-cholesterol levels below 35 mg/dl even though their total cholesterol was "normal." In fact, for women, low HDL levels are far more important than elevated LDL levels; nearly twice as many women with coronary artery disease have low HDL as those who have significant elevated LDL levels.

A low HDL-cholesterol level is a powerful predictor of future cardiovascular diseases. For every 1 mg/dl increase in HDL-cholesterol level, the risk of a heart attack or death from coronary artery disease is reduced by more than 6%. Yet, until a few years ago few healthcare providers paid attention to HDL-cholesterol levels. For more than four decades the healthcare establishment had focused on the quartet of elevated LDL-cholesterol, high blood pressure, smoking and a high-fat, high-cholesterol diet as the principal causes of cardiovascular diseases.

With the introduction of cholesterol-lowering statins and their aggresive promotion by pharmaceutical companies, LDL-cholesterol has been portrayed as the major culprit pushing HDL-cholesterol and most other risk factors to a less important status. The gravitational pull to LDL perpetuated by massive advertising directly to consumers has made statins blockbuster, multibillion-dollar drugs. To the delight of the big pharmaceutical companies (and the detriment of the public), elevated blood LDL-cholesterol has become synonymous with heart attack in the minds of the healthcare providers and the public at large.

Lowering blood levels of LDL-cholesterol by statins can reduce the risk of a heart attack or stroke in about 30% of those who take them. What about the other 70% who do not benefit from statins? Do we abandon them? Medical science has known for over 40 years that HDL-cholesterol protects the heart. But drug companies have no blockbuster HDL-raising drug, so there are few incentives to research and promote raising HDL for heart health. Yet, I've been advocating it for over 20 years. (In fact, my car's license tag over the same period has been HIGH-HDL!)

In the past few years, numerous studies have shown that although intensive LDL-cholesterol-lowering can arrest the progression of coronary artery disease, it does not shrink coronary plaques. Only significantly raising the HDL-cholesterol can actually reverse the process. But all HDL particles are not created equal; some are more heart-healthy than others.

Subclasses of HDL-cholesterol

The composition and size of all lipoproteins, including HDL, constantly change inside the bloodstream. They continuously barter and exchange components so that their sizes expand or shrink. HDL particles change almost nonstop, not only in the bloodstream but also within the wall of the arteries and inside coronary plaques.

Although HDL comes in several sizes, by and large two distinct types account for the majority of the mass of HDL: HDL-2, which is smaller, and HDL-3, which is larger. The most important difference between these two subclasses is that HDL-2 carries a special protein on its molecule, called apoprotein A1, which plays a crucial role in making HDL-2 cardioprotective. HDL-3 carries a different protein—apoprotein A2—which does not have the same cardioprotective role. In people without cardiovascular disease and normal HDL-cholesterol levels, more than 30% of their HDL particles are HDL-2. In contrast, people who naturally have very low HDL levels or those with coronary artery disease, almost always have very low levels of HDL-2—about 5% to 7% of their total HDL is made up of HDL-2.

What does HDL do to earn "The Good Cholesterol" label?

HDL particles are like tiny balls that carry several protein molecules along with cholesterol, triglycerides, other complex fat particles and potent antioxidant enzymes. Each one of these components plays a different role in heart-health. For example…

1. One of the most important functions of HDL-2 is carried out by one of its proteins, *apoprotein A1.* The liver makes LDL-cholesterol, which travels through the bloodstream, trespassing through the artery wall to cause havoc. Apoprotein A1 can extract LDL-cholesterol particles that are dumped in the wall of the arteries or within coronary plaques, and carry them through the bloodstream back to the liver for disposal. This process is aptly called *the reverse cholesterol transport,* and is one of our most important defenses against heart attack, stroke or peripheral vascular disease.

2. HDL-2 is the most potent antioxidant in the arteries, and dramatically reduces oxidation of LDL particles that are dumped in the subsurface of the arteries. Since LDL-cholesterol oxidation is a mandatory step in the development of coronary plaques, HDL-2 helps reduce plaque formation. The antioxidant function of HDL is carried out by its apoprotein A1 and an enzyme called paraoxanase.

3. HDL-2 particles act like sentries that guard and prevent LDL particles from going through the endothelium and into the subsurface of the arteries.

4. White blood cells and platelets are aggravated by oxidized LDL, and release toxic compounds with arterial wall plaques. These "inflammatory" compounds contribute to plaques' turmoil and eventual rupture. HDL-2 blocks activation of white blood cells and platelets, thereby reducing inflammation, within the plaques and reducing their vulnerability to rupture.

See page 45 for a summary of some of HDL's good deeds that have earned it the "good cholesterol" name.

Is HDL-cholesterol always cardioprotective?

One of the most common mistakes of healthcare providers is assuring their patients that their HDL levels are "normal," and that they don't have to worry about their high LDL-cholesterol. This erroneous assumption and the recommendations based upon it are dated and dangerous. I see these patients frequently in my practice! This creates a false sense of security, and makes it hard to convince them that their "normal" or even high levels of HDL do not always mean they are safe.

Although HDL is a potent antioxidant, like almost all other antioxidants, the hunter can become the hunted, and the antioxidant can become pro-oxidant. In many patients with diabetes, multiple coronary risk factors, or significant systemic inflammations that may cause an accelerated atherosclerosis—such as rheumatoid arthritis, systemic lupus or AIDS—the oxidant load within the bloodstream or coronary plaques is so intense that even the HDL particles become oxidized. These oxidized HDL particles are not only ineffective as an antioxidant, they paradoxically become oxidants themselves, and instead of retarding the oxidization of LDL-cholesterol, they contribute to it, further worsening the problem.

How does the "good" HDL become the "bad" HDL?

Coronary plaques are loaded with activated white blood cells, platelets and smooth muscle cells, which continuously spit out numerous inflammatory compounds that keep the turmoil within the plaques and their vicinity active. Nitric oxide (a cousin of nitroglycerine) is a powerful vasodilator that is produced by the cells lining the inner wall of the arteries (endothelium). Among their other misdeeds, some oxidants within active plaques break down nitric oxide, and further deprive the artery of needed protection. As if that weren't bad enough, some of these nitric oxide by products attack apoprotein A1 on the HDL-2 molecule, a process called nitration, transforming the HDL-2 into a turncoat pro-oxidant. The conversion of HDL-2 from good to bad is an enormously important issue not only in the management of people with cardiovascular disease, but also millions of people with elevated blood cholesterol who have not yet had a heart attack or stroke.

The majority of healthcare providers are not even aware of this phenomenon. I often see patients with a normal or even elevated HDL and multiple risk factors who have not been treated because, "My good cholesterol is very good—so I didn't need treatment for my bad cholesterol."

Should we routinely measure apoprotein A1?

In most cases, measuring HDL-cholesterol provides a reasonable guide for deciding the course of treatment. On occasion, tests to determine subclasses of HDL will provide some additional information. Similarly, in a few instances measurement of apoprotein A1 is helpful. Examples include people with co-existing major coronary risk factors; diabetics who usually have a high oxidant load; when both LDL and HDL are elevated. In people with moderate to excessive alcohol intake whose HDL-cholesterol levels are deceptively high, most of it is made up of the less cardioprotective HDL-3. So measuring HDL subclasses may be quite helpful.

Normal HDL-2 should be more than 30% of total HDL or greater than 15 mg/dl in men and greater than 18 mg/dl in women. The normal value for apoprotein A1 is greater than 100 mg/dl for both men and women.

What does HDL-cholesterol do?

- Blocks entry of white blood cells and cholesterol into the wall of the arteries, which reduces the risk of plaque formation

- Reduces oxidation and clumping of LDL-cholesterol particles by 50%

- Transports cholesterol from coronary plaques to the liver for disposal, hence it is a potent "reverse transporter" of cholesterol

- Helps to repair damaged lining of the arteries

- Reduces activation of platelet, so the risk of clot formation is reduced

- Improves coronary dilatation and blood flow through coronary artery*

- Is a potent antioxidant and anti-inflammatory within the wall of the arteries, reducing the risk of plaque rupture, which causes heart attack and stroke**

- All of this contributes to a significant reduction in the risk of heart attacks, stroke and peripheral artery disease.

*Levkau B et al. Circulation 2004; 110: 3355–59
**Ansell BJ et al. J Am Coll Cardiol 2005; 46: 1792–98

Why do some people have low HDL-cholesterol levels?

Low HDL-cholesterol level has multiple genetic, lifestyle or dietary causes…

- In many people, a low HDL level is in part due to a genetic defect in the production of HDL-cholesterol. For example, Japanese children consistently have higher HDL levels than their Western counterparts, an advantage that continues into their adult life. The more severe forms of HDL deficiency almost always have a familial and genetic component, and a family history of coronary artery disease in several members, usually under the age of 45.

- Regular, vigorous exercise can raise HDL-cholesterol by an average of 10% to 15%. On the other hand, sedentary people lower their HDL levels by 10% to 15%. A sedentary person who engages in regular, moderate-intensity exercise can increase HDL levels at times by 20% to 30%. For someone with an HDL of 30 mg/dl, a 10% to 20% increase is only an additional 3–6 mg/dl. Although every milligram increase in HDL level reduces the risk of a heart attack by 6%, 3–6 mg/dl are not enough to provide significant cardioprotection. When HDL is so low, these individuals will need additional means of raising it.

In people with naturally high levels of HDL-cholesterol (who obviously do not seem to have any genetic disorder impacting their ability to produce HDL), regular exercise causes a more pronounced increase in HDL-cholesterol levels, sometimes in excess of 20% to 30%. In contrast, the response to regular exercises in people with very low HDL-cholesterol is only 5% to 10%, even though these are the people who need higher HDL levels the most. Unfortunately, most of these people have one or more genetic abnormalities (mutations) in their HDL production, making them much less responsive to various dietary and lifestyle modifications.

- Abdominal obesity almost always lowers HDL by 10% to 20%. General obesity, however, is not necessarily associated with lower HDL levels. People with abdominal obesity and low HDL levels also have a high percentage of small dense LDL particles which are particularly atherogenic, making a bad situation even worse.

- Bad dietary habits can lower HDL-cholesterol by 10% to 20%. For example, consuming high-glyceric carbohydrates, especially sugar and starches, lowers the HDL production. A recent study among children and adolescents with elevated blood cholesterol levels showed that children who consumed too much carbohydrates had HDL-cholesterol levels that were about 20% lower than children whose carbohydrate intake was relatively low. In adults, limiting dietary carbohydrate intake to no more than 45% of total calories, while increasing monounsaturates, will frequently raise HDL-cholesterol by about 10% to 20%.

- Elevated blood triglycerides are usually associated with low-HDL-cholesterol levels. By lowering triglyceride levels, you can increase HDL by more than 20%. When the levels of blood triglyceride are high, the HDL particles unselfishly barter off some of their cholesterol to VLDL particles that carry a lot of triglycerides through the bloodstream. In exchange, VLDL particles donate or shed off some of their triglycerides to HDL particles. This internal exchange helps to somewhat lower the blood triglyceride level. At the same time the HDL-cholesterol level is lowered (by giving away its cholesterol).

  However, HDL-2 particles retain their apoprotein A1, but their work load is significantly increased because the large number of VLDL particles now act a bit like their step-sisters (LDL), and the poor HDL particles have to deal with them, too. This is a major problem associated with high levels of triglycerides. It's unfortunately often overlooked by healthcare providers. As triglycerides go down (with various interventions), the bartering process is reversed, allowing the HDL level to rise.

- Low-fat diets are still popular among many healthcare providers, nutritionists and dieticians who continue to use the American Heart

Rate of Coronary Artery Diseases by HDL Level

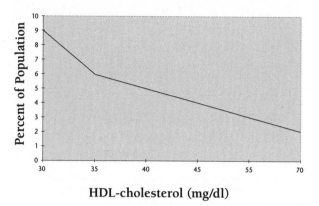

HDL-cholesterol (mg/dl)

Association's dated recommendations. Low-fat diets, especially those without monounsaturates or non-hydrogenated vegetable oils, also lower HDL-2 levels.

The public and healthcare providers have the misconception that changing your diet means going to a low-fat, low-cholesterol diet. This notion has had its "15 minutes of fame." It's not accurate, or helpful and may even be harmful. (Remember, it is the type, not the amount, of fat that is important.) Aside from the fact that a low-fat diet has no cardiovascular benefit and may increase the risk of stroke by 50%, a low-fat diet is the most common cause of diet-induced low HDL-cholesterol level.

Although saturated fats do not lower HDL levels (in fact, they may actually raise it), trans fatty acids lower it significantly. Deep fried foods, chips, french fried potatoes, cakes, chocolates, cookies, donuts, pastries, pies and snacks with a high concentration of trans fatty acids significantly decrease HDL levels.

A diet rich in olive oil (74% monounsaturates), nuts such as almonds and hazelnuts (84% monounsaturates), pistachios and walnuts (but not peanuts, cashews or Brazil nuts) and darker-fleshed fish (salmon, tuna) all help to raise HDL levels.

A glass of wine (or two) with dinner may also help raise the HDL by as much as 10–15 mg/dl. However, excessive alcohol intake may raise the HDL-3, and may paradoxically lower the much-needed HDL-2. This is an argument for drinking no more than one or two drinks.

- Smoking can lower HDL-cholesterol by more than 10%. Conversely, smoking cessation can raise HDL levels by 10% to 15% within a few weeks.

- Estrogen deficiency in post-menopausal women can lower HDL by 10% to 15%. On the other hand, oral estrogen replacement therapy can raise HDL by 10% to 15%. Estrogen skin patches, however, barely raise HDL-cholesterol levels (by two to five percent). Oral estrogen is effective because after absorption from the intestine it goes directly to the liver, where it stimulates the projection of HDL. However, estrogen patches provide only minute amounts of estrogen on a continuous basis, so very little estrogen reaches the liver to impact HDL production.

- Gender difference in blood levels of an enzyme produced by the liver called "hepatic lipase" is a significant contributor to lower HDL and higher LDL levels in men but not women (even after allowance is made for all other variables such as age, hormonal status and weight). The higher levels of this enzyme in men account for almost 97% of the gender difference in HDL levels. Intensive cholesterol-altering interventions can reduce blood levels of this lipase and raise the HDL levels.

- Long-term intake of steroid hormones, including cortisone-like compounds, anabolic steroids, testosterone, DHEA, and androsterone can lower HDL levels by five percent to 10%.

HOW TO RAISE YOUR GOOD HDL-CHOLESTEROL

- *Reduce:* Sugar and starches, margarines, shortening/cooking fat and deep-fried foods

- *Increase:* Seafood, especially dark-fleshed; olive oil; dark fruits and vegetables

- Excercise regularly, four to five times/week for 30-40 minutes each

- Stop smoking!

- Strictly control diabetes and elevated triglyceride levels

- Take niacin, 1500-2000 mg/day (under supervision of a healthcare provider)

- Statins (cholesterol-lowering drugs)

- Purified omega-3 fatty acid capsules, 2000-3000 mg/day

- Fibrates (triglyceride-lowering drugs)

- Alcohol, one to two drinks with dinner, if desired

What you should do

The best way to raise your HDL-cholesterol is to correct all the 10 factors that lower its levels in the blood. Among these, a sedentary lifestyle, abdominal obesity, elevated triglycerides, smoking and dietary habits are the primary culprits.

The Twenty Risk Factor Diet will help raise your HDL-cholesterol significantly. High glycemic foods (sweets and starches) invariably reduce HDL production. The single most important dietary factor that contributes to low HDL level is a low-fat diet. The liver requires the right kind of fat, such as monosaturates, even saturated fat, but not trans fat or vegetable fat (stick margarines, shortening or cooking fats) to produce HDL-cholesterol.

A recent Japanese study showed the benefit from daily consumption of about two tablespoons a day of cocoa powder. HDL-cholesterol increased by 24% and oxidation of LDL-cholesterol was significantly reduced. This antioxidant effect was partly due to production of a higher level of HDL (the most potent antioxidant in the artery wall) and polyphenolic antioxidants in cocoa. *Reminder:* That's dark chocolate, not milk chocolate (which contains shortening and the dreaded trans fats).

- **Know your TRF score**

A dietary plan based on the TRF scoring system (with TRF scores of 20 to 30 per day for all foods and snacks) fulfills all the dietary requirements for raising your HDL-cholesterol by 10% to 15%. The addition of one or two glasses of wine (or one or two cocktails) with dinner may contribute to a further 10% to 15% increase in HDL level.

- **Drugs to raise HDL-cholesterol**

Niacin, a member of the B vitamins (at doses of 1500–2000 mg/dl) is the most effective HDL-raising drug we have. Nearly everyone has side effects from niacin at high doses. They include skin rashes, hot flashes and rapid heart rate, which all subside in 15 to 30 minutes.

To minimize the risk, always start niacin at low doses of no more than 250 mg per day. The dose can be expanded by 250–500 mg every two weeks to reach the goal of 1000–1500 mg/every day in divided doses. This slow adaptive process taking four to six weeks will enable nine out of 10 people to tolerate niacin.

Important: Some useless "no flush" niacins are sold over-the-counter, but they do not raise HDL. Since many individuals with low HDL-cholesterol levels also have elevated LDL-cholesterol, the use of statins is an effective, double-edged approach to lower LDL levels and at the same time raise HDL by seven percent to 10%. Fibrates also can raise HDL levels by five percent to 10%, especially as triglyceride levels are lowered.

Some novel and effective HDL-raising drugs on the horizon may become available within a few years. *Torcetrapib* was a promising agent that could raise HDL-cholesterol by as much as 40% to 60% by partially blocking the exchange of its cholesterol with other lipoproteins. Unfortunately, data on undesirable side effects stopped its development. It is hoped that the molecule of this ascent can be altered to retain its HDL-raising, and eliminate its side effects.

In a recent study, five weekly intravenous infusions of a specially bioengineered apoprotein A1 resulted in a dramatic increase in reverse cholesterol transport, and early evidence of plaque regression. However, this type of treatment is very expensive and impractical, especially since it requires frequent, long-term intravenous treatments. *D-4F* is an investigational drug in development that mimics the functions of apoprotein A1, but importantly, it is able to withstand digestive enzymes so that it can be taken by mouth as a pill twice a day. The full clinical application of this drug, if its long-term safety can be established, is a few years away.

Risk Factor #6
Elevated LDL-Cholesterol

More than 50 years of research and countless well-conducted studies have shown high blood cholesterol levels of the "bad" LDL is a major risk factor for coronary artery disease, stroke and peripheral artery diseases. This association has been shown across all populations worldwide—in countries with low, as well as those with very high, prevalence of cardiovascular disease.

In general, when healthcare providers and the public speak of high cholesterol, they refer to

DOES EVERYONE WITH ELEVATED BLOOD CHOLESTEROL DEVELOP CORONARY ARTERY DISEASE?

Recently researchers reported the findings of a 25-year follow-up of 12,500 men between the ages of 40 and 59 years from seven countries (five European countries, the United States and Japan). Mortality from coronary artery disease correlated well with blood cholesterol levels across the board, even in countries with traditionally low rates of coronary artery disease.

At any given level of LDL-cholesterol, however, the risk of coronary artery disease and its complications varied among different populations. These findings illustrate why similarly elevated blood cholesterol levels among various populations do not necessarily impart similar risks or require similar interventions.

The relative sensitivity of different populations to cholesterol explains why universal cholesterol reduction rules are too simple. The corrolation of blood cholesterol levels to coronary artery disease applies to men and women equally.

Why is it that any given high blood cholesterol level in different populations confers different risk levels? This is not the case for diabetes, high blood pressure, high (or very low) levels of calcium, potassium or thyroid hormone. The answer lies in what I have been emphasizing: **There are 20 major coronary risk factors—not just one.**

The synergy among co-existing risk factors explains the differences. For example, people from the southern Mediterranean tend to be more physically active, eat very little trans fat, but consume a lot of seafood, olive oil and plenty of vegetables; they drink wine with dinner and have far less abdominal obesity or diabetes than northern Europeans or Americans.

In the United States, more than one hundred million Americans have elevated LDL-cholesterol levels exceeding the 100 mg/dl cut-off point. However, not everyone with an elevated blood cholesterol level develops clinically significant or symptomatic coronary artery disease; more than one-half do not. About 20 million Americans have advanced coronary heart disease, but at least an equal number have early or silent coronary heart disease.

Recent data suggest that among men over the age of 40 and women over 50, more than one-half have already developed significant coronary artery disease even they do not display the symptoms.

Approximately 80% (or about thirty-two million) of Americans with early or advanced coronary artery disease have elevated blood cholesterol levels. People with elevated blood cholesterol and coronary artery disease, however, nearly always have other co-existing risk factors as well.

elevated levels of LDL-cholesterol. Numerous studies have convincingly shown that as the LDL-cholesterol level goes up from an optimal level of less than 100mg/dl, the risk of cardiovascular events such as coronary heart disease (CHD), stroke and peripheral artery disease (PAD) progressively rise.

In the Multiple Risk Intervention Trial, 362,000 men were followed an average of six years. The death rate was 14 per 1,000 men whose overall cholesterol was 260mg/dl as compared to four per 1,000 whose cholesterol was 180mg/dl—more than three times higher.

What does LDL do?

Cholesterol is essential for human and animal life. Some is used to maintain the integrity of cell membranes, some is used to produce bile for food digestion and hormones, such as estrogen and testosterone. In fact, without adequate cholesterol, we would die.

Relation of Blood Cholesterol Levels to Age-adjusted Risk of Death for Coronary Artery Disease

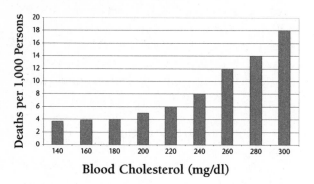

The function of LDL is to carry the life-sustaining cholesterol to various tissues and organs. But the human body only needs a small amount of cholesterol—roughly 30 to 40 mg/dl. When too many LDL-cholesterol particles travel through the bloodstream, inevitably some will trespass through the inner lining of the arteries, where they are oxidized, and set in motion a cycle that results in plaque formation.

Why do some people with high cholesterol levels have heart attacks and others don't?

Of course, not all 100 million Americans with elevated blood cholesterol are destined to have a heart attack, stroke or peripheral artery disease; more than half of them will. Not everyone who suffers a heart attack or any other major cardiovascular event has a significantly elevated LDL-cholesterol level. That's because cardiovascular diseases are nearly always caused by more than one risk factor. (The only exception is a genetic disorder affecting children and adolescents, in which blood cholesterol levels are over 400 mg/dl, and many of these youngsters develop severe coronary artery disease before age 20.) A person with multiple major (and minor) coronary risk factors has greater odds of developing

a cardiovascular event than someone with one or two risk factors. This has nothing to do with LDL.

There are other reasons, as well…

- *LDL particle size.* There are different types of LDL particles—large particles (type A) and small (type B). Generally, the large particles are less likely to trespass through the inner lining and land in the wall of the arteries. The small particles, however, readily pass through and settle in the wall of the arteries, where they quickly oxidize and contribute to the turmoil in the wall of the arteries. The small particles are more "atherogenic"—or more likely to cause plaque formation—than the large particles. Whether caused by genetics or diet and lifestyle factors, people with small, dense LDL particles are much more likely to develop coronary artery disease than those with larger LDL particles.

- *Number and "synergy" of risk factors.* Since coronary artery disease has many causes, the fewer risk factors you have, the smaller your risk of any cardiovascular disease. Moreover, the synergy among different coronary risk factors varies significantly. For example, elevated LDL-cholesterol alone may increase the 10-year risk of a cardiovascular event (such as angina, fatal or non-fatal heart attack, need for coronary artery bypass or angioplasty and stroke), by about threefold.

On the other hand, if the LDL particles are predominantly small (and therefore, more atherogenic), and the condition is associated with high levels of triglycerides and low levels of HDL, the risk goes up 10-fold. If we add in diabetes, the risk now goes up to 20-fold higher.

The potent synergy among different coronary risk factors suggests we must address all or

Relation between Total Blood Cholesterol and Rate of Death

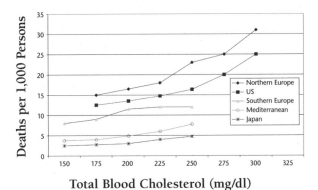

Total Blood Cholesterol (mg/dl)

as many co-existing risk factors as possible. Even more important is the timing—the sooner we start and the longer we keep all the risk factors under control, the better our chances are that we can prevent various cardiovascular events.

The tendency for the liver to overproduce LDL-cholesterol is often due to genetic abnormalities of liver cells. While you can't change your genetic makeup, you can alter the expression of these abnormal genes, blunt their role or block them altogether. The longer you wait, the more plaques will build and increase your risk of a catastrophic cardiovascular event.

I have never understood physicians who advise patients with risk factors to take a "wait and see" approach. The goal must be early intervention to prevent a cardiovascular event.

Fluctuations in blood cholesterol

Blood cholesterol levels always fluctuate from day to day or week to week. This is in part due to the constant bartering among various lipoproteins as they exchange cholesterol or triglycerides with one another. In addition to these continuous internal adjustments and fluctuations, a number of other factors can contribute to variation in blood cholesterol levels.

Recently I conducted a study among healthy hospital employees who were not on a

cholesterol-lowering drug or diet. Blood samples were taken on a weekly basis for four weeks and duplicate samples were sent to two different laboratories. More than 90% of the time, total cholesterol, LDL, HDL, and triglycerides varied by at least 10% during those four consecutive weeks. A person's total cholesterol level could be 200 mg/dl one week, and 220 mg/dl or 180 mg/dl another week, without any cholesterol-lowering intervention.

Because of the wide fluctuations in cholesterol levels from week to week, we can't always rely on one reading to judge an individual's cholesterol status unless they are very high or entirely normal. Similarly, you should not judge the success or failure of any cholesterol-altering diet or medication on the basis of one blood test, if the values are within 10% of either side.

Why do some people have high LDL-cholesterol?

Despite a common misconception, the LDL-cholesterol level has no significant correlation to dietary cholesterol. Millions of people who eat the typical Western diet loaded with fat and cholesterol have normal blood cholesterol levels. Conversely, millions of vegans (strict vegetarians who do not eat any animal products) have a diet that is totally cholesterol free but they do not have zero blood cholesterol. In fact, many of them have high blood cholesterol. Only animal products—as well as animal cells and tissues—contain cholesterol. Plants and plant products that include oils do not have any cholesterol.

So where does it come from? Humans and animals make cholesterol in the liver and some other organs. Think of a cow—the cow takes in perfectly healthy complex carbohydrates such as grass or corn and turns it into small molecules that reach the liver where they are reassembled into different compounds like fat and cholesterol.

Our bodies do the same thing. So, the vegans—in spite of their cholesterol-free diet, make their own cholesterol.

How much cholesterol the liver makes depends on various genetic signals the liver receives. Normally each liver cell has several receptors for LDL-cholesterol. As the particles reach the liver though the bloodstream, they recognize these receptors, and move in, whereby they are literally trapped, and brought inside the liver for disposal. The more LDL receptors per liver cell, the more LDL particles are filtered out, resulting in lower blood cholesterol. Unfortunately, millions of people have genetic abnormalities that will result in having very few or no functioning LDL-receptors.

Where do the particles go when there aren't enough receptors? The homeless LDL particles return to the bloodstream and keep the LDL levels high. The liver is also making more LDL, and sending it into the bloodstream, thereby increasing the blood cholesterol level.

In people who have normal blood cholesterol levels, each liver cell has two to four LDL-receptors at a given time, but the liver can numbers can be doubled when needed. Higher numbers of LDL receptors can remove a greater amount of LDL particles from the bloodstream, and help lower blood LDL-cholesterol level. But this scenario is not always smooth; many things can go wrong, including various genetic mutations in the LDL receptors, dietary and lifestyle behaviors or certain co-existing disorders, all of which can impact the role of the liver in controlling blood cholesterol levels.

LDL-cholesterol: Does particle size matter?

LDL particles come in two sizes: large particles, or type A, and small particles, or type B. The distinction is extremely important because the small type B particles can readily cross the inner lining (endothelium) of coronary and cerebral arteries, where they are quickly oxidized to initiate plaque formation. In other words, *they are more atherogenic*. However, the large type A particles are less likely to cross the lining of the arteries or become oxidized, so they are not as atherogenic as their smaller cousins.

WHY DO SOME PEOPLE HAVE "ATHEROGENIC" SMALL LDL PARTICLES?

- **Genetic predisposition** among persons with a family history of premature cardiovascular diseases before the age of 45
- **Elevated triglycerides for any reason:** Genetic, dietary or lifestyle
- **High glycemic index diet,** especially with frequent sweets and starches
- **Low-fat diets**
- **Foods containing high levels of trans fats** (stick margarines, shortening, cooking fat, deep-fried foods, sweets)
- **Excessive alcohol intake** (more than three drinks daily)
- **Sedentary lifestyle**
- **Abdominal obesity**
- **Insulin resistance or diabetes**
- **Elevated LDL-cholesterol**

The LDL particle size is enormously important in the development of coronary artery disease. People with a predominantly large variety (type A) are far less likely to develop coronary artery disease, even if their blood cholesterol levels are elevated. However, people with predominantly small, dense LDL particles (type B) have a higher risk of developing coronary artery disease, even when their blood cholesterol levels are "normal." The predominance of small, dense LDL particles, even with "normal" LDL-cholesterol levels, increases the risk of coronary artery disease by 300% to 500%. More importantly, among men with elevated LDL-cholesterol, type B LDL increases their risk of coronary artery disease by more than 600%.

Why do some people have small LDL particles?

Several factors contribute to having a higher proportion of small LDL particles, some genetic and others are due to dietary and lifestyle practices (see table…and figure…below). For example, as the blood triglycerides rise, the proportion of small, dense LDL particles increases progressively. Typically, when trigylcerides are under 100 mg/dl, most LDL particles are the large type A type. But as triglyceride levels exceed 300 mg/dl, the majority of LDL particles are the small, more atherogenic type B type. However, when triglycerides are between 100 to 300 mg/dl the distribution of type A or type B may be difficult to predict.

Particle size is also affected by diabetes or insulin resistance, abdominal obesity and sedentary lifestyle. In a recent study, Canadian researchers showed that having high blood sugar, high triglycerides and low HDL levels, a rather common, and predominant small, dense LDL particles raised the risk of coronary artery disease by 20-fold.

There is some good news: People with coronary artery disease who improve their LDL

The Relation of Dietary Fat Intake to LDL Particle Size

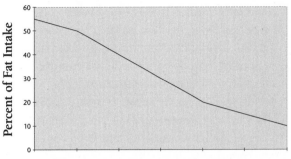

As the total dietary fat intake is decreased, a substantially higher percentage of LDL particles become smaller and denser (type B). Thus, very low-fat (and high-carbohydrate) diets often convert a type A (predominantly large LDL particles) to the more atherogenic type B (predominantly small, dense LDL particles).

particle size profile—going from B to A—show slower progression in their disease, and in some cases, may even stop it compared to those who continue to have predominantly small particles.

Regular exercise and weight in people with abdominal obesity loss can help improve LDL particle size. Strange as it seems, as less dietary fat is consumed, a greater number of LDL particles become smaller and more atherogenic. For instance, when about 30% of total calories come from dietary fat, approximately 40% of LDL particles are the artery-damaging type B type; when total dietary fat is reduced to only 10% of total food intake, more than two-thirds of LDL particles are small. This is another reason why low-fat diets have no values, in fact may be harmful, since they lower the good LDL, and in older persons may increase the risk of stroke.

Naturally low blood cholesterol vs. cholesterol-lowering

Not everyone with elevated LDL-cholesterol develops coronary artery disease—about 60% do. Yet the element of uncertainty—not knowing

LDL-Cholesterol Oxidation

One reason why small LDL particles are particularly dangerous is that they are very susceptible to oxidation as soon as they trespass into the wall of arteries. (Remember, a rusty nail, or an apple that turns brown when exposed to air, are examples of oxidation.) Oxidation of LDL-cholesterol is one of the earliest features of coronary artery disease—and has been seen in the walls of coronary arteries of infants as young as one month old. If it wasn't for this oxidation process of LDL particles, hardly anyone would have coronary artery disease or heart attack or other cardiovascular events.

Oxidized LDL particles act like aggressive combatants, whereas non-oxidized particles are more like unarmed soldiers. Trans fats found in stick margarines, shortenings and cooking fats make LDL-cholesterol more susceptible to oxidation (yet manufacturers of these products ceaselessly promote them as "all natural and cholesterol-free"). Trans fats-loaded products are also used by most fast food restaurants, another reason to avoid these eateries.

In contrast, monounsaturated fats, such as olive oil, not only reduce the number of small LDL particles, but also increase their resistance to oxidation. Even the often maligned saturated fats increase LDL particle resistance to oxidation.

exactly in whom, when and how it develops—makes cholesterol-lowering critical in the prevention of a future heart attack.

The high probability of benefit from reducing LDL-cholesterol outweighs the very low likelihood of treatment-related side effects, nearly all essentially minor or self-limiting. Since individuals with several risk factors have an extremely high risk of developing a major cardiovascular event resulting in disability or death, they must be more aggressive and start cholesterol-lowering as early as possible.

The heart-health benefits of cholesterol-lowering drugs, even when the LDL can be lowered by 40% to 60%, are limited to an approximately 30% reduction in heart attack risk. In other words, each one percent cholesterol reduction up to 30% is associated with one percent risk reduction. Any additional cholesterol-lowering beyond 30% does not appear to confer a significant further benefit, perhaps due to the impact of other co-existent risk factors. Direct measurement of LDL particle size is often not necessary, and can be estimated. In some cases, however, it is helpful to measure LDL particle size in people with; and may even be associated with some drug-induced side effects.

In the Multiple Risk Factor Intervention Trial study of 362,000 men without a previous history of coronary artery disease, the six-year risk of the disease in someone with a blood cholesterol level below 180 mg/dl was 70% less than the subjects whose blood cholesterol levels were 30% higher (greater than 260 mg/dl). In other words, for each one percent lower cholesterol, the risk of coronary artery disease was reduced by two percent. Why is there a 200% disparity in the risk of coronary artery disease among those who are fortunate enough to have naturally low blood cholesterol levels and those whose high blood cholesterol levels are brought down to normal with treatment?

Undoubtedly, long-term exposure of coronary and cerebral arteries to high levels of cholesterol may initiate and promote the process of coronary artery disease. For many people, 10, 20, or 30 years later the impact of cholesterol-lowering efforts may prove to be too little, too late. More alarming is the fact that the first manifestation of cardiovascular disease in one-third of all who have it is a fatal heart attack or stroke. Once atherosclerosis and coronary artery disease has set in,

WHAT SHOULD BE TESTED?

The typical cholesterol screening measures total blood cholesterol HDL, LDL, triglycerides and the total cholesterol-to-HDL ratio. However, additional tests may be required in some people.

A test that measures LDL's protein called apoprotein B100 may be advised for people who have...

- A family or personal history of premature cardiovascular disease
- Multiple risk factors and normal-to-slightly elevated LDL-cholesterol
- High triglycerides
- A family or personal history of premature cardiovascular disease
- Low HDL or personal cholesterol, even with "acceptable" LDL levels
- Diabetes, insulin resistance, or abdominal obesity

lowering cholesterol measures may slow down the progression of coronary artery disease in a third of treated individuals, and perhaps eventually produce some minimal regression in even fewer people. But these or any other measures cannot make the vessels normal again. Although lowering cholesterol reduces the risk of a heart attack by 30%, correction of other coronary risk factors provides a far greater additional protection.

The message here is my long-held slogan...

Think prevention, early action, multifactor intervention.

What does cholesterol-lowering do?

Cholesterol-lowering provides three distinct benefits. These benefits may not happen immediately or at the same time. Some occur within weeks, whereas other benefits require months or years of sustained treatment to have a tangible impact. In chronological order, the benefits are...

The immediate benefit

On average, approximately two percent to three percent of LDL particles in the blood are oxidized in the bloodstream. The number of oxidized LDL particles is much higher (up to 10%) in diabetics, in people with small, dense LDL particles and in people with a low antioxidant reserve, such as those with chronic infections or inflammations (rheumatoid arthritis, lupus or AIDS); malnutrition; a diet with high intake of trans fats, deep fried foods or with very little dark fruits and vegetables. By lowering LDL-cholesterol, along with measures to reduce the antioxidant load, fewer oxidized particles are produced in the bloodstream to cross into the arterial wall and start new coronary plaques or aggravate the existing ones.

Moreover, oxidized LDL particles contribute to dysfunction of the inner lining of arteries, making the barrier leaky and permissive so that more LDL particles can trespass into the wall of the artery.

On the other hand, with fewer oxidized LDL particles, the integrity and health of the inner lining of the arteries improves, making it less leaky and permissive. This improvement occurs within a few weeks of starting a cholesterol-lowering program. Conversely, when treatment is stopped, blood cholesterol level bounces back to high levels, which results in the return of endothelial dysfunction within two weeks. This rapid reversal illustrates the importance of long-term adherence to an effective treatment program. Other coronary risk factors, such as smoking, a sedentary lifestyle, high levels of lipoprotein(a), triglycerides or homocysteine and low levels of HDL-cholesterol, often sabotage the restoration of endothelial function, by lowering cholesterol without addressing the other risk factors.

The mid-range benefit: Coronary plaques stabilize

An elevated LDL-cholesterol level contributes to its progressive accumulation in the wall of coronary and cerebral arteries. As fat-laden plaques bulge, their protective cap becomes thinner and weaker compared to plaques that contain less fat and more smooth muscle cells or scar tissue. The accumulation of oxidized LDL particles or its breakdown by products creates an intense inflammatory process in the wall of the artery that is the hallmark of active and troublesome plaques.

Coronary plaques with inflammation and a thin cap are four times more likely to erode or rupture and cause heart attacks than plaques that are more fibrous, less inflamed and have a thicker cap. When the blood cholesterol level drops for a sustained period, very few or no further LDL deposits occur, and within six to 12 months the plaques become less inflamed, more stable, less inflamed and not as prone to erosions or rupture.

The long-term benefit: Shrinking of coronary plaques

Long-term cholesterol-lowering facilitates the removal of some fatty deposits from the wall of the arteries. This reverse transport of cholesterol out of the artery's wall is primarily the responsibility of HDL-cholesterol and requires adequate HDL-cholesterol level. As the cholesterol content of the plaques drops, they shrivel up slightly, contributing to the widening of the artery's lumen. The improvement or reduction of the size and bulging of coronary plaques is referred to as *regression*.

Regression is very time-dependent and, even after many years, may be in the order of only one percent to two percent. For most people, this regression in the size of coronary plaques amounts to no more than the thickness of two or three sheets of typing paper. In fact, regression of coronary lesions is not the main goal of cholesterol-lowering therapies; stability and less inflammation of the plaques, and sturdier TK are the prime objectives.

What you should do

If you have elevated blood cholesterol, with or without coronary artery disease, lowering your LDL-cholesterol helps to...

- Improve the endothelial function
- Reduce the development of new coronary plaques
- Stabilize the existing coronary plaque, by reducing inflammation within them.

- **Diet**

    The Twenty Risk Factor Diet provides you with the most sensible and unassailable nutritional plan to reduce your LDL-cholesterol level, decrease the number of small atherogenic LDL particles, and prevent the final assault on your arteries—oxidization of your LDL particles. Just as important, the TRF diet will help improve any other risk factors that you many have.

- **Exercise**

    A sedentary lifestyle increases your risk of coronary artery disease by 50%, along with significant increases in the risk of various cancers including breast, colon and prostate.

- **Aspirin**

    Low-dose aspirin (81 mg per day) can reduce your risk of a cardiovascular event by approximately 30%. This is an added benefit to cholesterol-lowering measures. And by improving the endothelial function, aspirin reduces the trespassing of LDL particles into the arterial wall.

PERCENT CHOLESTEROL-LOWERING BY SIX STATINS BASED ON DOSAGE				
Statin (mg/day)	**10 mg**	**20 mg**	**40 mg**	**80 mg**
Rosuvastatin (**Crestor**)	3–40	40–45	40–60	NA
Atorvastatin (**Lipitor**)	20–30	30–35	35–45	40–50
Simvastatin (**Zocor**)*†	20–25	20–30	30–35	30–40
Lovastatin (**Mevacor**)†	15–25	20–25	20–30	30–40
Pravastatin (**Pravachol**)†	15–20	15–25	20–30	30–35
Fluvastatin (**Lescol**)	15–20	15–20	20–30	25–35

*Vytorin is another cholesterol-lowering drug that is a combination of simvastatin and another agent, ezetimibe (Zetia). It is similar in potency to atorvastatin. Zetia is not a statin, but it reduces the intestinal absorption of cholesterol, and may lower LDL-cholesterol by 10% to 20%. By itself, Zetia is not an effective cholesterol-lowering drug and has no anti-inflammatory effect in or around coronary plaques, and should therefore be paired with one of the statins.
†Available in generic form.

Cholesterol-altering drugs

• Consider statins

Perhaps one of the most important developments in the past 20 years in the field of medicine has been the introduction of various statins—medications that can reduce blood cholesterol levels significantly and safely. All statins block the production of new cholesterol by liver cells and increase the number of LDL receptors, both of which lower the LDL-cholesterol by 30% to 60%. They also lower triglycerides in a dose-dependent manner by 10% to 30%, and increase the HDL by 5% to 15% (higher doses are not more effective). Statins reduce the inflammation in and around coronary plaques, so that they become less vulnerable to rupture, which causes heart attacks.

At present, six statins have been approved by the FDA and are available by prescription only. Three of them can be purchased as generics. There are subtle differences among these drugs with respect to their cholesterol-lowering potencies and other cardiovascular benefits. The chart above shows the LDL-lowering potency of these six drugs.

Sales of statin drugs are in the billions each year. Atorvastatin (Lipitor) alone is a $12 billion a year (worldwide) blockbuster. There is a great commercial interest in promoting these drugs. Statins are very safe drugs, which when used in proper doses, can effectively lower LDL-cholesterol levels in more than 80% of people. Even though they reduce overall risk of coronary artery disease by about 30%, and are ineffective in the other 70%, statins are the darling of pharmaceutical companies and healthcare providers because they are safe and effective in lowering blood cholesterol levels.

The nonstop promotion of statins to consumers and healthcare providers is so strong that is has completely masked their ineffectiveness to reduce cardiovascular deaths and disabilities in about 70% of people who take these drugs.

Lowering LDL-cholesterol alone is not the answer to our epidemic of cardiovascular disease. Statins cannot lower the risk of cardiovascular events in everyone, because unlike conditions with a single, identifiable cause, coronary artery disease has 20 major risk factors. Treating

---

CARDIOVASCULAR BENEFITS OF STATINS

Statins are the most effective agents for reduction of vascular inflammation. Statins...

- **Raise** vascular nitric oxide production, a potent dilator of coronary and cerebral arteries, thus improving blood flow and oxygen supply when needed
- **Raise** the HDL-cholesterol level
- **Raise** the number of LDL receptors in liver cells so they can trap more LDL from the bloodstream and bring them in for disposal, hence lowering blood LDL levels
- **Reduce** production of LDL-cholesterol by liver cells and lower blood LDL levels
- **Reduce** blood triglyceride levels
- **Reduce** oxidation of LDL-cholesterol so it would be less harmful
- **Reduce** inflammation and instability of vascular plaques so they resist rupture
- **Reduce** the size of plaques and improve blood flow
- **Reduce** the risk of clot formation inside the arteries
- **Reduce** the risk of heart attack, peripheral vascular disease, stroke and dementia (whether caused by repeated mini-strokes or Alzheimer's disease)
- **Reduce** need for stents or bypass surgery
- **Reduce** cardiovascular deaths and disabilities
- **Reduce** cardiovascular complications of diabetes and chronic kidney disease

---

a single risk factor, such as elevated LDL-cholesterol, will still leave 19 other foxes in the chicken coop! Coronary artery disease always requires a basket of interventions, and that's why we cannot and should not rely on statins, or cholesterol-lowering, alone!

What do statins do?

All statin manufacturers promote statins to reduce cholesterol and, by inference, to lower the risk of heart attack, stroke or peripheral vascular disease. They emphasize cholesterol-lowering because for decades the public has been led to believe that a high blood cholesterol level is the principal culprit. Statins have other benefits besides lowering cholesterol.

Coronary artery plaques, even at their earliest stage, contain a substantial amount of inflammation triggered by oxidized LDL particles. As the size and intensity of this inflammatory process continues, the plaques become more swollen and vulnerable to rupture. In fact, more than 80% of all heart attacks occur because these inflamed "vulnerable plaques" crack or rupture, allowing a small amount of blood to get into the subsurface of the artery. This blood quickly forms a small clot that rapidly snowballs into a larger and larger one (thrombosis), clogging the artery, sometimes within an hour or two. Without adequate blood flow, the affected part of the heart muscle is quickly and irreversibly damaged, producing symptoms of an acute heart attack. Statins are perhaps the most effective agents to reduce the inflammatory process within coronary plaques.

Who should take statins?

Although statins have many benefits beyond lowering cholesterol, they are now used only for cholesterol-lowering and reducing the risk of cardiovascular events. Even with this limited indication, statins are still significantly underused. Some people are reluctant to take any long-term prescription drugs, People often say, "I want to lower my cholesterol naturally," or, "I don't want to take some chemicals for a long time," or, "I want to stop it and see what happens." For most people, however, dietary and lifestyle changes alone are not enough to adequately lower cholesterol. Despite the best intentions, many people do not keep pledges to reduce cholesterol the "natural" way. Without adequate cholesterol-lowering and management of other major coronary risk factor, years of plaque buildup on the walls of arteries may continue untreated.

Statins are expensive drugs, even the generic versions. The massive number of deaths and disabilities each year from coronary artery disease and peripheral artery disease should leave no doubt that our current management of cardiovascular disease gets a failing grade. But doing nothing is even worse. An estimated 100 million Americans are uninsured or underinsured and have no prescription coverage. For them, spending $2–$4 per day for a statin is a problem. Since the cost of higher-dose statin pills is only slightly more than the lower dose pills, to reduce the cost I often prescribe the higher dose pills and ask my patients to cut the pill in half. (The minor variations in size do not make a significant difference for statins over time.)

Another problem is that the dose of statins may not be adjusted adequately to reduce blood cholesterol to optimal levels or to achieve some of the non-cholesterol-related benefits. Of course this is not always the fault of healthcare providers; more than one-third of people on statins take their pills haphazardly, or stop taking them altogether after a few months. Unfortunately, elevated blood cholesterol is most often a genetic, lifelong disorder that is aggravated by dietary and lifestyle miscues. A short course of treatment here and there almost always fails to accomplish anything, and may even trigger a heart attack soon after stopping these drugs. On the next page, I summarize who should take statins.

Are statin drugs safe?

All statins are reasonably safe drugs and have now been used by well over one billion people worldwide. They are among the best investigated drugs, both before and after their approval by the US Food and Drug Administration. As safe as they are, like any other drugs, they still have an occasional side effects.

The guidelines proposed here are distinctly different from the recent recommendations of the American Heart Association. In my view, their guidelines leave millions of Americans at high risk of catastrophic cardiovascular events. The AHA's 2007 update suggests using LDL-cholesterol-lowering if the LDL is higher than 130mg/dl with lifestyle therapy and if there are multiple risk factors and the healthcare

---

BENEFITS OF STATINS BEYOND HEART HEALTH

- **Reduce** risk of seven types of cancers (breast, colorectal, esophagus, liver, lung, pancreas and advanced prostate)
- **Reduce** risk of bone loss and osteoporosis
- **Reduce** joint inflammation in rheumatoid arthritis
- **Reduce** risk of relapse in multiple sclerosis
- **Reduce** severity of systemic lupus and AIDS
- **Reduce** in-hospital death rates from non-cardiovascular surgeries
- **Reduce** risk of transplant rejection

provider thinks that the risk of a cardiovascular event is high. Moreover, they suggest utilizing LDL-cholesterol-lowering if the LDL level is over 160mg/dl with lifestyle therapy and if there are multiple risk factors but the healthcare providers don't think the risk of a cardiovascular event is too high.

Can statins damage my liver?

Approximately one percent to two percent of patients experience a harmless leakage of liver enzymes into the bloodstream, which raises the blood levels of liver enzymes slightly. This effect is dose-dependent, and is almost always temporary, and does not mean or lead to liver injury.

Many people who have high blood cholesterol levels may also have pre-existing fatty liver (due to abdominal obesity, insulin resistance or diabetes and elevated triglyceride levels). These individuals often show frequent fluctuations in blood levels of liver enzymes regardless of any other drug they may take. Unfortunately, if these people also happen to be on statins, the first impulse of healthcare providers is to blame the statin and discontinue it.

When statins were first approved by the FDA in the mid-1980s, active liver disease was considered a "contraindication" to statin therapy.

Nearly every patient of mine with cholesterol abnormalities worries about liver side effects. The consumer advertising and patient information pamphlets perpetuate this phobia, with their disclaimers about liver damage. In my view their concern is not valid. In 2006, the Liver Experts Panel of the National Lipid Association on Statin Safety stressed the following...

- Asymptomatic increases in liver enzymes do not indicate liver dysfunction

---

WHO SHOULD TAKE STATINS?

- People with any cardiovascular disease and LDL over 70
- With diabetes and LDL over 70
- With chronic kidney failure and LDL over 70
- With Metabolic Syndrome and LDL over 70
- With multiple major coronary risk factors and LDL over 70
- With rheumatoid arthritis, lupus or AIDS and following heart transplant and LDL over 30
- With a family history of premature coronary artery disease and LDL over 100
- With one other major CAD risk factor and LDL over 100
- With no other major CAD risk factor* and LDL over 130
- Adolescents with familial type high cholesterol and LDL over 130

Statins reduce cardiovascular events by about 30%. We must not ignore the 70% risk from other major coronary risk factors!

Less than 5% of adults have no major coronary risk factors

- The current evidence does not support routine monitoring of liver function tests recommended by manufacturers

- Presence of chronic liver disease such as fatty liver, hepatitis, or cirrhosis, which affects 25 million Americans, should not be considered a contraindication for statin use.

However, many studies show that statins do not worsen pre-existing liver disease.

The chart on the next page summarizes the risk of developing severe liver toxicity from statin use compared with other life events, including some caused by other drugs.

Can statins damage my muscles?

Several large studies suggest that from one percent to four percent of people taking statins experience muscle aches, or "myalgia." But because muscle pain is so common, it's difficult to know whether it's really caused or aggravated by statin use. In four large studies, patients who took statins or placebo had similar rates of myalgia. In most cases these aches and pains are nothing more than an annoyance. But in a small number of people, myalgia may be significant and associated with muscle weakness that impacts the quality of life. For these individuals, it makes sense to stop the statin for a few weeks until the muscle symptoms disappear completely. Then resume the same or another statin at a lower dose and see if symptoms recur. If myalgia does not recur, the dose can then be slowly adjusted upward.

RISK OF SEVERE LIVER INJURY FROM STATINS COMPARED TO OTHER LIFE EVENTS	
• Statin-induced severe liver disease	1/500,000**
• Severe liver disease in background population	1/100,000
• Severe liver disease due to anti-inflammatory drugs	1/50,000**
• Risk of dying in a traffic accident per year	1/7,000
• Risk of crashing into a deer with car or motorcycle/year	1/200
• Risk of a car accident per year	1/70

*The five-year risk of a cardiovascular event in someone with coronary artery disease and untreated elevated LDL-cholesterol is 1 in 5, or 125,000 times greater than the risk of severe statin-induced liver injury! Gotto AM. Arch Intern Med 2003; 163: 657–59

**Rostom A et al. Clin Gastro Hepatol 2005; 3: 489–98

However, in people who experience significant myalgia associated with muscle weakness, which occurs in less than one percent of those on statins, a large majority may develop recurrence of their symptoms upon resumption of any statin. These individuals may require a few months of "drug holiday" in which no statin is used.

Myalgias usually involve large muscle groups, such as thighs, calves, upper arms and back. The myalgia may feel like a dull ache, a sharp or jabbing pain, or may just feel as if you had a hard workout. It usually always occurs on both sides of the body. Occasionally it may be asymmetrical or more severe on one side, especially when the lower back muscles are involved.

Statins can rarely cause neuropathy—damage to the peripheral nerves, presenting as weakness or burning sensation. Another very rare side effect of statins may involve tendonitis of the feet or shoulders. Here, too, it is often difficult to figure out whether such tendonitis would have occurred without the statins. Most neuropathies and tendonitis resolve when statins are discontinued for several weeks. Neuropathies, however, tend to recur soon after the resumption of all statins.

Coenzyme Q10 (ubiquinone) is an enzyme inside muscle and nerve cells that has a crucial role in internal energy use by both tissues. Although statins may reduce the production of this internal enzyme, supplemental coenzyme Q10 has not proven very effective in reducing the risk of statin-induced myalgia. Similarly, selenium, a trace mineral that is a major antioxidant component of many cells, including muscles, has not shown efficiency in myalgia or muscle weakness. Severe muscle damage, a condition called *rhabdomyolysis*, is a serious disease that requires prompt intervention. Fortunately it is extremely rare and occurs in less than one out of 15,000 persons

STATIN-INDUCED MUSCLE DAMAGE

- In four large studies, no difference was reported in musculoskeletal symptoms among statin-treated compared to placebo-treated subjects (muscle pain was reported by one percent to three percent).*

- Among 252,640 cases, the risk of severe muscle disease (called rhabdomyolysis) with a statin was about one in 15,000 persons per year.**

- When statins were combined with fibrates (a class of drugs used to lower triglycerides), the risk of muscle disease was one in 500 persons per year, especially among older persons, women, frail individuals, and those with kidney dysfunction or diabetes.**

- Mortality from statin-induced severe muscle disease is about one out of 85,000 persons on statins per year.**

*Gotto AM. Arch Intern Med 2003; et 163: 657–59
**Graham DJ et al. JAMA 2004; 292: 2585–90 more

taking statins. The table above summarizes the risk of statin-induced muscle disorder.

How much statin and which one?

The choice of a statin in the US (and to some extent overseas) is usually driven by the prescriber's habit or bias, insurance coverage for prescription drugs and the influence of direct-to-consumer advertising by statin manufacturers. The safety profile of all statins is very similar, but their potency varies significantly.

This is important because some people with elevated blood cholesterol levels, especially those with multiple mutations in their cholesterol production chain require the more potent statins. At present three generic statins are available in the US, and insurers frequently try to steer healthcare providers and the patients toward the generic statins. My preference is to prescribe the more potent rosuvastatin (Crestor) or atorvastatin (Lipitor) because they can lower LDL-cholesterol with lower doses and may be reasonably cost effective, especially when larger doses are prescribed. They may be cut in half.

The dose of statins should always be tailored to each individual to achieve cholesterol reduction goals. Several studies suggest that the best cholesterol-lowering results are achieved with taking the highest tolerated dose. Doubling a dose of statin does not mean a twofold benefit; instead, a larger dose often provides only a slight (10%–15%) further reduction in risks compared to lower doses.

A major problem with statin therapy is compliance; many patients do not take it on a regular basis, often for weeks or months. In fact, outside of research settings, in the real world of clinical practice, less than 50% of patients who take statins achieve "goal" (such as LDL-cholesterol-lowering) even on intensive, high-doses of statins therapy. This low success rate contributes to our failure to reduce cardiovascular events in people with high LDL-cholesterol, high blood pressure, and diabetes. Our success rate for achieving optimal control of all three diseases is less than 30%.

There are other concerns with over-enthusiastic reliance on high doses of statins. Even in a research setting, where people are monitored very carefully, about two-thirds of those taking high-dose statins do not experience any benefits from their long-term treatment. *What about these at-risk people?* Remember, there are 20 major coronary risk factors, not just one! In addition, intensive cholesterol-lowering does not mean or need maximal statin doses! The "*...concentration on drug treatment should not deflect attention from diet and lifestyle interventions that have the potential, even with moderate improvements, to reduce cardiovascular disease incidence by between 75% to 80%.*" (Sacks FMJAMA 2004;

291:1132-34) I don't think I could have said it more eloquently.

What about over-the-counter supplements to lower cholesterol?

Here is the market size: 100 million Americans with elevated blood cholesterol levels and over one billion people worldwide! What would you do if you were a supplement maker? Exploit this massive renewable market? The most heavily advertised products include garlic pills, ginseng, oyster shell products, herbal products, or policosanol, a newer compound, which is just as useless as the others. The range of misleading claims for these products is endless!

Recent double-blind studies have shown that after adjustment for dietary and lifestyle modifications, *Garlique*, a garlic extract promoted by paid testimonial of a celebrity, is no better than placebo in reducing blood cholesterol levels. Another study by Stanford University researchers showed that none of the three other garlic brands, including raw garlic, had any significant effect on LDL-cholesterol, HDL-cholesterol or triglycerides. (Gardner, CD et al. Arch Internal Med 2007; 167: 346–53)

Policosanol is an extract from various sources including sugar cane, wheat germ, rice bran or beeswax. It has been heavily advertised as a "natural statin" in various over-the-counter supplements. A recent double-blind, placebo-controlled study showed that even at high doses, policosanol extracted from cane sugar was no better than placebo in reducing blood cholesterol levels. *The bottom line:* No over-the-counter supplement, herbal or otherwise, lowers blood cholesterol level by more than a few useless points or has a true cardioprotective role!

What about oat products? Can they lower blood cholesterol?

The FDA made a big mistake when they agreed to allow cereal manufacturers to make the claim that certain oat products, in conjunction with a modified diet and lifestyle changes, can lower blood cholesterol levels. And ever since we have been bombarded with claims that a bowl of oats is the ticket to eternal life!

The truth is that if you eat three or more bowls of unsweetened oat products every day for three to six months, you may (or may not) lower your blood cholesterol by 5–7 mg/dl. The question is how many people are going to eat three bowls of oat bran every day for the rest of their lives to lower their cholesterol by a trivial 5 to 7 mg? Does it matter if you lower your blood cholesterol from 275 mg/dl to 270 mg/dl?

Elevated blood cholesterol is a major risk factor for coronary artery disease. Do not trivialize your health or your life by relying on advice from the TV or the internet.

Just as important, don't be satisfied with taking your statin and hoping for the best. Managing your blood cholesterol, lifestyle modifications recommended here, together with modifying as many major risk factors as possible.

Risk Factor #7
Elevated Triglycerides

Every dietary fat (saturated, monounsaturated or polyunsaturated) enters the bloodstream from the intestine as triglycerides—a mixture of three fatty acids. They serve the body both as the primary storage form of fat and as fuel for muscle tissue. Calories consumed from a meal that are not immediately used by tissues for energy are converted to triglycerides and transported, via the bloodstream, to fat cells to be stored for later use. Millions of people never use or burn this stored fat!

In addition to obtaining triglycerides through food, the liver also produces them by converting unused carbohydrates and, to a lesser extent, proteins. The liver dumps some of the triglycerides into the bloodstream at a rate dictated by various genes and by diet, lifestyle or other factors. When the body cannot use triglycerides, they accumulate in the bloodstream (as high triglyceride levels), the liver itself (fatty liver) or in fat cells (as obesity).

In the bloodstream, triglycerides can travel in their original form, or as Very Low Density Lipoprotein (VLDL) and Intermediate Density Lipoprotein (IDL). Both of these lipoproteins act very much like LDL, in that elevated levels increase the risk of cardiovascular disease. To make matters worse, high triglycerides tend to result in lower levels of "good" HDL-cholesterol and also contribute to the conversion of larger LDL particles to the more dangerous smaller-sized particles.

For many years elevated triglycerides were not even considered a coronary risk factor. Even today some healthcare providers still focus on LDL and ignore HDL or triglycerides. Yet, both VLDL and IDL assault the wall of coronary, cerebral and other arteries just as agressively as LDL-cholesterol. As a matter of laboratory convenience the VLDL and IDL are combined and reported as VLDL. Most laboratories do not directly measure these two lipoproteins; they simply calculate their blood level as one-fifth (20%) of blood triglycerides, often a reasonably accurate estimate.

Although triglyceride levels of less than 200 mg/dl are considered "desirable," this cut-off point should be lowered to less than 300 mg/dl. For example, in a 15-year study of 492 people with coronary artery disease, between the ages of 30 and 80, those with triglyceride levels of more than 100 mg/dl had twice the incidence of coronary events when compared with those whose initial triglyceride levels were less than 100 mg/dl.

In another study, researchers measured fasting triglyceride levels of 340 men and women who had had a heart attack. After adjusting for other coronary risk factors, people with elevated triglyceride levels had a 300% higher risk of another heart attack.

The Framingham Heart Study, the Paris Prospective Study, the Copenhagen Male Study, and 17 other population-based studies clearly show that an elevated blood triglyceride level is a significant independent risk factor for coronary artery disease.

The most common causes of elevated blood triglycerides are...

- A genetic predisposition, sometimes resulting in triglyceride levels that exceed 2000–4000 mg/dl.

- Insulin resistance, diabetes and abdominal obesity

- Sedentary lifestyle

- Excessive alcohol intake

- Excessive intake of high-glycemic carbohydrates/partially hydrogenated vegetable oils, such as stick margarine, shortening or cooking fats

- Excessive intake of fat

- Inadequate seafood intake

What you should do

The key to lowering triglycerides is diet and exercise-induced weight loss, especially for people with abdominal obesity. The most important aspect of a diet to lower blood triglycerides is to reduce intake of simple "sweet" carbohydrates (candies, cookies, cakes, pies, pastries, donuts, chocolates, jams, jellies, table sugar, carbonated beverages, honey and sweet fruits, such as raisins, dates and grapes).

Avoid complex carbohydrates that the body readily breaks down in the intestine and converts to sugar. They are bread, rice, pasta and potato. Sourdough or dark breads like pumpernickle bread, wild rice or whole wheat pasta in small portions are good alternatives.

- **Exercise**

The backbone of an effort to lower triglycerides is diet and exercise to lose weight, especially for people who have abdominal obesity. Even a small weight loss of five percent to 10% can play a big role in lowering elevated triglycerides and other heart disease risks.

Regular exercise complements and improves the effects of dieting by improving the body's ability to burn calories at rest. No matter your current level of activity, get some form of exercise every day, slowly increasing the duration and intensity of your workouts.

When dietary carbohydrates are 60% or more of your daily calories, your blood triglycerides can increase by as much as 20% to 30%, making a bad situation even worse. Since dietary fat ordinarily contributes 80% of blood triglycerides, people with high triglyceride levels should cut down all dietary fats. The exception to this rule is omega-3 polyunsaturated fats from seafood, which lower triglyceride levels by 20% to 30%.

Alcohol intake, especially by people with elevated triglyceride levels, can double to triple triglyceride levels. For people who do not have elevated triglycerides, one or two drinks will not raise the triglycerides.

- **Eat more seafood**

High doses of omega-3 fatty acids, present in fish such as mackerel, salmon and tuna, can lower triglycerides nearly as well as most prescription medication, and without the side effects.

Eat at least four servings of this "fatty" seafood each week. "White" fish such as flounder, tilapia, catfish, and rockfish doesn't contain high levels of omega-3s but they are preferable to beef or poultry. This dietary change alone should lower triglycerides by at least 20%.

Although eating dark-fleshed fish is best, an alternative is to take fish oil capsules two or three times daily (at each meal). Many fish oil capsules, however, contain other fish oils that are not omega-3s. In fact, most over-the-counter capsules have no more than 200mg–400mg of omega-3 per capsule. For example, the label of Nature Made fish oil capsules says "1,200mg"—but the fine print discloses that the serving size is two capsules. It further clarifies that only 300mg of the 600mg is actually omega-3.

Another brand, Nature's Bounty 1,000mg fish oil has even less—200mg omega-3 per capsule. So eight to 10 of these capsules equal one six- or eight-ounce serving of salmon. So start eating salmon!

Among over-the-counter fish oils, Solgar Omega-3 700 has a reasonably concentrated omega-3 fat content of about 600mg per capsule. Omacor, by prescription only, has 840mg of seafood omega-3 (EPA and DHA). Omega-3 fat from plants such as flaxseed oil does not lower triglycerides.

In the first few weeks of modifying your diet, eat at least four to five seafood meals per week and you may use a small amount of olive oil. This dietary change should lower your triglycerides by at least 20% to 30%.

Fortunately, most people with elevated triglycerides do not have very high levels. In these cases, abdominal obesity, sedentary lifestyle, insulin resistance or diabetes, excessive alcohol and poor diet readily account for their problem.

If you do not like seafood, take fish oil capsules enough to provide 2 to 4 gm of omega-3 fat per day as an alternative. This dose equals 10 to 20 fish oil capsules a day! Solgar Omega-3 700 or Omacor may be an easier choice. Be aware that many fish oil products contain impurities, including a high level of trans fatty acids. Another reason to eat seafood instead of fish oil capsules is that you may lose some weight and some abdominal obesity. That's due to having fish, instead of more fattening foods!

Fish oil capsules also have some unpleasant or annoying side effects, frequent fishy belching and breath. Do you really want to do that? In fact, most people who take fish oil usually take one or two capsules per day which is an inadequate amount of omega-3 fat, and gives them a false sense of security.

Because abdominal obesity contributes to insulin resistance and elevated triglycerides, even a five percent to 10% weight loss can be an essential part of lowering your triglycerides. Regular exercise complements and improves the efficacy of dietary intervention to lower triglycerides. It also helps with weight loss, abdominal obesity and insulin resistance.

Triglyceride-lowering drugs

There are several drugs with proven efficacy in lowering triglycerides, but they have certain side effects that may dictate the choice.

Niacin can decrease LDL-cholesterol and triglycerides, and raise good HDL, each by about 30%. But niacin—especially at high doses—can produce many side effects, including skin flushing, itching and redness, stomach upset, heartburn and headache. To avoid these problems, niacin should first be taken at low doses not to exceed 250 milligrams, two to three times daily. The dose can gradually be increased to 1,500 to 2,000 mg daily over several weeks.

Niaspan is another form of niacin that can be taken at the same time at night. Start at a smaller does and gradually increased this too, over a six-to-eight week period.

Fibrates are a distinct group of drugs that have significant triglyceride-lowering effect. They also raise HDL-cholesterol levels by 10% to 20% and have an anti-inflammatory effect in the wall of the arteries and coronary plaques. Gemfibrozil and fenofibrates are commonly used.

Gemfibrozil may cross-react with a number of drugs and should not be used by people with kidney disorders, elderly or frail persons, or with some statins such as rosuvastatin (Crestor) simvastatin (Zocor and Vytorin) because of a higher risk of myalgia. Fenofibrate can raise blood homocysteine by altering kidney functions, contributing to accumulation of homocysteine in the bloodstream.

Although fibrates significantly lower triglycerides in people with very high levels, they should be used along with omega-3 fat from seafood and often a statin. In most patients with moderately elevated triglycerides, control of underlying disorder, dietary and lifestyle changes, along with four to five seafood meals a week, or 2–4 gm/per day of seafood omega-3 will suffice. The fibrates are reserved for more severe cases.

Risk Factor #8
Age

Aging does not cause cardiovascular disease, but the diseases are associated with aging—after all, eight in 10 people who die from cardiovascular disease are older than 60. Similarly, cancer, diabetes and many chronic diseases are also associated with aging.

The main reason for the prevalence of so many age-associated chronic diseases is that long before we are "old," many risk factors have been ignored or inadequately treated. Even today, half of all people with elevated cholesterol or triglycerides, low HDL-cholesterol, diabetes, hypertension or other risk factors are inadequately treated or not treated at all. Years of exposure to multiple risk factors have set the stage for age-associated diseases. The diseases often begin when we are much younger and not wise enough to deal with them. After years of inadequate intervention and treatment, or no treatment, problems that could have been prevented instead result in deadly heart attack or stoke. And then we blame the aging process instead of placing the blame where it should go —the failure of our healthcare system!

Because cardiovascular disease begins in childhood, start taking steps to ensure a lifetime of heart health as early as possible. Children inherit coronary risk factors or gene mutations such as faulty LDL receptors. For these children, damage to coronary anteries may start silently and progress as they grow older.

Study: In a landmark study, autopsies were performed on nearly 2,900 young people who had died of various causes, not cardiovascular disease, between ages 15 and 34. One out of four teenage boys and one in 15 girls had already developed early signs of coronary artery disease, and among the 30 to 34 year-olds one out of two men, and one out of three women had evidence of early or advanced coronary artery disease. Arterial plaque was even higher in those who died in their 20s and 30s. This study confirmed that coronary artery disease begins well before the 40s or 50s, when its dangers become more apparent. In fact, another study of children between 10 and 14 revealed that more than half of them showed microscopic evidence of early plaque formation.

Another study from the University of California, San Diego, even showed that fatty streaks in the arterial wall may begin in fetuses (more so when the mother has high cholesterol).

Screening children and teens

Although screening adults for cholesterol and blood pressure or other risk factors is universally accepted, screening children and adolescents still generates an emotional debate. The controversy over cholesterol screening in younger people focuses on several concerns. Here are my responses…

1. *Measurement of cholesterol and lipoproteins is subject to inaccuracies.* As I have shown in my study (Mogadam M et al. Arch Intern Med 1990; 150; 1645–48), there are almost always fluctuations of about five percent to 10% in LDL and HDL and even greater than 20% in triglycerides from week to week. Such relatively minor fluctuations have not stopped us from screening adults and treating them for abnormal levels. No child or adolescent should be diagnosed with high cholesterol on the basis of a single measurement. Many factors can skew results of blood tests—acute illness, dietary changes (such as Halloween or birthdays, when more "junk" food is eaten), even getting tested right after intense exercise such as soccer, hockey or basketball.

2. *Children's "normal" cholesterol levels are unknown.* Not true. Optimal levels in children and adolescents are the same as those of older people—just like levels of sugar, sodium, potassium, calcium and kidney or liver function. Tests are all measured similarly across various age groups.

3. *Younger people with high cholesterol will not necessarily become adults with elevated cholesterol or have heart attacks.* Even using the currently accepted "normal" cholesterol levels, two out of three children and adolescents with elevated blood cholesterol will go on to have high levels as adults. The vast majority of children with abnormal cholesterol levels

will carry their disorder into adulthood. Almost all of these children with very high levels will. That's because these youngsters have familial or genetic reasons for their elevated LDL-cholesterol and triglycerides or low levels of HDL-cholesterol.

Conversely, among children and adolescents with normal blood cholesterol, only 20% to 30% go on to develop abnormal levels as adults; about 80% will maintain their normal cholesterol profile. The high probability of elevated cholesterol carrying over into adult life should be enough to call for vigorous screening and early preventive measures.

There is no doubt that abnormal cholesterol levels in childhood are more likely to cause cardiovascular disease in later years. But other factors play a role—obesity, smoking, lack of exercise, poor diet and more. Ignoring abnormal cholesterol levels in children and adolescents won't make them go away; they will pay the price with premature heart attacks, strokes and death.

Study: After studying 204 children and young adults who had died from non-cardiac causes, researchers found that the rate of advanced coronary lesions was already 13 times higher in those who had three risk factors (such as obesity, high cholesterol or a poor diet) compared to those who had no risk factors. No matter the age, abnormal cholesterol shouldn't be ignored.

4. *Screening children is expensive.* We spend money to discourage smoking, alcohol and drug use and to promote vaccines and seat belts. So facing an epidemic of coronary artery disease—the country's leading cause of death—why not spend a fraction of our healthcare resources to identify at-risk children? I believe that screening children should be a moral healthcare imperative and a social responsibility. Just as preventing youngsters from smoking, drinking or using drugs will save money and lives in the long run, so too will education about and prevention of coronary artery disease at an early age.

5. *Abnormal cholesterol in children is difficult to treat.* Like adults, children suffer no discomfort from cholesterol problems and unlike conditions like a sore throat or ear infection, treatment does not bring immediate or tangible relief or reward. So it is difficult to make a case for recommendations aimed at preventing a heart attack 20 or 40 years down the road. But that is precisely what we need. Instead of ignoring the problem, we ought to face it squarely, just as we deal with smoking, alcohol or drug abuse, obesity and depression in young people.

Managing high cholesterol in children is a family affair; it begins with educating and encouraging parents and other siblings to follow the guidelines suggested here. There is no doubt about the impact of dietary and lifestyle practices on children and adolescents. The evidence is overwhelming that humans are programmed from birth to like sweets and dislike bitter-tasting foods. Regrettably, parents often reward, bribe or console their children with sweets laden with invisible fat, most of which is saturated fat and trans fatty acids.

In a recent national survey, 80% of parents with children between the ages of six and 11 were familiar with the Food Guide Pyramid developed by the United States Department of Agriculture. Yet, fewer than half of them said that they followed the guidelines in preparing their children's meals. If parents set a good example and provide a sensible diet, it may help modify or alter the course of their children's cardiovascular health.

An easy way of changing the dietary pattern of youngsters is to change the family diet so that it is as close as possible to a TRF score of 30 per day.

Changing dietary preferences of a child, obese or not, should be handled with patience, reason and consistency, not emotionally or inflexibly. It may take a few months of fussing and griping before most youngsters gradually accept or adapt to a new diet, provided it is not rigid or punitive. Occasional treats ("junk foods") should not only make children happy, but also help them to better understand and appreciate their parents' reasonableness. Usually, the biggest problem is to convince the parents that they, too, need to change their dietary practices in order to make their youngsters' transition easier; this is often more of an obstacle than changing children's finicky or junk-eating habits.

Many meals served at school cafeterias are perfect examples of what children should *not* eat. Packing a nutritious meal at home for one or two youngsters is not very time-consuming. If they take time to shave, shower, fix their hair and dress for work, parents should have an extra few minutes to spend on their children's well-being and future health.

If they have a family history of premature cardiovascular diseases, children should be referred to a cholesterol specialist. Although, in the past, pediatricians shied away from treating children with this kind of problem vigorously, this is no longer acceptable or justified. Recent studies have shown that statins are highly effective and safe for adolescents and young people with high blood cholesterol levels.

What you should do

- *Try the Twenty Risk Factor (TRF) diet for your youngsters.* If you have children with abnormal cholesterol levels, the first step is to start them on a diet with TRF scores of less than 30 per day. This flexible dietary approach allows for a vast number of choices and also meets the goals of recommended dietary allowances for energy, protein, fat and various micronutrients. Such a diet will not interfere with the psychological or physical maturation of a child. More importantly, a diet based on TRF scores eliminates concern over levels of various fats, or cholesterol in a given food or snack.

- *Start with "mild" fish.* Since many children do not enjoy fish—especially if their parents

---

SHOULD CHILDREN BE SCREENED?

My recommendations are based upon over 100 published studies in the past decade. They provide a scientific basis for the screening of children and adolescents.

A complete lipid profile—screening for total cholesterol, LDL, HDL and triglycerides—should first be given to all children as early as age 10 (and repeated every five years) who have...

- A family history of coronary artery disease—especially if it occurred before age 55 in parents, grandparents, siblings, aunts, uncles or cousins

- Parents who have abnormal LDL, HDL or triglycerides

- A weight problem, especially abnormal obesity

- Any coronary risk factor, such as smoking, a sedentary lifestyle, diabetes, high blood pressure

As with adults, the ratio of total cholesterol-to-HDL should be less than 4-to-1, and preferably closer to 3.5-to-1. Children's cholesterol levels tend to fluctuate, like adults, over several weeks. If the test is abnormal, it should be repeated.

don't eat it frequently—starting children off with "mild" fish, such as flounder or lake trout, broiled or sautéed in olive oil, perhaps once or twice a week, may be a good strategy. Over the next several weeks, you can add tuna or salmon for one or two other meals.

WOMEN, AGING AND DISEASE

Cardiovascular disease is often viewed as a "man's disease," even though each year more women die of cardiovascular disease than men. In 2006, about 480,000 men died of cardiovascular disease, compared with 510,000 women. This is 13 times higher than the number of women who died of breast cancer. We have done very little to prevent cardiovascular diseases in men, and even less in women! Today more than half of women past the age of 50 have either early or advanced coronary artery disease.

In middle-aged women, symptoms of coronary artery disease or angina are often misdiagnosed as acid reflux, anxiety or musculo-skeletal disorders. The delay in diagnosis explains why women's coronary artery disease is frequently more advanced when it's diagnosed and is associated with more complications than in men.

The reason: An intentional bias by healthcare providers. A century ago, the average life expectancy was 47 and only one in six people lived to age 75. Today, the average life expectancy is 75 for men and 80 for women, and the world is rapidly getting "older." Yet most public awareness health programs—wearing seat belts, getting regular exercise and preventative health screenings—are directed at the young and middle-aged when they could benefit older persons as much, if not more. Fewer studies include men and women older than 65; and the findings of such studies are not quite applicable to older persons.

- *Consider professional help.* To reinforce and encourage children to follow the diet, periodic input and supervision by a healthcare provider may prove helpful. Healthcare providers should become familiar with the TRF system in order to avoid regressing into obsolete dietary recommendations. Remember that the purpose of dietary intervention is to reduce the risk of future cardiovascular disease and not merely to show a numerical drop in total or LDL-cholesterol levels so as to please the parents or pediatricians.

- *Encourage exercise.* Children should be encouraged to exercise preferably every day, or four to five times a week—getting at least 40 minutes of moderate to intense aerobic exercise. Team sports are a great alternative, since studies show that children who participate in such activities are less likely to take up smoking, drinking or drugs, or develop obesity.

- *Look at the family history.* If there's a family history of premature coronary artery disease, it's wise to have other familial risk factors looked at and treated.

A lipid clinic or cholesterol specialist with experience in pediatric disorders should be consulted—at least for the initial consultation or screening—for those under age 18 with a family history of cholesterol problems. Generally, youngsters whose overall LDL-cholesterol is lower than 160 mg/dl may respond to dietary and lifestyle modifications, at least initally, but those with higher levels will require statin therapy.

Blood cholesterol levels in older persons

Over the past several years, many studies have clarified the relevance of abnormal cholesterol values to cardiovascular diseases among older people. As people reach age 70 and beyond, blood levels of both LDL and HDL-cholesterol tend to go down. Nevertheless, for older people, acceptable cholesterol values are essentially the same as for their middle-aged counterparts.

Several studies show that after age 80, slightly elevated LDL levels are, paradoxically, associated with a lower risk of death than lower LDLs. Malnutrition, chronic depression, poor appetite, loss of teeth or sense of taste and smell will contribute to lower LDL-cholesterol levels.

Another reason why elevated LDL-cholesterol levels in persons over 80 do not seem to increase the risk of cardiovascular events is that, at this age, most of the LDL particles are of the large variety which are not so harmful. By this age, two out of three older persons with high cholesterol levels would have already developed atherosclerosis and may be on multiple drugs for treatment of other disorders. Unless they are otherwise healthy, an aggressive cholesterol-lowering along with all other medications, may not provide a significant benefit and could be burdensome in terms of cost and possible side effects.

The older person with high LDL-cholesterol and no apparent coronary artery disease may be in the group that is resistant to the negative impact of elevated cholesterol. Over time, the independent effect of each risk factor is overshadowed by other age-associated risk factors. Thus, in advanced age, the contribution of each risk factor tends to diminish, merge with, or be overshadowed by other risk factors.

The impact of high cholesterol is still significant between ages 65 and 80. In fact, one can argue that their window of opportunity to prevent a fatal or catastrophic cardiovascular event is much smaller than their younger counterparts. Thus, intensive cholesterol-lowering in these individuals is just as essential, if not more so, than in younger people. And yet studies show that relatively few people aged 65 to 80 who have high cholesterol take cholesterol-lowering medication. In one study of 500 people, only seven percent of those who were candidates for cholesterol-lowering medications were taking them; in another study of 5,888 people only 18% ever started these drugs—the other 82% who qualified for medication were never prescribed cholesterol-lowering drugs by their doctors. Why not?

What is especially troublesome is that as we age, low levels of HDL-cholesterol play a stronger role in coronary artery disease or death than does high LDL-cholesterol. At HDL levels between 35 and 49 mg/dl, the risk of coronary artery disease is increased by about 25% to 75%. But at HDL levels below 35 mg/dl, the risk of suffering a coronary event is more than 200% higher than it is at levels above 60 mg/dl. A low HDL-cholesterol level is also a significant risk factor for stroke and atherosclerosis of the legs in older persons.

In a recent study, 220 men with an average age of 64 and a history of coronary artery disease, were examined by ultrasound to detect thickening of the wall of their carotid arteries (the arteries in the neck that carry blood to the brain). Although LDL-cholesterol levels of these men were "desirable," their HDL-cholesterol levels were low (an average of 32 mg/dl). Despite their "desirable" LDL-cholesterol levels, more than 80% had significant atherosclerosis of their carotid arteries, a precursor of stroke. Several other studies have also shown a significant association between both elevated LDL-cholesterol and a low HDL-cholesterol level and the risk of stroke. The message is that there are 20 major coronary risk factors, and we should never focus on only one or two of them.

Recent data have shown that noninvasive measurements of the thickness of the wall of the carotid arteries using ultrasound provide valuable information about the future risk of a cardiovascular event in older persons. In a multi-center study, 4,476 men and women 65 or older without previous cardiovascular diseases were followed up for an average of six years. Those with the highest thickness of their carotid arteries at entry into the study had a risk of heart attack or stroke that was more than three times greater than older persons with the lowest thickness. In other words, vascular wall thickness is indicative of a silent or hidden atherosclerotic process that involves many arteries and not just the carotids.

What you should do

- *Have regular checkups.* Regular checkups become even more important as you age to determine if you have any evidence of atherosclerosis, poor blood circulation to your lower extremities, or coronary risk factors. Necessary blood tests should include LDL-cholesterol, HDL-cholesterol, triglycerides, blood sugar, kidney and liver function tests, along with homocysteine and a blood count check for anemia and a high hematocrit. Since the presence of an underactive thyroid gland in the elderly is quite common and may include elevated LDL-cholesterol or low HDL-cholesterol levels, you should also have a TSH test (the most accurate test to detect an underactive or overactive thyroid gland) every year.

An ultrasound measurement of the thickness of the carotid artery wall should be obtained in an older person with two or more coronary risk factors at least every two years. If you have developed thickened arterial walls, you will require a more aggressive treatment to reduce as many coronary risk factors as possible.

Treating abnormal cholesterol levels in the elderly should be considered together with any other medical problems. For example, elevated blood cholesterol level in an elderly person with dementia or multiple chronic diseases may not need treatment, whereas in an otherwise healthy person or one with coronary artery disease who is still functional and enjoys his or her life, it will require treatment.

As in all medical decisions, the management of cholesterol disorders in older persons must be individualized without regard to age. Treatment of cholesterol disorders in older persons are not appreciably different from those recommended for young or middle-aged persons. Rigid and impractical programs have even less relevance to older persons.

- *Regular exercise.* Older persons should begin new exercise regimens with low-impact, low-intensity workouts and advance slowly. In fact, if you do nothing else, exercising on a regular (daily) basis is the best thing you can do to reduce your risk of a disabling or fatal cardiovascular event by at least 50%. Recent data have shown that for this age group, mild to moderate weight training or resistance exercises not only increase strength by 25% to 100%, they also increase the bone density and lower the blood pressure and LDL-cholesterol. Even one set of 10 to 15 repetitions of eight to 10 different exercises several times a week may be adequate for some older persons.

- *Food for thought.* The adoption of the Twenty Risk Factor (TRF) diet with daily scores of about 30 provides older persons with varied choices and a dietary regimen that is suitable for managing almost any coexistent diseases. Almost all older persons should also take a low-dose aspirin (81 mg) and one multivitamin with minerals (but no iron) once or twice a day on a daily basis. The use of cholesterol-altering or other cardio-protective drugs requires judicious and thoughtful consideration for each person. In general, the approach to prevention or treatment of coronary risk factors of an older person should be the same as if they were in their 50s or 60s. In preventing coronary artery disease, we should learn to ignore birthdates.

We have come a long way since the heyday of smoking as socially acceptable behavior. I saw an old movie in which the doctor lit up a cigarette, took a deep satisfying drag and blew it over his patient. And this was during a physical exam! To my amazement, he offered one to his patient, right there in the exam room and assured him that "you're in excellent shape!"

Risk Factor #9
Smoking

In October 2006, the Centers for Disease Control had some sobering news. After years of steadily declining rates in smoking—prompted by continuous evidence of the overwhelming dangers of smoking—we seemed to have hit a wall. Smoking rates are no longer declining. One in five adults —more than 45 million Americans—continue to smoke. Teen smoking rates, meanwhile, had steadily climbed since the 1990s, contributing to the pool of adult smokers.

Smoking is the most extensively studied preventable cause of deaths and disabilities. The first preventable cause is sedentary lifestyle. Various health agencies including the American Cancer Society and the American Heart Association cling to old estimates that tobacco's annual death toll in the US is about 420,000. Although smoking-cessation rates have stalled, in the past decade America has had one of the world's lowest smoking rates; the highest rate is in Asia, where at least two in three men smoke. With changes in tobacco usage, and with better and earlier intervention in those suffering from tobacco-related diseases, the number of tobacco-related deaths in the US may be closer to 250,000 per year. It is, however, still an enormous preventable tragedy. For many years America has been the best "smoke-free" country in the world, so secondhand smoke is also far less of a problem than it was 30 years ago.

Smoking and longevity

In one 25-year study tracking the smoking and longevity of 50,000 Norwegians, heavy smokers (those who smoked one or more packs per day) were three times more likely to die in middle-age than nonsmokers—26% of women and 41% of men who died were middle age, compared with nine percent and 14% of those who had never smoked. In a recent study, the detrimental effects of smoking were greatest at earlier ages of smoking initiation, and in those who had smoked the longest. Conversely, the health benefits of quitting are most noticeable when it is done before age 40, instead of waiting until irreversible damage has occurred. Even those who kick the habit in their 50s or 60s can still reduce the risk of premature death, cardiovascular events or various cancers.

About 90% of smokers pick up the habit before they turn 18, and smoking rates among young people all over the world are on the rise. The trend is particularly disturbing in Eastern Europe, Asia and Latin America. This trend toward tobacco use at younger ages and for prolonged periods is a forerunner to an epidemic of tobacco-related disabilities and deaths throughout the world.

Smoking and cardiovascular health

According to the CDC, when everything else is considered—diet, lifestyle and other factors— smokers are two to four times more likely than nonsmokers to develop coronary artery disease, and twice as likely to have a stroke. Smoking increases stiffness of the arteries which contributes to high blood pressure.

Tobacco smoke contains over 1,200 chemical compounds, including at least 60 known carcinogens. However, many other compounds have yet to be identified or studied. Tobacco's chemical compounds also increase the antioxidant load of arterial plaques, making them more inflamed and vulnerable to plaque rupture, heart attack and stroke.

The cardio-toxic, carcinogenic and other harmful effects of tobacco are not limited to carbon monoxide and nicotine. Some other components of tobacco smoke are potent oxidants and carcinogens. Tobacco smoke alters many biological markers in the human body that can directly contribute to coronary artery disease.

Other toxic effects from smoking include...

- Increased oxidation of LDL-cholesterol

- Increased white blood cells, which contribute to inflammation processes within the plaque

- Increased fibrinogen, a potent clotting factor

- Increased stickiness and clumping of platelets, a high risk of arterial clots

- Spasm and constriction of the arteries, contributing to hypertension, angina and poor circulation to every organ from the brain to the lower legs

- Decreased "good" HDL-cholesterol level

Cigars, pipes, low-tar, low-nicotine cigarettes

Many cigar or pipe smokers believe they're smoking less harmful alternatives to cigarettes. True, cigarette users tend to smoke more often. But cigars and pipes contain more tobacco and it takes longer to finish one than several cigarettes.

Many cigar and pipe smokers claim that they do not inhale. But they do! Their blood nicotine levels (or urine cotinine level, a by-product of nicotine) is often as high as that of cigarette smokers. Cigar and pipe smokers inhale some endstream smoke (through the mouth) and a large amount of sidestream smoke (smoke in the air, through the nose), especially in rooms with poor ventilation.

Low-tar/low-nicotine cigarettes are not safer, either. Because the filters of these cigarettes have more or larger perforations than regular brands, they will mix the ambient air at a 75% to 25% ratio diluting the smoke. Many smokers seal off these perforations with their fingers and smokers tend to inhale more deeply to get their nicotine fix. This explains why smokers of "light" brands tend to develop cancers deep in the lung tissue, whereas smokers of regular brands tend to develop cancers in the bronchial tree.

Also, as saliva moves to and from the pipe stem and cigar butt into the mouth, it brings carcinogenic compounds into the mouth, and therefore, there is a high risk of oral and throat cancers among cigar and pipe smokers. Nicotine is readily absorbed from the mouth and the stomach while other compounds can cause irritation and cancers of the lips, tongue, oral cavity, larynx, throat, esophagus and stomach.

Decades of experience have clearly shown us that tobacco is harmful. The health and human cost of smoking is so staggering that it defies any estimate. The US tobacco industry agreed to pay $246 billion to the individual states over the next 25 years to compensate them for their anticipated tobacco-related health expenditures to Medicare and Medicaid recipients. But the cost of providing healthcare for all tobacco-related diseases (not counting an estimated 250,000 deaths annually) is many times greater.

Even shorter daily exposure to tobacco smoke, whether from cigarettes, cigars or passive smoking is unsafe. In a recent study, 225 men who had smoked only cigars for an average of 16 years were compared with 14,200 other men who had never smoked any tobacco products. Stogie smokers who averaged two cigars per day had an 87% higher risk of dying of cancer and an 89% higher risk of dying of various cardiovascular diseases. Is this a "safer" alternative to cigarettes?

A specific brain receptor for nicotine has been identified that controls the craving for nicotine and the frequent relapses after quitting. Undoubtedly many pharmaceutical companies will compete to find a drug that fools these receptors, and reduce or stop the craving for nicotine. That may help some solve one part of the psychological and biochemical aspects of smoking addiction and improve quit rates.

The message is: There is no safe tobacco, smoking or chewing varieties.

What you should do

You know the answer—quit! Yet, even though most smokers say they want to quit, fewer than 10% are successful in any given attempt. That's because no single method works for everyone, and it often takes several attempts. Even after quitting, there's a strong tendency toward relapse, because smoking is a chronic addiction.

Still, half of those who try more than once are eventually successful at quitting for good.

Nicotine replacement therapy

Nicotine replacement products are available in several forms—gums, skin patches that slowly release nicotine into the bloodstream, nasal sprays that provide nicotine through a mist, and inhalers that deliver a puff of nicotine vapor into the mouth and throat. No matter the delivery, these products provide nicotine to replace the addictive ingredient in tobacco smoke, to help cut cravings and avoid withdrawal symptoms.

The Food and Drug Administration has approved over-the-counter nicotine gums such as Nicorette and nicotine patches such as Nicoderm CQ and Nicotrol, because the majority of smokers

attempting to quit are unlikely to seek the services of a counselor or physician. Unfortunately, despite all the advertising, the six-month quit rates for users of these products is only about 10% to 20% —hardly a success story. For "healthy" smokers these products are safe in the short-term. For people with cardiovascular disease, it may be problematic to receive large amounts of nicotine delivered throughout the day with these methods, especially if they are continued for weeks or months.

Since the six-month quit rates for nicotine gums and patches are so low, some smoking counseling centers advocate a combination of both. Unfortunately, this dual approach has improved the quit rates by only an additional six percent to seven percent. Despite their relatively poor quit rates, the use of nicotine gums, patches, or a combination of smoking cessation aids and counselling may be one of the few options for those who have been unable to quit without a "nicotine fix."

Nicotine gum comes in two milligram and four milligram strengths. The higher dose is usually recommended more for those who smoke at least one pack a day. To use it...

- Rather than constant chewing like other gums, nicotine gum should be chewed slowly a few times to break it down, and then "parked" between your gums and cheek. This "chew and park" process is repeated for about 30 minutes,

Many states now operate telephone hotlines and organized groups for smokers who want to quit. To learn about offerings, contact your local or state health agency. You can also get information and telephone counseling by calling 1-800-QUIT-NOW.

or until the piece no longer releases a peppery taste.

- If you chew without parking, nicotine is released directly into saliva and swallowed. This can cause hiccups, heartburn, nausea or a craving for a cigarette.

- Avoid acidic beverages such as coffee, juices, and soda for at least 15 minutes before and after chewing. These drinks may contribute to stomach upset or nausea, and discourage you from using the gum.

Nictoine inhalers look like cigarettes, containing a cartridge that releases a puff of nicotine vapor in a measured dose. It is absorbed in your mouth and throat, but not your lungs. These products, available only by prescription, are cumbersome and expensive, and there is no evidence to suggest that they are any better than more practical aids like patches and gums. I have never prescribed these inhalers.

Nicotine patches look like large bandages that slowly releases a constant dose of nicotine into your skin—either for 16 or 24 hours, depending on the product. To use them…

- Typically, patches containing more nicotine are used for the first few weeks, then patches containing less nicotine are used. With some brands, after the initial higher-dose period, you stop wearing the patches. There is no evidence that the tapering method is more effective than abruptly stopping after the recommended time.

- Patches should be applied to clean, hairless skin between the neck and the waist, such as the upper arm, the shoulder or the back. Patch sites should be rotated to avoid skin irritation.

- Wear the patch all day. Do not apply and remove as a substitute for a cigarette.

Nicotine nasal sprays are often recommended for those who have not been able to quit using gums or patches. Unlike those other slow-release products, the nicotine in prescription sprays is quickly absorbed through the nose into the bloodstream, producing a "hit" like that of a cigarette. I do not recommend these sprays, especially because they often cause significant nasal irritation, require frequent dosing and are just too cumbersome.

Other therapies

Some studies suggest that hypnosis, acupuncture or psychotherapy might be helpful in quitting smoking. While many of these studies were poorly designed and have yet to prove long-term quitting rates, there is good evidence that support groups are beneficial. Some research shows that when coupled with a support group, smokers who use nicotine replacement therapy double their chances of successfully quitting, compared to using nicotine replacement therapy alone.

Prescription

Some studies have suggested that certain antidepressant drugs such as nortriptyline (Pamelor) and bupropion (Zyban, Wellbutrin) are helpful in smoking cessation. Due to side effects associated with larger doses, nortriptyline has not been used extensively for this purpose.

Two recent studies examined the efficacy and safety of bupropion at doses of 150mg–300mg per day for six to eight weeks. In one study of

Warning! Smoking cessation aids such as over-the-counter herbs and products obtainable through toll-free numbers or the internet are generally useless. Occasionally they are even dangerous. They are designed to take advantage of gullible and sometimes desperate consumers. Although an occasional smoker may be able to quit (a placebo effect), the failure rate is too high to justify spending money on these questionable products.

a smooth nicotine withdrawal. Interestingly, smokers who take bupropion are less likely to gain weight than with other approaches, mostly because bupropion seems to reduce the hand-to-mouth habit and to prevent snacking as a replacement for smoking.

The FDA approved varenicline (marketed in the US as Chantix by Pfizer Inc.) Chantix is the first nicotine-free drug approved by the FDA since bupropion. Two recent multicenter studies among smokers who were given Chantix 1mg twice a day for 12 weeks showed a significant

615 subjects, short-term quit rates were 40%. A year later, 22% of smokers who had taken bupropion for six to eight weeks still had not resumed smoking. As modest as these results seem, they are considerably better than those for other interventions. (Remember, the long-term quit rate for smokers using nicotine patches or nicotine gums is about 10%.)

In a second study of 893 people, a nine-week course of sustained-release bupropion was compared with a nicotine patch, bupropion plus a nicotine patch, and a placebo pill. The quit rates at 12 months were 15.6% for the placebo group, 30% for the bupropion group, and 35% for the group that received both bupropion and a nicotine patch. This study essentially validated the findings of the first one and confirmed that at least a third of smokers can be helped.

Bupropion (Zyban or Wellbutrin) is believed to work by targeting certain brain transmitters to reduce or stop nicotine cravings. It also minimizes irritability, depression and other emotional problems associated with quitting.

Although a single daily 150 mg dose of bupropion is adequate for most smokers, a heavy, long-term smoker may do better with 150 mg twice a day. The drug is started seven to 10 days before the actual quit date to ensure that enough of the drug has begun to act on brain cells; it is then continued for six to eight weeks to allow for

WHAT HAPPENS WHEN YOU QUIT

- *12 hours after quitting:* The carbon monoxide level in your blood drops to normal.

- *Two weeks to three months after quitting:* Circulation improves and lung function increases.

- *One to nine months after quitting:* Coughing and shortness of breath decrease; cilia (tiny hairly like structures that move mucus out of the lungs) regain normal function in the lungs, increasing the ability to handle mucus, clean the lungs, and reduce the risk of infection.

- *One year after quitting:* The excess risk of coronary heart disease is half that of a smoker's.

- *Five years after quitting:* Your stroke risk is reduced to that of a nonsmoker five to 15 years after quitting.

- *10 years after quitting:* The lung cancer death rate is about half that of a continuing smoker's. The risk of cancer of the mouth, throat, esophagus, bladder, cervix and pancreas decrease.

- *15 years after quitting:* The risk of coronary heart disease is that of a nonsmoker's.

quit rate of 44% compared to 18% for those who received a placebo and 30% for bupropion. Chantix is a nicotine pretender that fools the brain's nicotine receptors and minimizes nicotine cravings or withdrawal symptoms. One side effect of this drug is that may cause some nausea in about one in four smokers who take it—but it gradually goes away. Beyond that, so far, it seems to be a reasonably safe drug for quitting a bad habit.

Risk Factor #10
Kidney Disease

Kidney disease and cardiovascular problems often go hand-in-hand, with one impacting the other. People with diagnosed heart disease will often have variable degrees of kidney damage, just as people with kidney disease, even in early or mild stages, are likely to have a higher rate of coronary and cerebral artery diseases, which may contribute to heart attack and stroke. As the kidney dysfunction increases, the risk of a cardiovascular event increases dramatically.

One reason for this connection is that the two leading causes of kidney disease—high blood pressure and diabetes—are also major risk factors for cardiovascular disease. The kidneys also have a vast network of small arteries which are impacted by almost all other major coronary risk factors. Although we tend to focus on coronary or cerebral arteries, most other arteries also suffer from coronary risk factors to variable degrees.

As the body goes through its routine activities, a certain amount of metabolic end products enter the bloodstream. One major function of the kidneys is to remove these waste by-products by breaking them down into harmless compounds, or eliminating them via the urine. Thus, the kidneys' extensive network of blood vessels bring in the blood, have it filtered, and return cleansed blood back to the systemic circulation. In most cases of kidney dysfunction, the vessels in this vascular network do not relax or dilate appropriately, or remain constricted. This behavior mirrors the behavior of coronary arteries during the early stages of coronary artery disease.

In other words, kidney dysfunction is a consequence of a systemic vascular disease that included the kidneys' vascular network.

Even with mild abnormality in the kidneys' vascular network some protein (albumin) leaks in the urine. Many studies have show that urinary albumin level independently predicts the risk of cardiovascular events, because it's a clue of vascular disease.

In one important study tracking some 6,300 men for 27 years, as urinary protein levels increased, so did the risk of heart attack and stroke. This suggests that even early-stage kidney dysfunction needs to be addressed to reduce vulnerability to cardiovascular problems.

Chronic kidney dysfunction contributes to three other coronary risk factors...

1. Spasm of kidney arteries invariably reduces the blood supply of the kidneys, which increases blood pressure.

2. Since lipoprotein(a) is partially broken down in the kidneys, any slowdown in this process increases its levels in the blood.

3. Homocysteine, another major coronary risk factor, is a protein that is partially converted in the kidneys into a harmless protein. People with kidney dysfunction often have significantly higher levels of homocysteine, further increasing their risk of a cardiovascular event.

What you should do

Get screened. Even kidney disease that produces no noticeable symptoms translates to a proportionately higher risk of heart disease. One measure of kidney function is a test that collects GFR—glomerular filtration rate, which measures the kidney's ability to filter blood and produce urine. In normal persons, the GRF is about 80–90. A lower threshold of below 60 ml per minute reflects significant loss of kidney function.

Control blood pressure. As blood pressure increases, the arteries of the kidney develop more spasm, further impacting their blood supply. Any reduction in the kidneys' blood supply increases the blood pressure, perpetuating the vicious cycle.

In fact, intensive and strict control of blood pressure to lower than 120/80 mmHg is an essential step in reducing the progression of kidney dysfunction and risk of cardiovascular events.

Control all major coronary risk factors. A high level of LDL-cholesterol needs to be treated aggressively in anyone with even early-stage kidney dysfunction. Regrettably, many doctors still cling to 130 mg/dl as the so-called "normal" LDL level. As noted before, the acceptable LDL levels for people with cardiovascular disease, diabetes, multiple coronary risk factors, metabolic syndrome and kidney dysfunction should be less than 70 mg/dl.

In addition to adhering to principles of the Twenty Risk Factor Diet and appropriate exercise, a statin drug is nearly always required to lower LDL-cholesterol to below 70 mg/dl. Blood levels of lipoprotein(a) and homocysteine should be checked periodically and treated appropriately along with any other co-existing risk factor.

Take aspirin and eat fish. Since elevated lipoprotein(a) or homocysteine raises risk of an arterial blood clot, you should take one low-dose aspirin (81 mg) per day and eat at least four servings of omega-3-rich seafood each week. Both are effective at lowering this clotting risk.

Note: People with coronary artery disease should periodically have a urinary albumin level test (an inexpensive test available at almost all laboratories) to detect any underlying kidney dysfunction.

Risk Factor #11
Chronic Inflammation and Infection

Here's an important risk factor in heart disease and stroke about which many people—including healthcare providers—are unaware. In fact, the majority of healthcare providers overlook these major risk factors and don't discuss the associated cardiovascular risk with patients who have these diseases. Some chronic infections, such as sinusitis, periodontitis or chronic bronchitis contribute to the release of inflammatory compounds that trigger a mild systemic inflammatory response involving the arteries and various joints. This inflammatory overload may increase the risk of a coronary event by 30%.

AIDS not only contributes to this systemic inflammatory process, it also impairs the body's response to such inflammatory assault. The consequence is more overwhelming and triggers an accelerated form of coronary and cerebral artery disease that increases the risk of a cardiovascular event by more than threefold.

Inflammation is the body's response to any tissue injury. When you catch a cold or slash your skin, the obvious signs of inflammation—redness and swelling—are evidence that your immune system is doing its job: white blood cells (WBCs) attack the invader and enter the site of damage to repair the damage and allow healthy cells to thrive and replace damaged or dead cells. In the process, WBCs release certain inflammatory compounds, some of which escape into the systemic bloodstream. If the local damage is repaired, tissue healing occurs, and the inflammation goes away. However, in certain circumstances, the inflammation is not handled by body's immune system and a chronic, smoldering inflammatory process sets in.

There are 30 different types of white blood cells. Unfortunately, sometimes "activated" white blood cells produce toxic and cell-damaging compounds (called cytokines), which may contribute to unintended consequences such as rheumatoid arthritis, lupus and coronary and cerebral artery disease.

When LDL particles infiltrate into the subsurface of the arteries, WBCs release oxidizing cytokines, clumping them together to "gobble" them up. Eventually they burst and release oxidized LDL by products into the arterial subsurface. These by products trigger an intense inflammation and more WBCs pour in to defend against it. Unfortunately, the defenders once again turn into offenders, and the cycle goes on. Debris made up of oxidized LDL by-products, numerous white blood cells (dead and alive), smooth muscle cells, collagen fibers, calcium, and iron pile up in the subsurface of the artery. This inflammatory junk pile is coronary artery plaque. Without the inflammatory turmoil within the wall of the arteries, no one would ever develop coronary and cerebral plaques or suffer a heart attack or stroke due to their rupture.

Inflammation elsewhere in the body is more or less the same; sometimes it does not involve the inner wall of coronary or cerebral artery. Instead, it occurs in various joints, as is the case with rheumatoid arthritis or blood vessels elsewhere in the body or other tissues such as systemic lupus.

In rheumatoid arthritis, for instance, WBCs feast on synovial joint cells; in systemic lupus, hungry white blood cells attack kidney and skin cells. Regardless of the site of inflammation, some cytokines produced by WBCs eventually enter the bloodstream and travel to coronary and cerebral arteries, where they accelerate the process of

plaque formation. In fact, having rheumatoid arthritis causes an accelerated inflammatory response that can cause significant plaque formation —and arterial blockage—within a few short years. This explains why people with chronic inflammatory or infectious diseases (such as AIDS) have high rates of cardiovascular disease and often have heart attacks or other serious events in their 30s and 40s.

In a study from Cornell University in New York, a group of patients with rheumatoid arthritis was compared to healthy people of the same age, who did not have rheumatoid arthritis. Carotid artery ultrasound study was also done in both groups. The results showed that persons with rheumatoid arthritis had a threefold increased risk of carotid artery plaques (a surrogate for coronary artery plaques) compared to people without arthritis. The risk was even higher in persons younger than 50 years of age, a clear reflection of the accelerated course of atherosclerosis in these cases. Unfortunately, some recent drugs used for this disabling joint disease or systemic lupus can also backfire and perpetuate this fast-track process.

More than three million Americans have rheumatoid arthritis or systemic lupus, two of the so-called "autoimmune diseases" in which white blood cells release cytokines and other chemicals to cause a constant state of inflammation. Many of these patients are under age 50, prompting them into a premature state of cardiovascular disease. Millions of people also have other chronic inflammatory conditions or infections, such as AIDS, sinusitis, periodontitis or Chlamydia pneumoniae (lung) infection. These at-risk people require early and aggressive treatment, not only for their "primary" inflammatory disorder, but also for every co-existing coronary risk factor.

AIDS is a worldwide issue affecting millions of men and women, most under the age of 40. At this age, the risk of heart attack should not be high, but people infected with HIV have a significantly higher risk of developing coronary artery disease at an accelerated pace. To compound the problem, one of the most effective classes of antiviral drugs, called *protease inhibitors*, further increase the risk of heart attack among HIV-infected persons by 16% per year of use. Thus, the risk is doubled after six years of continuous treatment (Friis-Møller, V et al., *N Eng J Med* 2007; 356: 1723–35).

Recent data have shown a moderately higher risk of cardiovascular events among individuals with periodontitis. How does some "low grade," chronic gum infection cause heart attacks? As noted before, chronic infection sites produce and release into the bloodstream various inflammatory compounds that increase the oxidant load at distant organs including coronary and cerebral arteries. However, people with chronic periodontitis may also have some unhealthy lifestyles, dietary and hygienic practices, or a less proactive approach toward screening for and treatment of cardiovascular risk factors, which contribute to their higher risk.

What you should do

Strict and long-term control of all inflammation and infections. Because the local source of inflammation (for example, joints in rheumatoid arthritis) is where inflammatory compounds are produced, every effort must be made to reduce joint swelling and inflammation so that very little or no cytokines can escape into bloodstream. In the case of AIDS, which is a chronic systemic infection, vigorous treatment of HIV is essential to reduce the risk of accelerated coronary artery disease. Frequent measurement of LDL, HDL, triglycerides and homocysteine levels and vigorous treatment of these risk factors will help prevent the accelerated cardiovascular disease.

Diet. The Twenty Risk Factor diet is even more important for anyone with an inflammatory condition or infection. Eating four to five seafood meals a week rich in omega-3 fatty acids offers a significant anti-inflammatory effect, locally at the site of primary inflammation, and systemically. Also important is replacing vegetable oils, fats and margarines that are high in omega-6s, which contribute to and fuel the inflammatory process, with olive oil, which has 74% monounsaturates which can actually slow down the inflammatory cascade.

Weight management. Intra-abdominal fat cells produce numerous inflammatory compounds, and they stimulate the liver to do the same. Special attention should be paid to losing as much of your abdominal obesity as possible.

Statins. Recent studies have shown that these drugs also reduce activation of WBCs and cytokine production within the arterial wall and elsewhere. Moreover, several studies have shown a significant reduction in the inflammation of joints in persons with rheumatoid arthritis who take statins.

Treating all chronic infections and inflammatory diseases requires the help of specialists such as infectious disease physicians, or rheumatologists, who can assess your need for directed therapy with medications and other approaches. The sooner you seek help, the lower is your risk of a catastrophic cardiovascular event.

Risk Factor #12
High Blood Pressure

High blood pressure, or hypertension, is defined as regular blood pressure readings more than 120 mmHg (systolic, top number) over 80 (diastolic, bottom number). It currently affects at least 80 million Americans—one in three adults under 50 years of age and more than half of those over 50. Its incidence is soaring, both in the US and elsewhere. By 2025, hypertension will affect more than 1.5 billion people worldwide, a 60% increase from current incidence rates. What are the implications?

High blood pressure has a wide range of causes, including kidney disease, sedentary lifestyle, abdominal obesity, diabetes, narrowing of the artery of one or both kidneys, certain tumors of adrenal glands, poor dietary practices and being underweight at birth. More than 80% of all hypertension is due to these factors.

The other 20% may not have any of these risk factors, at least not initially. Hence, this hypertension is called "essential," a confusing term that should be dropped from healthcare providers' vocabularies. "Undetermined cause" hypertension is more rational, because as we investigate these cases, many will be found to have one or more reasons for their hypertension. In fact, recent studies have shown that people with this form of disease often have genetic abnormalities in enzymes or other compounds that regulate blood pressure. Such defects or mutations result in dysfunctional or nonfunctional enzymes that regulate blood pressure.

Malnutrition during fetal life can also affect the formation of elastin, a substance that plays a major role in pliability and dilating ability of the arteries. Developments in molecular biology and DNA technology give hope that we are getting closer to discovering every cause of hypertension. These developments also provide incentives for the pharmaceutical industry to find targeted drugs that can be matched to individual needs.

Blood pressure dangers

Blood pressure is the force of the blood pushing against the walls of the arteries. Each time the heart beats—generally about 70 times a minute while at rest—it pumps blood into the arteries. Your blood pressure is at its highest when the heart beats, pumping the blood, which is the systolic pressure. When the heart is at rest, between beats, blood pressure falls. This is the diastolic pressure. Blood pressure changes throughout the day. It increases more when you are excited, nervous or physically active.

What is a normal blood pressure?

Although there is solid and compelling evidence that blood pressure greater than 120/80 mmHg is abnormal for people of all ages, male or female, most people and healthcare providers still use 140/90 mmHg as their yardstick. Why? The best answer is the least logical—habit! It is well known in the medical profession that the translation of scientific evidence into clinical practice takes a long time, sometimes up to 17 years for positive evidence to be adopted and put into practice.

WHITE COAT WARNING

Blood pressure may fluctuate noticeably day-to-day and sometimes even on the same day. This so-called "unstable hypertension" (as opposed to consistently high blood pressure) may be attributed to the "white coat effect"—the belief that blood pressure may increase because of the anxiety of a doctor's appointment.

The problem is, if the anticipation of seeing a healthcare provider can raise blood pressure, the real time and real-life encounters of everyday life may also provoke the same hypertensive response. Since blood pressure is not monitored continuously, these abnormally high readings may be the norm... and "normal" blood pressure numbers could be the exception.

What's the take-home message? Don't shrug off high readings at the doctor's office...and take note of an important study known as the US Physicians' Study. After tracking more than 55,000 men with no history of hypertension for almost six years, researchers found that systolic readings—the top number—are generally the best predictor of cardiovascular risk. This study, published in *American Journal of Hypertension*, found that for each 10 mmHg increase in systolic pressure, the risk rose about 1.5 times in men between ages 39 and 49, and about 1.13 times in older men.

Do not ignore unstable hypertension. Its effects (intermittent streams of blood lashing against the plaques in the coronary and cerebral arteries) can significantly increase your risk of heart attack and stroke if left untreated.

That long delay is unfortunate, because a report reviewing data collected in 61 previous studies —tracking one million men and women— showed that even slight changes in blood pressure can have major consequences. The risk of dying from stroke doubles with each 20 mmHg increase in systolic pressure *or* 10 mmHg increase in diastolic pressure above the optimal 115/75 reading. A report by the Joint National Committee on preventing and treating high blood pressure notes a doubling in other cardiovascular risks with the same 20/10 mmHg increase.

In a recent study of 8,960 middle-aged Americans, the risk of cardiovascular disease among those with blood pressure of 120-129 systolic, and 80-85 diastolic was 80% greater compared to optimal blood pressure of less than 120/80. Even more important, among those with so-called "high normal" blood pressure—a massive group of millions of Americans fall into this category—whose systolic blood pressure was 130-139 and diastolic was 85-89, the risk increased by 230% (2.3-fold)! Among African-Americans and obese persons, with "high normal" blood pressure, the risk of cardiovascular events (such as fatal or nonfatal heart attack or stroke, need for stent or bypass surgery) was more than 330% (3.3-fold). However, a vast number of these hypertensive people go untreated. Some of them will develop heart attack or stroke, and some will die or become disabled.

Why do so many people with hypertension go untreated, or inadequately treated? You may ask the same question about cholesterol, diabetes, homocysteine or any other coronary risk factor. The answer is that many healthcare providers still won't treat the blood pressure until it is above 140/90. However, a more important factor is that most people don't check their blood pressure to see if they have hypertension. Even when prescribed the appropriate antihypertension drugs, often patients do not take them on a regular or long-term basis.

About one in three hypertensives have what's called "nocturnal hypertension," in which their blood pressure may not be high during the

WHAT'S NORMAL?

As a general rule, "normal" optimal blood pressure is considered anything less than 120/80…and therein lies the problem. Too often, people with so-called "normal" or "high normal" blood pressure (130–139 for systolic and 85–89 for diastolic) are inappropriately assured they have nothing to worry about—and no attempt is made to lower their blood pressure.

Yet a study published in the *American Journal of Medicine* finds the risk of cardiovascular disease is 2.4 times greater among people with "normal" readings who are African-American, obese, and/or diabetic, compared to others in this 120/80 range. Compared to others with "high normal" levels, the risk is between 3.3 and 3.5 times higher in these high-risk groups.

morning—when they may see their doctors—but tends to increase in the afternoon or at night. This condition may account, at least in part, for some cases of nighttime heart attacks and strokes. Clearly, these people cannot get proper treatment if their blood pressure readings are only taken in the daytime. Therefore, it is important to have random late afternoon or nighttime blood pressure readings at home or at your neighborhood drugstore to make sure you don't have nocturnal hypertension.

In addition, the blood pressure recorded on the right arm is frequently somewhat higher (at times by 20 to 30 mmHg) than the left arm. The reason is that the diameter of the artery that branches off from the aorta and goes to the right arm is sometimes larger than the left (rarely is it the other way around). Since higher blood pressure on the right is your true blood pressure, you should always ask your healthcare provider to check it on both sides.

Long-term hypertension can cause small "mini-strokes" which may lead progressively to dementia. In a long-term French study, doctors treated 1,238 hypertensives vigorously with two or three drugs. A comparable number of patients were treated less vigorously (with one antihypertensive drug). Those treated vigorously had 50% lower risk of dementia than the "control" group who were treated less vigorously.

It's estimated that about 20 new dementia cases could be avoided for every 1,000 hypertensives treated more aggressively with multiple drugs for at least five years. Numerous studies have already shown a clear link between having high blood pressure and a greater risk of eventually developing memory loss. In a 20-year study of 999 older men, Swedish investigators also found a significant link between hypertension and dementia. Since there is no effective treatment for dementia, controlling high blood pressure as early as possible becomes even more imperative.

For some hypertensives, identifying and treating the underlying cause may cure their disease. For most others, however, hypertension may remain a lifelong disorder that requires dietary and lifestyle changes and, often, daily use of medication.

Blood pressure, like blood sugar or blood cholesterol, is not a constantly stable, flat-line marker; it fluctuates from day to day or even hour to hour. Often, during a visit to a physician, blood pressure may go up by 10 to 20 mmHg, and if repeated within 10 to 15 minutes, it may go down to its unprovoked level. Although the anticipatory anxiety over what the doctor might find may contribute to this "white coat syndrome," you or your doctor should not dismiss it outright or assume "I was just a bit nervous." If this anxiety is enough to raise your blood pressure, it may very well be that other stressful events throughout the day will do likewise. However, since your blood pressure is not continuously monitored throughout the day, you don't know that, nor does your doctor. It is for this reason that I always ask my patients with "white coat" hypertension (any value higher than 120/80) to check their blood pressure in the morning and in late afternoon (or after coming home from work), on Monday, Wednesday and Friday, for two weeks. Share these 12 readings with your healthcare provider to decide if you have hypertension, and if so, what to do about it.

What you should do

Know your blood pressure. Every time you see a healthcare provider, have your blood pressure checked. If it is more than 120/80, don't dismiss it because your doctor said it is okay. It is not, and it is your health and your life. Check it several times over the next two weeks, both in the morning and late at night. Two-thirds of those with systolic blood pressure of 120-130 will develop higher blood pressure, exceeding 140 mmHg within two years. In the meantime, your ignored high blood pressure has brutalized the arteries of your brain, your eyes, your heart and your kidneys for two years. Do not accept your doctor's recommendation to "watch it." You need intervention to control and lower your blood pressure, not a security guard!

Diet. The Twenty Risk Factor Diet provides you with a rational, varied and practical approach to lower your blood pressure, and help control other co-existing coronary risk factors. Most Americans consume much more sodium than they need. This includes salt added to meals, but also the salt in prepackaged and frozen foods or canned soups and vegetables. Salt restraint is especially helpful in so-called "salt responders" that include seniors, African-Americans and people with abdominal obesity or a body mass index of 30 or more.

Exercise. Numerous studies have documented the blood-pressure-lowering effects of regular aerobic exercise. Ideally, you should get 30 to 60 minutes of moderate (such as brisk walking) to vigorous (running, bicycling, etc.) exercise most days.

Quit smoking. Need another reason? The nicotine causes blood vessels to stiffen and constrict, makes the heart beat faster, which raises blood pressure, especially in heavy smokers (more than one pack per day).

Limit alcohol. Although one or two drinks with dinner can lower blood pressure by relaxing the arteries, higher alcohol intake, especially if it is done on a regular daily basis, may raise blood pressure. As a rule, if you drink, limit alcohol to no more than one or two drinks per day. (One drink is measured one can of beer, one glass of wine, or one ounce of liquor.) If you find your blood pressure increases with alcohol, it's best not to drink at all.

DIASTOLIC BLOOD PRESSURE COUNTS

- In one study involving 19,000 men and women with hypertension, researchers found that a diastolic number over 85 increased risk of heart attack by 35% and risk of stroke by 45% compared to a diastolic number of 80 or lower.

- Another study, tracking nearly 125,000 people in China and Japan for about seven years, found that for each five-point drop in diastolic pressure, stroke risk decreased by 40%. (Overall, those with the highest blood pressure faced 13 times the risk of stroke compare to those with the lowest readings.)

- In the largest study to date—involving 450,000 people tracked an average of 16 years—the risk of stroke was deemed five times higher with a diastolic reading of 120 compared to 75. For the hypertensives studied, the risk of stroke was five times higher for people from 44 to 65, while the risk for persons over 65 was two times higher. This study confirms that the danger of high blood pressure is not confined to older adults, but is a danger to all.

ANTIHYPERTENSION DRUGS

There are many safe, effective blood-pressure lowering medications, and many hypertensives are prescribed more than one. *The classes include...*

- *Diuretics* that help the body get rid of extra sodium and fluid so blood vessels don't have to hold so much fluid
- *ACE* (angiotensin-converting enzyme) *inhibitors* that block an enzyme necessary to produce a substance that causes blood vessels to constrict.
- *ARBs* (Angiotensin II Receptor Blockers), a newer sibling of ACE inhibitors
- *Beta-blockers* that block the effects of adrenaline and lower heart rate
- *Alpha-blockers* that help blood vessels relax
- *Calcium channel blockers* that keep blood vessels from constricting by blocking calcium from entering cells
- *Combinations:* These drugs combine an ACE inhibitor with a calcium channel blocker, diuretic or beta-blocker.

Despite the entrenched notion, there is no direct correlation between blood pressure lowering effects of a drug and its ultimate benefit—reducing the risk of heart attack, stroke or other complications caused by high blood pressure. That's because some drugs may lower blood pressure but increase insulin resistance, adversely impact LDL-cholesterol or particle size or alter platelet function to increase risk of clot formation. Some calcium channel blockers may actually cause fluid retention in some people even though they may still lower the blood pressure.

For most people, a combination of a diuretic and an ACE inhibitor or ARB may be good first-line drugs. These drugs can reduce thickening of the walls of tiny arteries, protect kidney function and improve heart muscle health. However, your healthcare provider should be allowed to match your need to any available antihypertensive drug. (At last count, I found over 270 of them!)

Buy yourself a blood pressure monitor. There are many reasonably priced, digital monitors at your neighborhood drugstore or department stores.

Do not buy a wrist or finger monitor. They are inaccurate and virtually useless. Always buy monitors with arm cuffs.

Risk Factor #13
Elevated Lipoprotein(a)

Lipoprotein(a), commonly known as Lp(a), is a specific class of lipoprotein that is an independent risk factor for cardiovascular disease. Lp(a) is particularly harmful because it consists of an LDL molecule and a coronary unfriendly protein called apoprotein(a), which makes the whole molecule even worse than LDL. In addition to the effects of "bad" cholesterol, Lp(a) provokes the formation of microscopic clots within coronary plaques. These small clots play a major role in progression of coronary plaques and greater risk of a heart attack.

In one study, when coronary plaques were surgically removed from 72 heart disease patients, all specimens contained Lp(a). However, more troublesome, perhaps, was that in 90% of these samples, white blood cells had surrounded the Lp(a) particles. White blood cells contain certain enzymes that weaken plaques, making them more vulnerable to rupture. When a plaque cracks or ruptures, it allows blood to seep into the plaque and form a clot that gradually expands and eventually clogs up the lumen of the artery within an hour or more. Eighty percent of all heart attacks follow the rupture of a relatively small, non-obstructing plaque.

In a recent study, researchers used ultrasound probes inside a coronary artery, the most accurate test to detect coronary plaques and their sizes and to measure the behavior and progression of coronary plaques. Among individuals with elevated lipoprotein(a), coronary plaques grew in size at a greater rate and were more fatty (which makes them more likely to burst and rupture) than in those with optimal lipoprotein(a) (Hartmann, M et al., *J. Amer Coll Cardiol* 2006; 48: 446–52).

Recent studies have shown that kidney dysfunction slows down the breakdown of lipoprotein(a), resulting in accumulation (high levels) of Lp(a) in the bloodstream. In some cases of lupus (a systemic autoimmune disease) and rheumatoid arthritis, Lp(a) is also elevated. Although Lp(a) levels higher than 30 mg/dl are abnormal, recent studies have shown a threshold of 60 to 65 mg/dl as the levels at which Lp(a) becomes quite harmful. This finding also explains why, in some studies, slight elevation of Lp(a) was not found to be particularly harmful.

Several recent studies suggest that elevated lipoprotein(a) increases the risk of stroke by more than threefold, especially among men. In an eight-year study of 32,826 women in the US Nurses Health Study, elevated lipoprotein(a), especially when associated with high fibrinogen (a clotting factor made by the liver) increased the risk of fatal or nonfatal heart attacks by more than threefold.

Routine cholesterol profile tests do not include lipoprotein(a), so it needs to be requested and tested separately. The size of apoprotein(a) molecule, the coronary-unfriendly protein carried by Lp(a), is genetically determined and may vary from one person to another by as much as two and one-half times.

The size of apoprotein(a) changes its danger to the heart's health. People who inherit the gene that produces smaller molecules tend to be impacted more than those who have the larger versions. Women tend to have medium-sized to larger version of apoprotein(a), whereas men tend to have the smaller versions. African-Americans usually have the largest types, so that they are not negatively impacted even when their blood lipoprotein(a) levels are two to three times higher than the normal levels. The new technique to measure Lp(a) bypasses the confusion created by apoprotein size, but this technique is not widely available at most laboratories. Therefore, ask your healthcare provider to request in the prescription order that your blood sample be sent to the most reliable laboratories. With the new technique, Lp(a) level for everyone—young, old, male, female and various ethnicities—should not be more than 60 mg/dl.

What you should do

Lp(a) is largely unaffected by diet. However, there are some exceptions...high intake of omega-3 rich seafood can lower elevated Lp(a) about 10% but most important, seafood omega-3 fat (not plant omega-3) significantly reduces the clot-forming risk associated with high levels of Lp(a).

Conversely, trans fatty acids found in margarine, shortenings, cooking fats and deep-fried items can raise Lp(a) levels by 10%—providing yet another reason to avoid these dangerous fats.

Elevated Lp(a) is far more damaging to your arteries when LDL-cholesterol is also high, because of the added harm of both combined. Therefore, you should lower your LDL-cholesterol to under 100 mg/dl. Similarly, because homocysteine also increases the risk of clot formation, the combination of these two risk factors particularly increases the risk of a cardiovascular event.

Consider medication. Only niacin, at doses of 1,500 to 2,000 mg per day, can lower Lp(a) up to 30%. *Warning:* Estrogen-replacement therapy in women can also lower Lp(a) up to 20%. Thyroid hormone (for those who have underactive thyroid) can lower Lp(a) by 10%–20%.

Risk Factor #14
Family History of
Cardiovascular Disease

At least half of the 20 major coronary risk factors I've presented are fully or partially inherited disorders. In fact, more than 80% of people with coronary artery disease have at least one inherited factor that interacts with other nonhereditary risk factors. Some major risk factors—such as smoking, diet, exercise habits, or abdominal obesity—may not have a direct genetic component, but they are strongly influenced by family environment. Regrettably, very few people in the US and most of the developed countries are raised in a heart-healthy family environment.

Some genetic disorders are easy to detect—provided they are looked for—and their impacts are well-known. Elevated LDL-cholesterol and triglycerides, low HDL-cholesterol, early or advanced diabetes, and hypertension can all be assessed with simple tests. Other factors such as elevated lipoprotein(a), homocysteine, and fibrinogen, or small, dense LDL particle size need more sophisticated testing. Other genetic or family factors, such as certain enzymes and receptors, etc., also play a role, but the contribution of these novel factors is rather small, since the 20 major risk factors outlined here account for well over 95% of all cardiovascular events.

Genetics and cardiovascular risk

Over the past decade, we have greatly increased our understanding about how genetics—and more specifically, mutations in human genes—affect cardiovascular health. *For example…*

- *HDL-related genetic abnormalities:* Some people have a family history of low levels of "good" HDL-cholesterol, a significant risk for heart attack. In addition, some inherit HDL particles that do not have the right kind of antioxidant activity to reduce the risk of oxidative damage that exacerbates cardiovascular risks. (See Risk Factor #5.)

For instance, genetics play a role in levels and activity of paraoxonase enzymes, which normally act as a detoxifier. In a recent study, researchers removed from rodents the gene responsible for producing the paraoxonase enzyme. Without this enzyme, HDL-cholesterol particles lost their antioxidant capacity and failed to protect LDL particles from oxidation. Remember, LDL particles become harmful only after they are oxidized.

- *LDL-related genetic abnormalities:* More than 400 different genetic mutations in LDL receptors have already been discovered. Depending on the number and type, these mutations can impede—from slightly to severely—the liver's ability to entrap and remove LDL-cholesterol from entering the bloodstream. Since all of these mutations result in elevation of LDL-cholesterol levels, we do not need to test people for these inherited disorders.

- *Apoprotein E-related genetic abnormalities:* Aside from apoprotein A and B (see the ABCs of Coronary Artery Disease), other apoproteins (from C to H) have various roles in cardiovascular health. Apoprotein E—also referred to as apo E—and its subgroups (apo E2, E3, and E4; apo E1 is extremely rare) have a significant role in a person's response to dietary fat and cholesterol.

Depending on which genetic form of apo E a person receives from each parent, there could be six variants or "isoforms" of apo E: E2-2, E2-3, E2-4, E3-3, E3-4, E4-4. People who have apo E4-4 (one E4 from each parent) are cholesterol and saturated fat responders. This means that after eating a fatty meal, containing a high "dose" of cholesterol, their blood cholesterol levels increase nearly three times as much as those who have the apo E2-2. People with apo E4-4 also show a more dramatic fall in their blood cholesterol level in response to cholesterol-lowering measures. On the other hand, those with apo E2-2 or 3-2 typically have much lower cholesterol levels to begin with, and their blood cholesterol levels don't fluctuate much from day to day. Thus, the apo E status of an individual goes a long way toward explaining why some people with "terrible" eating habits do not have raised blood cholesterol levels or develop coronary artery disease.

The role of apoprotein E has become even more important over the past decade with the discovery that apo E4 plays a significant role in predisposing people to Alzheimer's disease. In fact, testing for apo E variants is a helpful screening for those with a family history of Alzheimer's disease in a close family member under the age of 60-65. The finding of apo E-4, especially E4-4, might indicate a higher risk for developing Alzheimer's, and should prompt those who test positive to become more proactive with preventive measures.

What you should do

Check the family history. When a parent develops cardiovascular disease before age 45, it's a strong indicator of multiple genetic mutations—and perhaps strong warning that aggressive preventative measures in the offspring may be needed. Premature cardiovascular disease in a parent before the age of 50 carries a significant likelihood that some of these mutations may be passed on to children.

The development of premature cardiovascular disease (heart attack, angina, coronary stents or bypass surgery, stroke and peripheral artery disease), or any major coronary risk factor, such as high cholesterol, in a sibling is also a

There is a valid tool to calculate your risk of a future heart attack. The goal is not to frighten you but to highlight your risks and encourage more preemptive intervention. Because you are saddled with a genetic burden, it does not mean you are helpless or unable to do anything about it.

Almost all of these inherited disorders are treatable. Just as you have to apply your brakes before, not after a car accident, you need to prevent the heart attack or stroke before, not after, the fact. Since familial or genetic-related cardiovascular events commonly occur at a much younger age, you need to start correcting all your risk factors in your teens and twenties, or *as early as you can.*

strong clue that there are genetic, inherited mutations in the family, even if the parents have not had premature cardiovascular events.

In a recent study, 2,500 men and women with average age of 49 were followed up for eight years. During the follow-up, the risk of heart attack or other cardiovascular event was 45% higher in those who had a sibling with cardiovascular disease, compared to those whose siblings had no cardiovascular disease. Thus, the sibling's cardiovascular disease may be a sign of either dormant or unrecognized genetic mutations or predisposition to cardiovascular disease in other family members. Parental or sibling cardiovascular disease, especially when it occurs before the age of 45, is a powerful indicator of multiple "genetic hits" (mutations). Although the family history carries a significant likelihood that some of these mutations may be transferred to one or more offspring, it is not obligatory that every family member will indeed inherit these mutations.

Thus, the presence of one or more major coronary risk factors or premature cardiovascular disease before the age of 50 in one or more first-degree relatives is a strong indicator of an inheritable, familial disorder. This familial predisposition usually is through one or more major risk factors that can be identified with appropriate tests. If you have such a strong family history, even in the absence of other personal risk factors (such as abdominal obesity, diabetes, smoking, a sedentary lifestyle), you must be thoroughly evaluated. Intervention must be started early and carried out as consistently as possible.

Because the impact of genetic factors is lifelong, short-term interventions provide very little or no protection. Lowering your homocysteine or blood cholesterol for two months, or treating hypertension and diabetes for six months cannot be expected to offer lasting protection against coronary artery disease and its catastrophic complications. Once a genetic predisposition has been established, you need to adopt an intervention and treatment program for the long-term. If you have any family history of premature cardiovascular disease, or major risk factors, your siblings and children over age 10 should also be tested.

Risk Factor #15
Elevated Levels of
Blood Homocysteine

Homocysteine is a protein, not a fat. We all have homocysteine in our blood, but the kidneys usually maintain it at a normal level. About half of it is broken down and eliminated in urine as harmless by-products. The other half is converted to an essential amino acid called "methionine" with the help of folic acid (vitamin B-9) and vitamin B-12.

Although deficiencies in these vitamins can interfere with the operation of this pathway and result in overaccumulation of homocysteine in the bloodstream, this accounts for only a small percentage of people with high blood levels of homocysteine. Other factors that contribute to elevated levels include aging, especially when associated with poor nutrition and low levels of folic acid or vitamin B-12; chronic kidney disease; eating too much red meat (although seafood helps lower homocysteine levels); and taking "sulfa" drugs—which can raise the homocysteine blood level by 30% to 50% during treatment. The levels go down rather quickly when these drugs are stopped.

Still, the primary cause of high homocysteine is genetics, accounting for about 90% of all cases. A recent discovery suggests that about one in 10 people in the US and Great Britain have an inherited defect in the enzyme responsible for the breakdown of homocysteine, making them genetically vulnerable to elevated levels.

Is elevated blood homocysteine a cardiovascular risk factor?

In the past 20 years, over 1,000 studies in human and laboratory animals have shown that elevated blood homocysteine increases oxidant load and arterial inflammation, contributes to the dysfunction of endothelial (inner) lining of the arteries, which is a prerequisite for plaque formation, and significantly increases the risk of cardiovascular diseases, especially stroke, peripheral artery disease and dementia. However, three recent *flawed* studies have reported that *modest* homocysteine-lowering in patients with *mildly* elevated blood homocysteine, who also have advanced cardiovascular disease or multiple other major risk factors, may not reduce the risk of cardiovascular events. These reports have contributed to confusion among healthcare providers and the public as to whether elevated homocysteine should be considered a major cardiovascular risk factor.

Since we often pay more attention to the sound bites than the substance of any issue, many healthcare providers look at a paragraph or two of an article, and blindly accept the sound bites of the abstract. In this case, many physicians mistakenly assure their patients that they don't need to have their homocysteine levels checked, or if they had been taking folic acid (vitamin B-9) and vitamin B-12 to lower their homocysteine, they should stop taking them. Almost every week I see these patients, whose primary care physicians or cardiologists have given them this poor and, in my view, harmful advice.

Here are some reasons why these studies were flawed, and, actually documented the harmful role of high homocysteine in cardiovascular disease…

1. None of these studies was designed to see if lowering blood homocysteine reduces the risk of a future cardiovascular event. They were designed to see the effects of folic acid (vitamin B-9) and vitamin B-12 on randomly selected individuals with previous cardiovascular regardless of their homocysteine level. Since many of these individuals may have had other cardiovascular risk factors, giving a small number of them with mildly elevated blood pressure an antihypertension drug is not going to show a dramatic change in outcomes.

2. The homocysteine levels in those who had their blood levels tested only mildly elevated, and were lowered only slightly. Some still had elevated levels at the end of the studies. As is the case with lipoprotein(a), there is frequently a threshold below which the harm is not that significant. Here, too, very mild elevation of homocysteine may not necessarily increase the risk of a cardiovascular event when other major risk factors are also involved. However, it does not follow that high levels of homocysteine are harmless, especially when they are greater than 15–20 micromol per liter.

3. In fact, in one of the studies (HOPE-2 Trial), folic acid-treated cases had a 28% lower risk of nonfatal strokes and a 24% lower risk of all strokes than the group who were given placebo. Even more compelling, in the placebo group, those who had moderately to severely high homocysteine levels (the kind of patients I see) had an 85% higher risk of cardiovascular events compared to those with normal homocysteine levels! A recent study of patients with chronic kidney failure, who often have high homocysteine levels, also showed that homocysteine-lowering with folic acid reduced the risk of stroke by more than 50%.

4. Nearly all those who were treated with folic acid or received placebo had preexisting cardiovascular diseases or multiple major coronary risk factors requiring treatments. Since co-therapy of multiple risk factors has synergistic effect, the true benefit of each individual intervention is diluted. Thus, on a background of multiple co-existing major coronary risk factors, the individual contribution a slightly elevated LDL-cholesterol, blood pressure or homocysteine may not be readily apparent. However, it does not follow that very high LDL-cholesterol, blood pressure or homocysteine are innocent bystanders and should be ignored.

5. Our knowledge about the harmful impact of smoking, not wearing seat belts, or lead in drinking water has never been tested in double blind, prospective controlled studies. Yet, we accept the vast number of well conducted observational, clinical and laboratory studies, which have consistently shown harm. The conclusions of a few flawed studies of giving folic acid and vitamin B-12 to everyone with cardiovascular disease whether they have high levels of homocysteine or not, do *not* negate the vast amount of compelling data

accumulated over the past two decades showing that a high blood homocysteine level is a major cardiovascular risk factor, and particularly increases the risk of stroke, peripheral vascular disease and dementia. Many healthcare providers still do not treat, or grossly undertreat millions of people with hypertension, elevated LDL-cholesterol, or low levels of HDL-cholesterol, metabolic syndrome and abdominal obesity. This pervasive neglect is not based on lack of evidence, but lack of knowledge. Homocysteine is another neglected major coronary risk factor.

In a recent study, among young women between 15 and 44 who had developed strokes, homocysteine levels above 11 micromol per liter were associated with a 300% higher risk of stroke. Taking into account other risk factors, such as blood cholesterol level, blood pressure and smoking, did not change this strong association. In the Women's Health Study of over 28,000 postmenopausal women, an elevated homocysteine level more than doubled the risk of cardiovascular events. The impact of an elevated homocysteine level is even more severe when people have high blood pressure or are smokers.

FAST FACTS: HOMOCYSTEINE

- Women are twice as likely as men to develop cardiovascular problems because of elevated homocysteine.

- In both sexes, there is strong evidence that risks steadily rise in line with homocysteine blood levels.

- Normal homocysteine level should not exceed 9 micromol per liter.

- Elevated homocysteine levels raise the risk of heart attack, stroke, phlebitis, dementia and osteoporosis.

WHO SHOULD BE SCREENED FOR HOMOCYSTEINE?

Anyone with the following conditions
One or more major coronary risk factors

- Any cardiovascular disease

- A family history of premature cardiovascular disease

- Phlebitis (blood clots) in the legs, lungs or elsewhere

- Chronic kidney dysfunction

- A family history of dementia

If you fall into any of the above categories, ask your healthcare provider to test your blood homocysteine level. If your values are greater than 9-10 micromol/liter, you should be treated. Do not settle for "watching it."

Treatment of high homocysteine requires a combination of folic acid (1-4 mg) along with vitamin B-12 (1 mg) on a daily basis. More than 70% of people would have a good response to this combination. However, 20%–30% of people may be

HOMOCYSTEINE LEVELS AND ALZHEIMER'S DISEASE

Recent studies have shown that elevated blood homocysteine levels significantly increase the risk of Alzheimer's disease.

Investigators at the University of Oxford looked at 164 patients aged 55 or older with a diagnosis of Alzheimer's disease. They were found to have significantly higher blood homocysteine along with lower folic acid and vitamin B-12 levels than the control population (without Alzheimer's disease).

With simple, practical, and very inexpensive measures (such as daily supplementation with folic acid, B-12 and B-6), many people may potentially prevent this catastrophic disease or slow down its rapid deterioration.

folic acid-resistant. This is because commercial folic acid (not the natural folic acid in fat and vegetables) is not an active substance; it has to go through four steps in the liver to become "activated." Most of those who do not respond to folic acid have certain genetic mutations in the enzymes responsible for converting folic acid to its active form. At present, activated folic acid and vitamin B-12 is available by prescription. *Example:* each tablet contains 2.5 mg folic acid, 2 mg vitamin B-12 and 25 mg vitamin B-6. Folic acid-resistant individuals should be placed on activated folic acid.

What you should do

Although folic acid and vitamin B-12 supplements are usually required to treat elevated homocysteine, some deeply colored fruits and vegetables —spinach, asparagus, oranges, broccoli and bananas—as well as most fortified cereals, are good sources of folic acid and B-12. However, the amount of folic acid and vitamin B-12 in foods is always inadequate to significantly impact homocysteine levels.

Risk Factor #16
Negative Affect

Negative affect or emotions, including what I call "the HAD syndrome" (Hostility, Anger and Depression), are present in at least 10% of US adults. Several studies have shown depression rates in people hospitalized for coronary artery disease to be more than 20%. A recent report from the US Department of Health and Human Services summarized 17 studies showing that depression following a coronary event increased cardiac deaths by threefold. More recent studies have shown that persons with various chronic diseases such as cardiovascular disease, cancers, chronic lung disease, etc., have HAD rates ranging from 30% to more than 50%.

Depression is very common after coronary artery bypass surgery; one in two individuals has clinical depression. The majority of these cases are either unrecognized or inadequately treated (Whooley, MA et al., *JAMA* 2006; 295:2874-81). In an international study of 25,000 men and women, who had had a previous heart attack, depression or HAD was just as strong or even a stronger risk factor for a subsequent heart attack as other major coronary risk factors (Yuduf, S et al, *Lancet* 2004; 364; 937-52).

Some studies show that negative emotions produce distinct physiologic reactions, such as changes in blood pressure, heart rate or constriction of coronary arteries and increased clotting ability of the blood. Certain hormones or other substances may also be released that influence other risk factors.

For example, a certain breed of mice susceptible to hardening of the arteries responds quite differently to a high fat, high-cholesterol diet when the mice are subjected to various stresses. Coronary plaques similar to those in humans were found far more often in mice housed five to a cage than in mice housed in their own cages. Further, people prone to negative emotions are more likely to practice unhealthy habits, such as smoking, drinking, poor eating, a sedentary lifestyle, and frequently neglect their other health issues including coronary risk factors.

Negative affect has two components...

1. Acute, short-term symptoms such as frequent episodes of sadness, depression or anger even over trivial matters.

2. Chronic, long-term symptoms, which may range from a pessimistic outlook, cynicism and defensiveness to outright hostility and rage (traffic, family, work), a "bad attitude" and persistent depression.

Hostility, anger and depression have the most potent impact on coronary artery disease. Contrary to popular belief, type-A personality itself does not raise risk of coronary artery disease. In a large, nine-year follow-up study from Finland, people with high hostility scores were three times more likely to die from cardiovascular diseases than those with low scores. Depression and hostility affect heart rhythms, increase blood pressure, alter blood clotting, elevate insulin and lower HDL-cholesterol levels. They may also result in chronically high levels of stress hormones such as cortisol and adrenaline. The "stress factors" released in the bloodstream also lower HDL-cholesterol, increase blood triglycerides and homocysteine levels, and cause spasm of coronary and cerebral arteries.

The recent Baltimore Epidemiological Catchment Area Study showed that persons with at least one episode of major depression were approximately two to eight times more likely to have a heart attack than those without such a history. Among those 18 to 44 years of age, who had no history of depression, only one percent developed heart attack during the 13-year follow-up compared to eight percent of those with a history of at least one major depression. In the 45 to 64 age group, the heart attack rates were eight percent and 17% respectively.

In a 40-year follow-up of male medical students who graduated from Johns Hopkins University, the risk of heart attack among those who had experienced an episode of clinical depression was more than twice those without a history of depression. Adjusting for other risk factors, such as age, smoking, hypertension, blood cholesterol levels, obesity, level of physical activities and family history of heart attacks, did not change these findings.

Two recent studies also showed that negative affect increases the risk of stroke by as much as 60%. Even the risk of cardiac arrest (after a heart attack) was 30% higher in mildly depressed persons than in those without a previous history of depression. Among those with more severe chronic depression, the rate of cardiac arrests was even greater at 77%.

Unfortunately, negative affect is quite prevalent in people who have already developed coronary artery disease, affecting nearly half of this group. In a Belgian study, researchers tracked more than 300 men and women between the ages of 31 and 79 who had coronary artery disease. They found that subjects with depression had a death rate that was more than four times greater than the death rate for those who did not have depression.

What you should do

Negative emotions, such as depression, hostility and anger, are treatable disorders—but the first step is to overcome a common hurdle and acknowledge that there is a problem. Once you are willing to seek help, a sympathetic physician, psychiatrist or other healthcare provider can make a lifesaving difference.

Although combination therapy of counseling and antidepressant medication is usually advised for those with depression, a recent randomized Canadian study showed that certain antidepressants, such as citalopram (Celexa) or sertraline (Zoloft), plus clinical management (regular office follow-up visits) were highly effective in persons with coronary artery disease and depression. However, the researchers found no benefit for interpersonal psychotherapy (Lesprance, F et al., *JAMA* 2007; 247: 367–79). Still, many people with "HAD Syndrome" will require cognitive therapy, life coaching or other interpersonal psychotherapy because usually they have a well-entrenched emotional and affective disorder that cannot be treated by pills alone.

Don't rely on over-the-counter products. Despite their exaggerated claims of efficacy, herbs such as St. John's wort and kava-kava have no significant impact on negative affect, especially among people who have already suffered a cardiovascular event. These people need genuine, effective care, and questionable herbal therapy is not the solution.

Eat more seafood. Studies show that omega-3 fat concentration in red blood cells is significantly lower in people with depression than in nondepressed patients. This suggests that depressed people likely eat less seafood than others do.

The human brain contains the highest concentration of omega-3 fat than any other organ. Thus, a low omega-3 fat concentration of red blood cells is a strong surrogate for lower concentration of these fats in the brain. Numerous studies from the US, Scandinavia and Japan have shown that frequent seafood consumption significantly reduces the depression scores. For people who do not eat dark-fleshed seafood (salmon, tuna, mackerel), two to four seafood omega-3 capsules such as Solgar's Omega-3 700 are reasonable substitutes.

Numerous studies show regular, frequent exercise, four to five times a week for 30-40 minutes each, can reduce the depression and anxiety score by more than 50%. Other means of improving coping skills, such as yoga, meditation, learning to play a musical instrument or joining social clubs, may also be helpful.

Risk Factor #17
Too Many Red Blood Cells

People often assume that having rosy cheeks is a sign of good health. Unfortunately, a reddish face can be a sign of excess red blood cells in the bloodstream. Other factors that may make the face and cheeks appear overly rosy include excessive alcohol intake, obesity, chronic lung disease, hemochromatosis (a disorder in which iron accumulates in the blood, liver, brain, pancreas and skin) and too much sun exposure.

Normally, there are approximately 4.5 to 5.5 million red blood cells per cubic milliliter of blood. For most people, the volume of red blood cells that settles at the bottom of a test tube (called "hematocrit") is between 42% and 45% of the whole blood volume (the remainder is the serum or plasma). In people with too many red cells, or "too much" blood, the hematocrit can comprise up to 50% to 52% of the blood.

In people with hematocrit greater than 47%, the blood flow in the arteries slows down, and vital organs may not receive adequate amounts of oxygen. Poor oxygen delivery is especially troublesome during times when our bodies require more oxygen, such as during vigorous exercise or at times of emotional or mental stress.

Healthy coronary or cerebral arteries are resilient enough to adapt partially and accommodate overcrowding by red cells. However,

> If you feel prolonged sadness, frustration, impatience, defensiveness, aggressiveness, explosive anger or depression, or feel as if you have hit bottom, please talk to your doctor.
>
> People with negative affect nearly always have biochemical abnormalities in the brain. Many safe and effective drugs are available that can dramatically improve these chemical imbalances and bring equilibrium to the brain's neurotransmitters. Negative affect is essentially a neurotransmitter-deficiency disease, much as diabetes is an insulin-deficiency disease. Ignoring it or not taking a lifesaving drug to help control your disease will not make your problem disappear.

arteries affected by atherosclerosis (hardening of the arteries) become stiff and lose their ability to dilate and accommodate this overcrowding. The volume of red blood cells accounts for approximately 70% of the blood viscosity or "thickness." Any increase in hematocrit can significantly increase blood viscosity, making blood flow through smaller arteries more difficult.

A simple, inexpensive blood test that is frequently done on most patients, called CBC (Complete Blood Count), measures hematocrit and hemoglobin. However, CBC is done primarily to see if someone is anemic (has too few red blood cells) or low hemoglobin and hematocrit. To my amazement, I see patients with hematocrits of 49%–52% who have never been told that their CBC is abnormal. Do we do this with high blood sugar, cholesterol, calcium or potassium? No, we don't. So why ignore the higher hematocrit? The answer is inattention and/or lack of knowledge.

In addition to rosy cheeks, other possible signs of too many red cells include bouts of dizziness, confusion or forgetfulness; sudden changes in vision; impotence; shortness of breath or high blood pressure. High hematocrit also increases risk of having mini-strokes, which can eventually result in dementia. This is because the viscous and thickened blood cannot flow easily through small brain arteries, clamp together and choke off blood flow to brain cells. When this process continues, more and more brains cells are lost, eventually contributing to cognitive decline and dementia.

Several studies have shown that the risk of coronary events increases progressively as the hematocrit is raised from 42% to 48% and beyond.

When the hematocrit exceeds 51%, the risk of cardiovascular mortality increases nearly nine times compared to those with a hematocrit below 44%.

In a large study of 39,922 patients with unstable angina (frequent chest pain due to coronary artery disease), the risk of adverse events (heart attack, need for stent or bypass surgery, hospitalization) within a 30-day period was 50% greater in those with high hematocrit (Sabatino, MS et al., *Circulation* 2005; III: 2042-49). In the same study, being severely anemic (a hemoglobin less than 8 g/dl or hematocrit less than 24%) increased the risk of an adverse cardiovascular event by threefold. Being moderately anemic (a hemoglobin 8–10 g/dl or hematocrit of 24%–28%) increased the risk by twofold. In other words, like every other biological marker, too much or too little are problematic.

For more than a decade, we have known that the 10-year risk of cardiovascular death can triple with high hematocrit levels or elevated hemoglobin—levels over 17 g/dl as determined in another blood test that measures total red blood cell pigment. (Normal hematocrit values are 40%–44% and for hemoglobin 12–14 g/dl.)

What you should do

Whenever you have a CBC (Complete Blood Count) done, ask your healthcare provider what your hematocrit and hemoglobin levels are. You can also request to have a copy of your blood tests so you can look at them yourself. If your hematocrit and hemoglobin levels are high, then your doctor should evaluate you for all possible causes of elevated hematocrit.

Obesity, smoking and excessive drinking can all contribute to elevated hematocrit. If you take a multivitamin supplement, choose one that doesn't include iron if you are male or a post-menopausal woman. High iron intake can raise hematocrit levels.

Donate blood. One of the most effective and the quickest way of reducing your hematocrit is to donate a unit of blood. This act of goodwill may not only save your life, but also the life of someone else! Once your hematocrit reaches 42%–44% range, you should consider donating blood every three to four months to prevent your hematocrit from creeping up again.

Some blood banks are reluctant to accept donations from people with severely high hematocrit; in these cases, they may simply do a "blood letting" in which the removed blood is discarded. This procedure is generally covered by medical insurance.

Risk Factor #18
Abnormal Blood Platelets or High Fibrinogen Levels

An acute heart attack results from a blockage in vessels supplying blood to the heart. This occurs when a plaque in the arterial wall suddenly breaks apart or ruptures and forms an open wound. Blood platelets and a potent clotting protein called fibrinogen rush to the wound and form a very tiny clot—called a "thrombus"—at the injury site. Within moments, the tiny clot snowballs into a larger and larger thrombus that sometimes, within an hour or two, can clog up the lumen of the artery and obstruct blood flow to the heart. Without this vascular injury and the subsequent clumping of platelets and its interaction with fibrinogen, a heart attack would not occur.

To initiate and sustain clumping, platelets produce a substance called "adhesion protein," which helps platelets stick together and to the inner lining of the artery. This adhesion protein becomes active when it meets certain compounds in the plaque, such as oxidized LDL-cholesterol. The activated adhesion protein makes platelets especially "sticky." The more sticky platelets are, the more likely they are to clump together and bind with fibrinogen and the greater is the risk of arterial blockage.

Recently two inherited variations of platelet adhesion protein have been identified that make platelets much more likely to clump and stick to the arterial wall. Persons with these abnormalities—called "platelet polymorphism" —have a high risk of developing premature heart disease. A minor difference or mutation in the DNA of these platelets causes a sixfold increase in the risk of coronary events among people under 60 years of age.

What you should do

Platelet count and blood fibrinogen level. If you have a risk of coronary artery disease, have a complete blood count (CBC) along with other blood tests that measure your cholesterol, sugar, etc. A platelet count is a component of CBC, as are hematocrit and hemoglobin. The fibrinogen blood level should also be tested periodically to assure you do not have a high level. Normal fibrinogen levels range about 200 to 300 mg/dl. A

> Vein clots, referred to as phlebitis, have relatively few platelets but plenty of fibrinogen and trapped red blood cells. The tendency to develop phlebitis is often increased significantly when the blood flow through the veins, especially in the legs, is slowed down. This can occur in varicose veins or during long periods of inactivity such as long flights, recovery from a broken leg or hip, hospitalization, major surgeries and certain illnesses.

A LOW-DOSE ASPIRIN CAN SAVE YOUR LIFE

There's compelling evidence that aspirin therapy—which is safe, effective and costs pennies a day—can save countless lives. Yet...

- Only half of Americans with coronary artery disease currently take aspirin, making it far underutilized. In a recent study, the death rate at six months following a heart attack was twice as high in those not taking aspirin compared to those taking it.

- More than one in three healthcare providers don't take aspirin themselves...and even fewer recommend aspirin therapy to their patients.

- Aspirin use among African-Americans, who have a high risk of fatal heart attacks and stroke, is especially dismal. Only 35% of men and 13% of women who would benefit from aspirin therapy utilize it.

ASPIRIN AND YOUR HEART

Aspirin costs pennies per pill—but is priceless for your cardiovascular health. Not only does aspirin reduce the risk of coronary and cerebral thrombosis (clot formation), but it increases blood circulation and oxygen supply to the heart muscles by improving function of the artery's inner lining.

In fact, aspirin's heart healthy benefits are so compelling that every man over age 40 and every woman over 50 should take a low-dose, 81-milligram aspirin every day, and boost this regimen to a full-dose 325 milligram dose once a week. Of course, for those few people —less than 5%—who are allergic to aspirin, clopidogrel 75 mg is a reasonable, but more expensive, substitute.

Ideally, choose uncoated aspirin. The risk of stomach irritation is low and it is a faster-acting version than the popular enteric-coated aspirins. Uncoated aspirin is absorbed in the intestines within 30 to 40 minutes, compared to the three to four hours it takes coated types to be absorbed. The faster absorption is critical for patients who experience angina; for them, chewing the coated aspirin well before swallowing it improves its absorption rate.

Obese persons should double the dosage —and take 162 milligrams daily; that's two "low-dose" aspirins daily to achieve adequate platelet response.

The downside of aspirin: It may cause one case of minor bleeding per 1,000 cases per year of usage from the stomach, nose or as skin bruising.

---

normal platelet count is about 150,000 to 250,000 platelets per milliliter.

Testing for platelet polymorphism is not routinely available, and is not necessary in everyone unless there is a history of previous blood clots (phlebitis), or a family history of premature cardiovascular disease, including heart rate irregularities such as atrial fibrillation.

Aspirin therapy. The purpose of aspirin therapy to prevent heart attacks is to reduce platelet stickiness. Even in low doses—80–100 milligrams per day—aspirin destroys an enzyme inside platelets called "COX-1" that activates platelets' adhesion protein. Because red blood cells also activate platelets, it is helpful to boost the dose to 324 milligrams one day a week.

In adults with or without a history of coronary artery disease, low-dose aspirin can reduce the risk of a heart attack by about 30%. This is as good as that of most currently available cholesterol-lowering drugs. However, aspirin is not a replacement for statins or other risk factor modifications. It is one among many other interventions.

Seasonality of heart attacks. Heart attacks are nearly 50% more common in winter than

ASPIRIN AND WOMEN

In the past, doctors were reluctant to recommend aspirin therapy for women as often as for men. However, recent studies show that aspirin, as well as other risk factor modifications, are just as effective in women as in men (Nicholls, SJ et al., *J Am Coll Cardiol* 2007; 49: 1546–51).

In one study, researchers from Johns Hopkins University School of Medicine compared platelet response in 571 men and 711 women. The results showed that the impact of low-dose aspirin was essentially the same.

In the Women's Health Study, of nearly 40,000 women over six years, low-dose aspirin reduced the risk of stroke by 24% compared to a placebo.

In another study, older women taking low-dose aspirin each day were one-third less likely to have a heart attack than others—a similar benefit to that of men.

No matter your gender, aspirin is a simple and effective way to reduce your risk. Aspirin also reduces the risk of colon cancer by 30%.

ASPIRIN vs. ANTI-INFLAMMATORY DRUGS

If you're taking nonsteroidal anti-inflammatory drugs (NSAIDS), such as ibuprofen (Advil, Motrin) or naproxen (Aleve), make sure to take aspirin at least two to three hours beforehand—ideally, in the morning with breakfast. That's because NSAIDS compete with aspirin for the same "docking" sites inside platelets. When taken together, NSAIDS prevent aspirin from entering platelets to block COX-1, and essentially defeat or negate the aspirin's cardioprotective benefit.

Those who have high platelet counts need a thorough evaluation by a hematologist (blood specialist) and may require specific, targeted treatment. The liver produces fibrinogen, but its production is reduced by frequent consumption of dark-fleshed seafoods, which contain several times more omega-3 fat than whitefish or shellfish. Olive oil and hazelnut oil are excellent choices, but for not cooking or searing at high temperatures.

in summer. These variations are seen despite geographic and climatic differences, so escaping to the Sunbelt for the winter does not alter the pattern. In fact, studies from Australia, whose seasons are the reverse of ours, have also shown that fatal or nonfatal heart attacks are 20%–40% more common in its winter and spring than during other times of the year.

These seasonal variations are partly due to the shorter duration of light per day, lower levels of physical activity, negative affect, higher incidence of respiratory infections and low consumption of seafoods in winter. However, they are also due to changes in platelets that enhance their clumping and stickiness. Here, too, both aspirin and omega-3 polyunsaturates from seafood provide considerable protection.

Seafood omega-3 fats. Another effective way to improve the function of your platelets, make them coronary-friendly and lower your fibrinogen is to increase your intake of omega-3 fatty acids from seafood. This requires an average of three to four seafood meals per week over a long period of time. You should not cook seafood with vegetable-sourced fats.

Manage stress. In addition to other good reasons to manage stress for better cardiovascular and overall health, British researchers have shown that during periods of stress, higher levels of platelets are suddenly released into the bloodstream. This is another reason why heart attacks can occur during stressful periods.

Risk Factor #19
Obstructive Sleep Apnea or Chronic Lung Disease

The ability to breathe easily, no doubt, affects heart health. In obstructive sleep apnea, breathing is briefly and repeatedly interrupted during sleep. (The word "apnea" literally means "without breath.") This occurs when the upper airways prevent airflow into the lungs despite efforts to breathe. It's a chronic disease that affects about 2% of middle-aged women and 4% of all middle-aged adults. Recent studies suggest that the true rates of sleep apnea may be many times higher in most people, and as high as 30%–40% in obese persons. Obstruction of the upper airways by structural abnormalities in the nose, soft palate, tongue or throat is often compounded by fatty deposits around the throat and larynx in obese persons.

Obstructive apnea creates two problems: fragmented sleep and lowered levels of oxygen in the blood; each can contribute to poor oxygenation of heart muscle, brain and other organs. It also causes chronic fatigue, memory and mood disorders, and because of daytime drowsiness, a greater risk of accidents. More than 18 million American adults have sleep apnea; the majority also have multiple coronary risk factors, including abdominal obesity, high blood pressure, insulin resistance or diabetes, high cholesterol levels and may be smokers or heavy drinkers—all factors that increase the risk of heart attack, stroke and heart failure.

Certainly, repeated episodes of poor oxygenation of the heart and brain—called "hypoxia"—contribute to the high risk of heart attack and stroke. Ultimately, the co-existence of other risk factors significantly increases the risk of various cardiovascular events. In one four-year study of 697 people, researchers determined that sleep apnea doubled the risk of stroke, independent of other factors; but severe apnea more than tripled death from stroke or other causes.

In a Swedish study of middle-aged men and women, over a seven-year follow-up, 16.2% of those with sleep apnea developed coronary artery disease compared to 5.4% of those without sleep apnea (threefold higher risk). However, effective sleep apnea treatment reduced the risk by almost two-thirds (Peker, Y et al., Eur Respir J 2006; 28: 596–602). What this important study demonstrated was that early and effective treatment of sleep apnea is essential to reduce catastrophic cardiovascular events.

Sleep accounts for a third of our lives and plays a crucial role in enabling us to be awake and perform tasks during our wakeful hours. Sleep also plays a significant role in our emotional and physical state. In addition to being a serious and life-threatening disease, sleep deprivation, an immediate consequence of obstructive sleep apnea, also wreaks havoc with quality of life and dramatically increases daytime sleepiness, poor performance and concentration, and risk of various accidents. Fortunately, the available treatment options can significantly improve the sleep quality and long-term cardiovascular risk. Early diagnosis and treatment is the crucial determinant of prognosis.

What about chronic lung disease?

Chronic lung disease is not just the consequence of tobacco abuse. Poorly treated asthma or bronchitis caused by repeated bacterial infections that include Chlamydia pneumoniae, miners' lung disease, silicosis and sarcoidosis also impede oxygenation of the heart, brain and kidneys.

Chronic lung disease also hinders any meaningful physical activity. In addition, people with chronic lung disease have an oxidant overload that negatively affects the cardiovascular system. Thus, they have a high risk for cardiovascular events particularly stroke and heart failure.

In a recent study, nearly 78,000 patients undergoing cardiac testing were followed up for about three years. Among patients with no known history of coronary artery disease, those with shortness of breath had four times the risk of sudden death from cardiac causes than those who did not have shortness of breath. Even after adjustments for any cardiac abnormalities, there was still a tripling of cardiac events among subjects with shortness of breath. Being short of breath, due to chronic lung disease, poor cardio-responding fitness, anemia, or any other cause, is a major risk factor for cardiovascular events.

What you should do

Aggressive treatment. Obstructive sleep apnea is not just a simple sleep disorder; it's a serious and life-threatening disease that needs multi-specialist help. Because of several co-existing risk factors, see a nose and throat specialist, a pulmonologist (lung specialist), an internist and a sleep disorder specialist (neurologist). However, your primary care physician or internist should manage this multi-specialist interaction.

Obstructive sleep apnea is often treated with a continuous positive airway pressure device (CPAP). This mask fits over the nose and/or mouth, and gently blows air into the airway to help keep it open during sleep. This method of treatment is highly effective, but some consider the mask uncomfortable. A second line of treatment includes oral appliances, which reposition the lower jaw, tongue and upper airway, surgery to remove excessive tissue from soft palate, or correcting deviated nasal septum. In general, these approaches are most helpful for mild disease or heavy snoring.

Since a significant number of people with sleep apnea are obese, weight loss is a major factor in reducing the severity of sleep apnea. Avoid alcohol, which makes the upper airway breathing muscles relax; and sleep on your side with two firm pillows, rather than your back or abdomen.

Stop smoking. Tobacco use worsens sleep apnea and, obviously, chronic lung disease. Regular exercise, meanwhile, helps boost lung capacity and function.

Risk Factor #20
Low Birth Weight

A low weight at birth (less than five pounds) and during early infancy is associated with higher risk of certain diseases in adulthood, including heart disease, stroke, high blood pressure, obesity, diabetes and kidney disease.

There are several possible explanations. Malnutrition or under-nutrition during pregnancy or in a child's first year of life can…

- Contribute to lower production of a compound called elastin which plays an important role in the pulsation and dilation of arteries. A deficiency in elastin makes arteries stiffer and less likely to dilate properly when needed. Arterial stiffness is a major contributor to hypertension, kidney dysfunction, stroke and heart attack.

- Cause mutations in many genes. These may remain dormant for years and contribute to cardiovascular diseases.

- Affect insulin-producing glands in the pancreas. Some studies suggest that these glands do not fully mature in adults who were underweight when they were born, or as infants. This may explain why type 2 diabetes is more common in adults whose birth weight was less than five pounds.

In one recent study from Scotland, more than 12,000 children born between 1950 and 1956 were tracked during adulthood. Researchers discovered that the risk of coronary artery disease after age 40 was twice as high in people whose birthweight was less than five pounds compared to those born weighing more than eight pounds. Furthermore, the risk of stroke was even steeper —it was three times higher for those who had low birth weight than for those with higher birth weight.

Low birth weight is often related to health and other factors affecting pregnant women. Some of these factors include poverty, poor education, lack of family or social links, smoking, drinking, drug abuse and inconsistent prenatal care. These factors can affect the nutritional status and health of the mother and the fetus she carries.

The association of low birth weight and coronary artery disease is independent of other cardiovascular risk factors. Many studies have shown that malnutrition in the fetal stage and infancy can result in the later development of several chronic diseases. Other risk factors in adult life expedite and worsen the impact of low birth weight on coronary artery disease.

What you should do

Take extra precautions. If you were underweight at birth, chronic diseases are not inevitable. Nor

---

LOW BIRTH WEIGHT AND DIABETES

In the US Nurses Study, which included more than 69,000 women, birth weight of less than five pounds was associated with an 83% higher risk of diabetes.

WHAT WE SHOULD DO

Sadly, famine and malnutrition in many areas of the world will have a devastating impact on the future health of many populations. For the public health around the world, I believe that we should support efforts to prevent fetal and childhood malnutrition in order to reduce the risk of diseases in future generations, especially in poor or underdeveloped countries where very few can afford the cost of caring for their sick.

---

are they inherited. They occur on an individual basis and are not necessarily passed on to subsequent generations or even to your siblings. They are random events that occurred during your fetal life.

If you did have a low birth weight, you should be tested for coronary risk factors periodically and treated vigorously to preempt or modify the impact of each risk factor.

Even if you don't have any major risk factors yet, adopt a healthy lifestyle (including a diet based on the Twenty Risk Factor system, exercise, weight control, no smoking, etc.) to minimize the health impact of your low birth weight.

Many healthcare providers are unaware that low birth weight is a major risk factor for coronary artery disease, heart attack, stroke, hypertension, diabetes and kidney or thyroid diseases. All of these are serious diseases with serious complications. Readers who had low birth weight or were underweight as infants should bring this to the attention of their physicians and request screening for these diseases from time to time. 🍏

3

DEBUNKING DIETARY MYTHS

Should You Really Fear Dietary Cholesterol?

Cholesterol is a pearly fat that is present in animal flesh and animal products such as dairy products and eggs. Contrary to a common misconception, dietary cholesterol accounts for only 10% to 30% of blood cholesterol. The other 70% to 90% is made from the breakdown by-products of carbohydrates and proteins, mostly in the liver.

Humans and animals function like efficient factories. They take in various nutrients, including carbohydrates, proteins and fat, break them into smaller compounds, and reassemble them as fat, cholesterol, hormones or other biological compounds.

Although most cells in the body need cholesterol for survival, dietary cholesterol is not essential. This explains why strict vegans can have perfectly normal functioning bodies, and may have normal or even high blood cholesterol levels, without intake of any cholesterol from outside sources.

For the past 30 years, many nutrition gurus and zealots have targeted dietary cholesterol for extinction, but their reasons are usually due to emotion and misinformation rather than scientific merit. For the past 20 years, I have persistently argued that cutting back dietary cholesterol to less than 200 mg per day is neither practical nor relevant to cardiovascular health. Although 100 million Americans have elevated blood cholesterol levels, dietary cholesterol is not the main culprit in the majority of cases. The other nearly 200 million Americans who have "desirable" cholesterol levels are not all strict vegetarians. Many vegans have elevated blood cholesterol and suffer heart attacks, at only marginally lower rates than nonvegetarians.

> Cattle eat no cholesterol, get very little saturated fat from hay or feed, and have a diet that is rich in complex carbohydrates. Yet, cattle grow to huge sizes and have plenty of saturated fat and cholesterol in their fat, meat and milk. Chickens also have a rigid vegetarian diet, their eggs are not fat-free or cholesterol-free.

> From the nutritional standpoint, dietary cholesterol is unnecessary. It entered our diet about 2½ million years ago when *Homo erectus,* our distant ancestor, began eating meat. But dietary cholesterol is not necessarily harmful or bad.

Many studies over the past two decades have shown that long-term, low-cholesterol diets are unlikely to have a significant impact on lowering blood cholesterol levels or the risk of heart disease. For every 100 mg reduction in dietary cholesterol intake, there is an average decrease of only 2–4 mg in blood cholesterol. So for most people, lowering their dietary cholesterol from 400 mg per day to 200 mg only lowers their blood cholesterol by 4–8 mg. This result is too trivial to justify the fuss surrounding dietary cholesterol.

Researchers at Stanford University conducted a randomized study of four diets popular with overweight women: Atkins (very low-carb and very high-fat), the Zone (low-carb), LEARN (similar to the current American Heart Association recommendations) and Ornish (strict, very high-carb, very low-fat and nearly cholesterol-free). After one year, the Atkins dieters had lost about 10 pounds compared with six pounds for the Ornish dieters, five pounds for those following the LEARN program, and four pounds for those following the Zone. However, the Ornish dieters, who were on a strict vegetarian diet with very little fat and practically no cholesterol for one year, lowered their bad LDL-cholesterol by only 4 mg/dl! The decline in LDL-cholesterol among other dieters was negligible.

Our bodies have two ways to control the buildup of dietary cholesterol. First, the intestine absorbs only 30% to 50% of dietary cholesterol. A large dietary load of cholesterol can overwhelm the absorptive capacity of the intestine and lower the absorption of dietary cholesterol even more. This explains partly why the blood cholesterol level of one 88 year-old man was perfectly normal, even though for nearly 20 years he consumed about 25 eggs per day, about 6000 mg of dietary cholesterol daily!

Second, every liver cell has special receptors that facilitate the entry of LDL-cholesterol so that it can be converted to other necessary compounds.

In many people dietary cholesterol does not raise blood cholesterol levels. These individuals are referred to as "cholesterol nonresponders." Their defensive systems—the liver and the intestines—work effectively to cope with dietary cholesterol load. For example, the man who ate 25 eggs every day for nearly 20 years not only reduced his cholesterol absorption to less than 10% but also trapped and disposed of more LDL particles by doubling or tripling the number of LDL receptors in his liver cells.

"Cholesterol responders," on the other hand, have impaired defense systems, resulting in an elevated blood cholesterol level. Often the problem is not the number of LDL receptors but the inability of these receptors to function properly. Since LDL receptors are primarily made up of proteins, even a minor genetic alteration can render them useless, or far less effective. Nearly 400 different defects in LDL-receptors have been identified, each affecting the ability of these receptors to various degrees. Individuals with these mutations of their LDL-receptors are almost always cholesterol-responders (their blood cholesterol goes up with dietary cholesterol and saturated fat intake).

A high number of LDL receptors (six to eight receptor sites per cell) will trap and remove more LDL particles from the blood circulation, thereby lowering blood cholesterol levels. When the liver cells do not or cannot produce LDL receptors, the "homeless" LDL particles stay in the blood circulation and keep the blood cholesterol level high.

It is estimated that nearly 70% of the US population are cholesterol nonresponders; their blood cholesterol levels do not rise significantly in response to high cholesterol intake. The other 30% are cholesterol responders. Blood cholesterol level will not rise significantly after eating two eggs or a shrimp dinner even in cholesterol responders. The kind of fat accompanying dietary cholesterol has a significant impact on how the body responds to a given cholesterol load. The absorption of cholesterol may be hindered by other dietary components, including fruits, vegetables and legumes containing plant sterols (cholesterol look-alikes). Certain shellfish also contain cholesterol look-alikes that, like their plant counterparts, decrease the absorption of shellfish's cholesterol from the intestine.

A recent study examined the risk of coronary artery disease in middle-aged men of Japanese ancestry living in Japan, Honolulu and San Francisco. Their dietary cholesterol was essentially similar. The Japanese men had dietary cholesterol intake of 464 mg per day, compared with 545 mg per day for Japanese Hawaiians, and 533 mg per day for men of Japanese ancestry living in San Francisco.

Death from coronary artery disease was two times higher among Japanese living in Hawaii and nearly three times higher among those living in San Francisco than among those residing in Japan. The key dietary difference among the three groups was their intake of saturated fat and trans fats. The intake of dietary saturated fat was significantly different at 7%, 13%, and 16% of total fat intake for the Japan, Honolulu, and San Francisco groups, respectively. The Japanese-Americans in San Francisco consumed much more trans fat from deep-fried foods and snacks prepared with margarine or shortening. The San Franciscans were more like to be sedentary than their counterparts living in Japan.

Eating any nutrient excessively is unhealthy and may be harmful. The constant publicity and concern about dietary cholesterol has created much confusion among the public. Saturated and trans fats are a bigger problem than cholesterol. People avoid eggs when in fact eggs are nearly the perfect food, especially for children and older persons. Often people avoid eating shellfish, when any shellfish (except squid which has

a high concentration of cholesterol) is preferable to chicken, turkey or any other meat. The food oil industry has further added to the anti-cholesterol campaign by perpetuating the myth that margarines and shortenings are healthy alternatives to butter—which they most certainly are not!

No scientifically valid evidence suggests that moderate dietary cholesterol intake of 300 mg to 400 mg per day—particularly when the food is prepared with olive oil, hazelnut oil, canola oil or other nonhydrogenated vegetable oils—contributes to cardiovascular diseases. In fact, if you have a low level of HDL-cholesterol, severe dietary cholesterol restrictions may contribute to further lowering of HDL levels, increasing your risk. A single meal, or a day, or even a week of dietary "indiscretion" in which cholesterol exceeds a certain arbitrary limit would not cause irreparable harm to coronary arteries or provoke a heart attack. Instead of drastically cutting back dietary cholesterol, the smart way to go is to reduce saturated fats and trans fatty acid, replacing them with monosaturated fats, such as olive oil.

Most important, following the Twenty Risk Factor Diet (TRF), described in Chapter 4, obviates the need for any concern over cholesterol or fat content of foods, because these variables have already been calculated into the TRF scores.

Saturated Fat (SFA): Not Always Evil

For decades, dietary saturated fats and cholesterol have been cited as major factors in our epidemic of coronary artery disease. In fact their role in causing any cardiovascular disease is limited. It is true that in response to frequent consumption of saturated fats, approximately one-third of the population may show a seven percent to 10% rise in blood cholesterol levels, the "saturated fat responders." On the other hand, in two-thirds of the population blood cholesterol levels either do not change or increase very little with saturated fat consumption. They are called "saturated fat nonresponders." However, aside from their cholesterol-raising effect, some saturated fats may cause other mischief.

How do saturated fats raise blood cholesterol levels?

The free cholesterol within liver cells dictates whether liver cells produce new LDL receptors and how much is produced. Since saturated fat cannot bind onto cholesterol particles, liver cells receive a good amount of free cholesterol and shut down their production of LDL receptors. With fewer LDL receptors around, LDL particles return to the bloodstream and raise the LDL level.

For several hours following a fatty meal with butter, cheese, stick margarines or shortening (which all contain high concentrations of saturated fat or trans fatty acids), blood levels of triglycerides may rise by more than 60%. This may interfere with the normal function of the arteries. Moreover, high triglyceride levels can also decrease the good HDL-cholesterol level by more than 50%.

One undesirable effect of saturated fats is that they increase the tendency of blood platelets to clump together and adhere to the inner lining of the arteries, setting the stage for a heart attack or stroke. Therefore, excessive amounts of saturated fat have four undesirable consequences: they (1) raise blood levels of the "bad" LDL-cholesterol; (2) raise triglyceride levels; (3) lower the "good" HDL-cholesterol; and (4) promote clot formation, which may result in a sudden heart attack or stroke.

Are saturated fats always harmful?

Saturated fats are not always harmful or coronary-unfriendly. In fact, saturated fats play an important role in maintaining the health and integrity of the vascular system and other organs, including the brain and the liver. This virtue of saturated fat may be due to its resistance to oxidization. This property is shared by monounsaturated fats but not polyunsaturates or trans fatty acids.

Not all saturated fats are equally bad. Stearic acid, which accounts for nearly one-half of saturated fat in most lean meats, acts very much like monounsaturates and is not unfriendly to your heart. This helps explain why lean red meats do not raise blood cholesterol levels. That's why they are included in the Twenty Risk Factor Diet.

Although many consumers think that coronary-unfriendly saturated fat comes only from animal sources, a large amount of dietary saturated fat is derived from plant sources. Coconut and palm kernel oils, for example, contain the highest concentrations of saturated fatty acids (92% and 82%, respectively), most of which are coronary-unfriendly.

It's commonly thought that cocoa butter or dark chocolate contains harmful saturated fat. But their predominant fat is a healthy saturated fat known as stearic acid that behaves like a monounsaturated fat.

A recent Japanese study showed that using about two tablespoons of cocoa butter powder (26 grams) daily for 12 weeks, caused HDL-cholesterol levels to increase by 24%. There was also a significant decrease in LDL oxidation, partly due to higher HDL-cholesterol, which is a potent antioxidant, and partly due to polyphenolic antioxidants in cocoa butter.

Another study from Germany also showed that regular consumption of cocoa butter reduces the blood pressure by about 5 mm and also makes platelets less sticky. The reason for the beneficial effect of cocoa or dark chocolate is that it's a rich source of potent antioxidants and polyphenols which improve the functioning of the endothelial cells of the arteries, hence relaxing the arteries to lower blood pressure. The main polyphenols of cocoa and dark chocolates are *procynanidins*.

Does saturated fat have any other benefits? Recent studies suggest that saturated fat may actually protect liver cells against damage caused by alcohol. So, it is possible that certain saturated fats can be used to treat acute alcohol-induced hepatitis in humans. This might also explain why alcohol taken with meals is less likely to cause liver damage. However, no adequate studies at this stage show whether the benefits of saturated fat seen in experiments with animals can be duplicated in humans.

Saturated fat also plays a major role in protecting the integrity of the brain's arteries. That is because saturated fats, lecithin and other fats reduce the fragility of smaller brain arteries, so that they would resist rupture and hemorrhage into the brain, causing stroke. Recent studies have shown that very low-fat diets are associated with a 50% higher risk of stroke.

Monounsaturated Fat: The Heart Protector

A vast body of scientific evidence has consistently confirmed the long-term safety and health benefits of monounsaturated fats.

The beneficial effect on brain function of monounsaturated fat and the omega-3 polyunsaturates found in seafood may be partly due to

A recent study of 5,632 Italians, from 65 to 84 years of age, showed that for those who follow a typical Mediterranean diet, higher intake of monounsaturated fat was associated with a significant protection against age-related cognitive decline. Another study, however, showed that high consumption of vegetable source polyunsaturated fats was associated with cognitive impairment. A diet that had high fish consumption, very much like a high-monounsaturated fat diet, improved elderly cognition.

incorporation of these fatty acids into brain cells, making them healthier and less prone to oxidization or natural cell-death. These fatty acids also reduce the risk of repeated "mini-strokes," which can slowly destroy a substantial part of the brain's cortex, causing dementia that may mimic Alzheimer's disease.

Does this suggest that we should all increase our dietary fat? Does reducing the risk of stroke compensate for a slightly higher risk of heart attack from increased dietary fat? Obviously, it depends on the type of fat. There are five times as many deaths from coronary heart disease than from stroke. On the other hand, increasing monounsaturated fat and omega-3 polyunsaturated fat from seafoods, while decreasing saturated fats (to less than seven percent energy intake) and trans fatty acids (preferably none), lowers the risk of both coronary artery disease and stroke —a win/win situation.

A 14-year follow-up study of more than 80,000 female nurses in the United States showed that replacing five percent of energy from saturated fats with energy from unsaturated fats (monounsaturated fat or nonhydrogenated polyunsaturated fat) would reduce the risk of coronary artery disease by 42%. Replacement of 2% of energy from trans fatty acids (margarine, shortenings and cooking fats) would reduce the risk even more—by 53%.

By signaling the liver cells to produce more LDL-receptors and bringing in a much larger amount of LDL particles, monounsaturates actually reduce the blood LDL levels by approximately 10%. But they also help to raise the HDL-cholesterol by the same percentage.

Both monounsaturated fats and polyunsaturated fats are readily incorporated into LDL particles. LDL particles enriched with monounsaturated fat are remarkably resistant to oxidization, an essential element in the initiation and progression of coronary artery disease. This is the exact opposite of what trans fats do. By reducing the oxidization of LDL-cholesterol, monounsaturated fat provides enormously important protection against cardiovascular diseases. This benefit is even more relevant to diabetics whose LDL particles have a greater tendency to become oxidized.

Long-term use of monounsaturated fat can reduce the risk of a stroke by as much as 50%. The importance of dietary fat in stroke prevention was recently reported in a 20-year study of 832 men from the Framingham Heart Study. These healthy individuals were between 45 and 65 years of age at the beginning of the study. The study showed that men who had the highest total dietary fat, dietary monounsaturated fat, or even dietary saturated fats—but not polyunsaturates or trans fats—had a stroke risk one-half to two-thirds lower than those who followed a very low-fat diet. A similar inverse relationship between dietary fat intake and stroke risk was reported among both Japanese living in Japan and Japanese living in Hawaii. Other experiments with animals support the stroke prevention role of dietary fat.

Why should a high-fat diet cause atherosclerosis in large arteries (the heart's coronary arteries and the carotid arteries in the neck that carry the blood to the brain) while it protects smaller arteries of the brain? In humans, only 10% to 15% of all strokes are caused by large vessel disease or clogging of carotid arteries. The other 85% to 90% are due to small vessel disease within and around the brain tissue. Numerous studies suggest that the brain's small arteries require sufficient amounts of fat to maintain their integrity and pliability so that they do not crack or rupture readily, especially during periods of emotional or physical stress.

Olive oil: The oil for everyone

Olive oil is not a vegetable oil; it is a fruit oil containing 72% to 74% monounsaturated fat. It is also a rich source of many antioxidants and phenolic compounds that enhance its healthfulness. There are different types of oil on the shelf...

- Extra virgin olive oil from the first pressing is always preferable and more healthful and a rich source of cardioprotective and anti-carcinogenic compounds.

- Virgin olive oil (second pressing) does not contain as much flavor, color and antioxidants or other phenolic compounds as the extra virgin oil, but it is still a wonderful and healthy oil.

- Extra light, light or plain olive oil is extracted from what is left after the second pressing. In this third pressing, the manufacturers often use steam pressure or other techniques to remove the oil. This olive oil is mostly stripped of its personality, antioxidants and anticarcinogenic phenolic compounds, but it still contains 72% to 74% monounsaturate and is still superior to all other vegetable oils like corn oil, soybean oil and safflower oil, which have only a small amount of monounsaturated fat.

> *Helpful*: Olive oil at high heat smokes more quickly than vegetable oils like canola or corn oil. For sautéing or searing food at high temperatures, especially indoors, canola oil (which has about 57% monounsaturated fat) can be substituted. Canola oil lacks the antioxidants present in virgin or extra virgin olive oil.
>
> While hazelnut oil has the highest concentration of monounsaturated fat (about 78–82%) and very low levels of saturated fat (about seven percent), it is expensive and impractical for everyday cooking.

OLIVE OIL: WHAT DOES IT DO?

Reduces the LDL-cholesterol

Reduces triglycerides

Raises the HDL-cholesterol

Esterifies dietary cholesterol; helping lower the bad LDL-cholesterol level

Reduces oxidization of LDL-cholesterol and DNA damage in various tissues*

Reduces the risk of cardiovascular disease

Reduces insulin resistance and diabetes

Reduces the risk of breast, colon and prostate cancer

Is less likely to cause obesity than vegetable oils and fats

Has a more than 3000-year clinical history of safety and versatility!

*Native or unoxidized LDL particles are far less harmful than when they are oxidized in the bloodstream or inside the wall of the arteries.

But no matter which olive oil you prefer, from the most exotic to the ordinary, it is a versatile oil for everyone and all occasions.

What olive oil does is distinctly different from other monounsaturated fats, which makes olive oil unique. Its phenolic compounds (present in high concentration in extra virgin olive oil and to a lesser extent in virgin olive oil but with very little or none in the light varieties) provide many benefits. A recent joint European study showed that the LDL-lowering, HDL-raising, triglyceride-lowering and reduction in LDL were proportionately greater with higher phenol compounds in olive oil. The advantage of using light olive oil is that it has no taste or aroma and is very much like other cooking oils. People who object to the taste of olive oil, can use extra light olive oil for a wide range of baking and cooking purposes, including muffins or cookies.

Olive oil, of course, contains fat, and each gram of fat contains approximately 10 calories. This is important for people with weight problems. Fat cells cannot differentiate between calories from corn oil, butter or olive oil. Each gram of fat is still 10 calories to a fat cell, no matter

where it comes from. If those calories are not burned, they will be stored in fat cells, adding to body weight. In obese persons, any dietary program must focus on reducing total energy intake (calories) from all sources—especially fats and carbohydrates. The idea is to replace all other fats (cream, butter, vegetable oils, margarine or shortening) with olive oil. Adding olive oil to a rich, fat-laden Western diet serves absolutely no purpose, and by contributing to obesity, may even be harmful. A teaspoon of olive oil in the salad dressing cannot counteract an unhealthy load of saturated fats and trans fatty acids in a steak and fries dinner, not to mention the fat-laden dessert.

Many foods served at Italian or French restaurants in the United States have extremely high TRF scores. These menus have no resemblance to, and share none of the benefits of, a genuine Mediterranean diet.

The discovery of LDL receptors and how they work to regulate blood cholesterol was so important in understanding the role of blood cholesterol in cardiovascular diseases that two American scientists, Drs. Joseph Goldstein and

Michael Brown, were awarded the Nobel Prize for Physiology and Medicine for their pioneering research in this area.

What is a free cholesterol?

When cholesterol is absorbed from the intestine, a single molecule of fatty acid may attach to it, a process called "esterification." Esterified cholesterol particles are no longer the "free" cholesterol the liver cells are interested in. Thus, the liver cells begin to look for cholesterol elsewhere and produce more LDL receptors to bring in what they need. Dietary saturated fats and trans fatty acids cannot attach to cholesterol particles. Consequently, plenty of free cholesterol reaches the liver cells, quenching their needs, so they stop producing LDL receptors. Blood cholesterol goes up as a result of this LDL receptor deficiency. Monounsaturated fats and polyunsaturated fats readily attach to cholesterol particles, leaving very little free cholesterol to reach liver cells. Thus, liver cells produce more LDL receptors to trap LDL-cholesterol particles from the bloodstream, lowering the blood cholesterol.

The interaction of monounsaturated fat with dietary cholesterol can be used to our advantage. For example, omelettes prepared in olive or canola oil have very little effect on raising blood cholesterol levels. In contrast, omelettes prepared with butter or stick margarine (which may contain up to 30% saturated fat and as much as 10% to 20% trans fatty acids) may raise blood cholesterol level. Similarly, shellfish, such as clams, oysters, or shrimp, prepared in olive oil, do not have a significant impact on blood cholesterol levels. Given the choice, you should always choose olive oil!

Polyunsaturated Fat

We see the term "polyunsaturated fat" on food labels every day. It is helpful to know what these fats are, what they do, and how to interpret all the publicity surrounding vegetable oils, margarine and shortenings.

The molecule of all fatty acids resembles a charm bracelet. The chain or rope of the bracelet is made up of carbon atoms lined side by side to which hydrogen atoms are attached like charms on a bracelet. Fatty acids may have as few as three or as many as 25 carbons in their chains. Those with three to five carbons are called "short-chain"; those with six to 11 "medium"; those with 12 to 20 are "long"; and those with 20 or more carbons in their chain are referred to as "longer-chain" fatty acids.

The most important structural distinction of fatty acids is whether both sides of their carbon atoms are fully occupied by hydrogen atoms. If they are fully occupied or "saturated," they are called saturated fatty acids. Otherwise, they would be "unsaturated." In the latter, carbon atoms have one less hydrogen atom dangling from them. This unsaturation forces the carbons missing a hydrogen atom to form a double bond (shown as=) with each other. The number of double bonds, and their positions along the chain of fatty acids, is enormously important and changes the entire character and function of fatty acids.

> You can buy ground meat that has seven percent or 10% fat and mix it with a tablespoon of olive oil to prevent it from getting too dry on the grill. This not only improves the taste (fat is a major taste enhancer) but also makes your hamburger more healthful. Similarly, you can sauté your fish, chicken or vegetables in olive oil instead of butter, shortening or corn oil. If you are a diabetic, or have low HDL-cholesterol, increasing monounsaturated fat should be an essential part of your dietary changes.

When all the carbon molecules are fully occupied (they have *single bonds*), the fatty acid is saturated.

When the carbon molecules are not fully occupied (they have *double bonds),* the fatty acid is unsaturated.

If one carbon molecule is unsaturated, the fatty acid is *mono*unsaturated. If more carbon molecules are unsaturated, the fatty acid is *poly*-unsaturated.

Oleic acid, the principal fatty acid of olive oil, canola oil and hazelnut oil, has 18 carbons in its chain with one double bond. Thus, oleic acid is called a monounsaturated fatty acid. Linoleic acid, the main fatty acid of many vegetable oils such as corn, safflower, sunflower and soybean has two double bonds. Linoleic acid and all other fatty acids with two or more unsaturated carbons are called polyunsaturated fatty acids.

Nearly all fat molecules are called fatty acids because they are in reality very weak acidic compounds with a COOH at one end. But when they join together or to other compounds, they lose their acidic status.

What are omega-3 and omega-6 polyunsaturated fats? They are two distinctly different types of polyunsaturated fats with vastly different roles in human health.

The heart-friendly fatty acids in seafood are omega-3 polyunsaturated fatty acids with 20 or 22 carbons in their chains. This type of fatty acid is not present in any plant and can be produced in the human body only in minimal amounts. Omega-3 fats are referred to as essential fatty acids, meaning that they must be supplied from outside sources. Linolenic acid is an 18 carbon omega-3 polyunsaturated fat, present to varying degrees in certain seed oils such as flax seed, canola oil, soybean and Persian or English walnuts. A small amount of this plant-source omega-3 (no more than one percent to two percent) may be elongated and converted into longer-chain fatty acids. In people who do not eat any seafood, this may be their only source of omega-3 polyunsaturated fat.

Omega-6 polyunsaturated fats are plentiful and present in all vegetable oils or fats, including margarine, shortenings and cooking fats. The usual dietary intake of omega-3 polyunsaturated fat in the United States and many Western countries is about one-half to two grams per day, compared with 20 or more grams per day for omega-6 polyunsaturated fat. Before the 1940s, the ratio of dietary omega-6 to omega-3 was 4 to 1, but because of the abundance of vegetable oils and fats in our foods, the ratio has increased to 20 to 1.

The most important benefit of vegetable oils, but not vegetable fats, is that as a replacement for dietary saturated fats and trans fats they can help lower blood cholesterol level by about five percent to seven percent. This is because omega-6 polyunsaturated fatty acids can bind to dietary cholesterol whereas saturated fatty acids cannot and trans fats do not bind with dietary cholesterol.

The vegetable oil industry has been promoting their products as "100% cholesterol-free and 100% natural" and heart-healthy for decades. So consumers have accepted these promotions, aided by flawed communications from the health establishments. Aside from a small LDL-lowering effect, the case for increasing dietary omega-6 polyunsaturated fat is weak and very difficult to justify. American diets and those of many developed countries have contained unacceptably high levels of transfat, the majority of which are vegetable fats. So it is doubtful that vegetable oils have provided any heart health or cancer fighting benefit. Unlike monounsaturates, which have a 3,000-year history of safety combined with proven heart-protective benefits, omega-6 polyunsaturated fat has a short history with many unanswered questions.

Major concerns about omega-6 polyunsaturated fat include…

- Dietary omega-6 polyunsaturated fat will lower HDL-cholesterol by approximately 5 percent to 10%. Lowering the HDL, especially in people whose level is already low, is a major step in the wrong direction.

- Omega-6 polyunsaturated fat is more susceptible to oxidization than saturated fats or monounsaturates. The oxidized LDL contributes to coronary artery disease. This concern is especially troublesome with margarines, shortening and cooking fats, which all contain trans fat.

A recent study of 393 men with elevated blood cholesterol levels showed that dietary omega-6 polyunsaturated fat, without supplementation with antioxidants such as vitamin E, was the most important determinant of LDL susceptibility to oxidization.

- In people with elevated LDL-cholesterol levels, it makes no sense to add anything even "all natural and cholesterol-free," to their diet that can increase oxidization of their cholesterol. Increased oxidization of LDL-cholesterol, and the resulting damage to various tissues (oxidative stress), is even more troublesome in diabetics who already have a greater tendency for cardiovascular diseases. Diabetics should actually reduce dietary omega-6 polyunsaturated fat (all vegetable oils, margarine and shortenings) as much as possible and replace them with monounsaturates, which stabilize their LDL particles and decrease oxidative stress.

Unfortunately soybean and other vegetable oils provide about 20% of all calories from food. We should reduce this by half and replace it with olive oil.

Repeated heating of omega-6 polyunsaturated fat at high temperatures, such as deep frying at home or fast food restaurants, degrades these fats and produces harmful oxidized by-products which diffuse into our foods.

Recent studies have shown that consumption of foods containing degradation products of previously heated omega-6 polyunsaturated fat makes the endothelium (inner lining) of the arteries dysfunctional, a precursor to coronary artery disease. Pretreatment of individuals consuming these products with antioxidant vitamins C and E blocks or decreases the endothelial dysfunction caused by repeatedly heated fats.

What about "designer" margarines?

Recently margarine manufacturers in the United States, following the lead of European countries, have marketed soft margarines with very little or no trans fatty acids. Some of these spreads (such as Benecol and Take Control) also contain plant additives that can reduce the absorption of cholesterol from the intestine. For example, each serving of Benecol contains 1.5 gm of stanol (extracted from pine). Several studies have shown that stanol, 3 grams per day in divided doses and taken with food, can lower blood cholesterol by five percent. So multiple servings, everyday, for a long time are needed to achieve this minor cholesterol-lowering benefit.

Other newer spreads contain different kinds of plant additives. For example, Take Control contains a plant sterol (chemically different from stanol) derived from soybean. It is less efficient in cholesterol-lowering than stanol. None of the plant additives has any impact on HDL-cholesterol or triglyceride levels.

Most "designer" margarines have less total fat and calories (and more water) per serving than the conventional margarine spreads. They also have substantially less saturated fat and no trans fatty acids, making them a sensible substitute for other spreads, even though they are more costly.

Other margarines, shortenings and cooking fats

For several decades, the vegetable oil industry has been converting liquid vegetable oils into solid fats by adding hydrogen atoms to the polyunsaturated oils. This chemical process essentially changes the character of the original undiluted oils, making the new products unhealthy.

The process of partial hydrogenation is very imprecise. All fat molecules in the oil are not hydrogenated uniformly. In fact, only 30% to 50% of the fat molecules are hydrogenated, meaning they accept additional hydrogen atoms. Moreover, hydrogen atoms are added to fat molecules in a random fashion along the chain of fatty acids. The process is very much like adding one or more charm pieces, at random, to a bracelet. When the job of adding new pieces is completed, not many bracelets would be alike. Similarly, during partial hydrogenation, at least 20 different new fatty acids (or "isomeres") of the original fat are produced. Each one of these new fat molecules may be different from the others depending on where and how many new hydrogen atoms have been added to the original fat molecule.

If the added hydrogen atoms are all on one side of the fatty acid chain, the fat is called a "cis fatty acid." However, if the hydrogen atoms are distributed on both sides of the chain, the new fat is called a "trans fatty acid."

Hydrogenation processing can also produce harmful saturated fats. During hydrogenation of vegetable oils, small amounts of three saturated fatty acids (arachidic, behemic and lignoceric) are produced. These substances are all coronary-unfriendly, even in small quantities.

What makes trans fatty acids distinctly different from cis fatty acids is that the cis varieties

> ### SIDE EFFECTS OF VEGETABLE OILS
> ### (OMEGA-6 PUFA)
>
> - Reduce HDL-cholesterol
> - May increase blood pressure
> - Increase oxidization of LDL-cholesterol and endothelial dysfunction
> - Promote blood clotting
> - May increase the risk of gallstone formation
> - Can suppress the function of T-lymphocytes and decrease immune response
> - May be carcinogenic in some animals, especially breast, colon and prostate cancers

(such as fatty acids in natural vegetable oils) are "wiggly" and flexible at their double bonds, and therefore are liquid. On the other hand, the double bond in the molecule of a trans fatty acid is not wiggly and keeps the chain stiff, which contributes to keeping these fats solid at room temperature. These partially hydrogenated new fats now act a lot more like saturated fat than the polyunsaturated fat they used to be. In ruminating animals such as cows, sheep, goats, deer and camels, a small amount of trans fat is produced by bacterial action in their rumen. Some of this trans fat will eventually appear in their flesh and milk.

The popularity of vegetable oils and fats has been one of the most successful (and in my opinion regrettable) manipulative dietary campaigns. The most charitable judgment on vegetable oils is that they may have been relatively harmless. Mounting evidence suggests that high consumption of vegetable fats, in particular hard margarine and cooking fat, containing trans fats, are as harmful as the butter they replaced in many diets.

Some hard margarines and shortenings may have as much as 30% saturated fatty acids to go along with 20% to 30% trans fatty acids, making them as unhealthful as, or even worse than, butter or cream.

Should you switch?

Is switching from butter to hard, stick margarines and shortenings jumping from the frying pan into the fire? The answer is "yes." Although liquid, nonhydrogenated vegetable oils like corn and soybean oil in small amounts are reasonably safe, my recommendation is to use olive oil for all your needs. However, canola oil is a reasonable alternative. But if you crave butter on your toast, you can use a small amount of soft, tub margarine with low concentrations of, or preferably no, trans fatty acid (such as Benecol, Brummel & Brown Spread, Smart Balance, Take Control). Mayonnaise, stick margarines, shortenings and cooking fats have the convenience of long shelf life but are hazardous to your health.

Trans Fatty Acids: No Redeeming Value

In the 1930s a process was developed to make liquid oils more solid. Partial hydrogenation of liquid fats (by adding hydrogen atoms to them) made these oils solid at room temperature and also less likely to become rancid. It also increased their shelf life. The resulting oils are known as trans fatty acids. But partial hydrogenation creaters highly undesirable trans fats with many side effects.

There are two types of trans fatty acids. The first are naturally occurring trans fats produced by animals incorporated into their milk and flesh. It is present in very small amounts (usually about one percent to two percent of total fat) in milk products and in the meat of cattle, sheep, goat and buffalo. Low-fat milk or lean red meats have a negligible amount of trans fats. The major naturally occurring trans fat is vaccenic

acid, which is not as harmful as elaidic acid, the predominant industrial trans fat.

In 2004, Denmark banned the use of partially hydrogenated fats from the Danish food staple. Germany, Netherlands, Norway and Spain followed the example of Denmark. And what did the US government do? The US government capitulated to food industry lobbies and the Food and Drug Administration merely required food manufacturers to add trans fatty acid content of their products to nutrition information labels in 2006!

In a further capitulation, foods and snacks that contain up to 500 mg of trans fats per serving are allowed to list the trans fat content as zero! This ignores the fact that most people don't eat just one serving of trans fatty foods like cakes, cookies or chips! At fast food places, many customers eat several servings of deep-fried foods, side dishes and cookies. These meals usually contain several grams of industrial-strength trans fatty acids and yet they are permitted to be called "trans fat free." Now the food manufacturers can still claim that their products contain "zero trans fat," and the consumers are left in the dark about what they're eating.

At present a serving of McDonald's Chicken Nuggets and large french fries in New York City has approximately 10 to 12 grams (10,000 to 12,000 mg) of trans fatty acids compared with the same two items served by McDonald's restaurants in Denmark or Spain that have zero and less than 3 grams, respectively. If you add some cookies, your trans fat intake skyrockets to around 14 to 15 grams of trans fatty acid! Does this make any sense? I am troubled that Europeans can offer healthier choices than we do in America.

On average, Americans consume six to eight grams of industrial trans fatty acids per day. Pregnant women or nursing mothers who frequently eat sweets and deep-fried foods expose their fetuses or infants to high levels of trans fatty acids. It is conceivable that such exposures may contribute to the high prevalence of early coronary lesions and diabetes in children and adolescents in the United States.

Why are trans fatty acids hazardous?

Partially hydrogenated fats are promoted as "natural," but they are chemically processed by adding hydrogen atoms to the original liquid oils, so they are industrial fats and cannot be called "natural." We have long known that processed vegetable fats with trans fats are far worse than the butter they were designed to replace. Like tobacco, they are "grandfathered" into our dietary staple.

But trans fats have several troublesome effects…

A large body of evidence suggests that by reducing consumption of trans fat by only half and replacing it with monounsaturates (olive oil, canola oil or nuts such as almonds, hazelnut, pistachios and walnuts), the number of heart attacks in the US can be reduced by more than 40,000 each year.

By following the sensible food safety policies of Denmark, and eliminating industrial trans fat from our food and snacks, we could lower the number of heart attacks by more than 100,000 per year.

Until then, all foods and snacks containing trans fat should carry a label, like tobacco products, that reads, "This product may be hazardous to your health when used as directed!"

Many Americans consume more trans fatty acids than four to six grams per day, especially those who have switched to margarines and shortenings for diet reasons. Stick margarines, on average, have more than 20% trans fatty acids. The amount may range from 19% to 49%). Many tub or soft margarines contain about 15% trans fatty acids (and some have as much as 28%). Commercial shortenings (used in baking pastries, cakes, cookies, croissants, nuts and in cooking and frying) consistently have a much higher concentration of trans fatty acids, averaging more than 30%.

Many food manufacturers have begun to reduce or eliminate trans fats from products like popcorn and potato chips. But, many products, especially snacks on the grocery shelves, continue to have high levels of these undesirable fats Remember, "zero trans fats" does not necessarily mean zero; it may mean up to 500mg per serving.

☞ **WARNING:** *Avoid any food or snack that has "partially hydrogenated oil," shortening or cooking fat, regardless of what the nutrition label says.* Trans fatty acids have no nutritional virtue and are far worse for you than any existing edible fat.

Omega-3 Polyunsaturated Fat: Is Seafood the "Right Stuff?"

Over the last decade, several hundred studies have examined the beneficial health impact of seafood omega-3 polyunsaturated fat (omega-3 PUFA). Seafood omega-3 polyunsaturated fats lower triglycerides by as much as 30%. In fact, in many people with very high triglyceride levels, fish oil is one of the most effective triglyceride-lowering "drugs," and is much safer than currently available drugs.

Some convincing studies about the benefits of seafood

The results of a six-year study of 45,000 male health professionals (ranging in age from 45 to 70) were recently reported. Each man was free of cardiovascular disease at the beginning of the study. In the six-year follow-up, there were 25%

TRANS FATTY ACID CONTENT OF SELECTED FOODS

Food	% TFA Range	Grams TFA Per Serving
Beef*	4 (2 to 5)	0.20 (3½ oz)
Benecol Spread	Trace	Trace
Butter*	4 (2 to 7)	0.4 (½ oz)
Chicken	1 (0.5 to 1.5)	0.04 (3½ oz)
Cookies	18 (4 to 36)	1.5 (one piece)
Cooking Oils, Soy, Etc.	12 (1 to 13)	1.5 (½ oz)
Fish	0	0
French Fries	21 (3 to 34)	4 (large)
Hamburger*	4 (3 to 5)	0.5 (serving)
Potato Chips	13 (0 to 40)	1.5 (serving)
Pork	0.2 (0.1 to 0.3)	0.01 (3½ oz)
Shortenings	37 (34 to 44)	5 (½ oz)
Smart Balance	0	0
Stick Margarine	27 (19 to 49)	3 (½ oz)
Take Control Spread	Trace	Trace
Tub, Soft Margarine	17 (11 to 28)	2 (½ oz)
Whole Milk*	3 (2.5 to 3.5)	0.20 (3½ oz)

*TFA are produced in the rumen by fermentation and absorbed from the intestine of these animals. Eventually, these TFA appear in their meat and milk.

HARMFUL EFFECTS OF TRANS FATTY ACIDS

Increase blood levels of the bad LDL-cholesterol

Increase blood levels of triglycerides

Decrease blood levels of the good HDL-cholesterol

Make LDL particles smaller (which are more harmful than larger LDL particles)

Increase oxidization of LDL (making it more harmful) and HDL (making it less helpful)

Increase the risk of heart attack, stroke and sudden cardiac deaths (by two to three fold)

Increase the risk of obesity and diabetes (have contributed to worldwide epidemics of obesity and diabetes, especially among younger people)

Increase the risk of breast, colon and prostate cancers

Increase the risk of asthma (and have contributed to the epidemic of asthma in children)

Have no nutritional value, can be easily replaced with other fats that do not contain trans fatty acids fewer cardiac deaths among those who had eaten at least some fish each week compared with those who had eaten no fish at all.

In another study, more than 20,000 male physicians were followed up for 12 years. The results showed that consuming seafood only once per week reduced the risk of sudden cardiac deaths (the majority due to arrhythmia or irregular heart rate) by 50%. This finding was identical to another study from Seattle, Washington, which showed that eating just one serving of a fatty fish per week (equivalent to two to three nonfatty fish meals) reduced the risk of sudden cardiac arrest by 50%. With higher seafood consumption (three to four times per week), the risk of cardiac arrest was lowered by 70%.

In a recent Italian study, more than 11,000 men and women who had had a heart attack within the previous three months were randomly given one gram of fish oil (containing a relatively small amount of omega-3 polyunsaturated fat) or no fish oil. They were followed up for an average of three-and-a-half years. Participants were also given "blood thinners" (anticlotting agents) and other drugs, and were put on a Mediterranean diet. The results showed that the group that received a small amount of fish oil had an additional 15% lower risk of fatal or nonfatal heart attacks or strokes.

The longest study of omega-3 polyunsaturated fat was recently reported by the investigators of the Chicago Western Electric Study Group. In this study, 1,822 men, aged 40 to 55 and free of cardiovascular disease at the start, were followed up for 30 years. The data showed that the risk of sudden or nonsudden deaths from heart attack was 44% lower among those who ate an average of more than eight ounces of fish per week compared with those who did not eat any fish. Although studies dealing with the impact of omega-3 polyunsaturated fat on women's health are not as extensive as those for men,

the results of available studies show a nearly identical response.

The box on page 120 summarizes the findings of some of the most extensive studies done today, and shows the dramatic, life-saving impact of eating several seafood meals a week.

The vast benefits of seafood omega-3 PUFAs are dose-dependant, meaning that the more you consume, the greater the health benefits. An occasional deep-fried seafood or tuna fish sandwich drowned in mayonnaise offers no health benefit.

The most recent data (2007) from the US Physicians' Health Study also showed a dose response between lower risk of colorectal cancer. In men who ate fish one to two times weekly, the risk reduction was 13%; for those who ate fish two to five times a week, the risk was reduced by 20%, and for those eating seafood five times a week, the risk reduction was 40%. Similarly the risk reduction for other cancers, phlebitis and osteoporosis were also dose-dependent.

To obtain the peak heart health and cancer preventive benefits, eat at least three or four seafood meals a week, two of them preferably dark-fleshed fish (which have higher concentrations of omega-3 PUFAs). Seafood's benefits are seen among all populations, diverse ethnic groups, and even among people who habitually consume a large amount of seafood such as the Japanese.

This study and many other studies on animals have documented that consumption of omega-3 polyunsaturated fat from seafood reduces the vulnerability of heart muscle to serious arrhythmias and cardiac arrest. That's important because more than half of all coronary deaths are due to cardiac arrhythmias and cardiac arrest.

Omega-3 polyunsaturated fat from seafood provides one of the most effective measures against coronary death. In fact, at present, no single drug or combination of currently available anti-arrhythmia drugs can match the life-saving

FATTY ACID COMPOSITION OF SEAFOOD*
(Grams/3.5 oz)

Fish	Fat	SFA	MUFA	Omega-3 PUFA	Cholesterol
Bass, Striped	2.3	0.5	0.7	0.8	80
Bass, Freshwater	2	0.4	0.7	0.8	60
Bluefish	4.5	1	2	1	59
Catfish	1.3	0.4	0.5	0.3	58
Cod	0.7	0.1	0.1	0.3	43
Flounder	1	0.2	0.3	0.4	46
Haddock	0.7	0.1	0.1	0.2	58
Halibut	2.3	0.3	0.7	0.4	32
Herring	6	2	2.8	1.8	60
Mackerel	11	3.3	4	2.7	70
Perch	1	0.2	0.2	0.4	76
Pike	1.2	0.3	0.3	0.4	86
Pollock	1	0.2	0.2	0.5	71
Rockfish	1.5	0.4	0.5	0.4	44
Sablefish	11	3.5	5	1.7	50
Salmon, Chinook	7	2.0	3.5	1.7	66
Salmon, Coho	6	1.3	2.2	1.5	45
Sea Bass	2	0.5	0.4	0.4	42
Shark	1.9	0.3	0.4	0.5	44
Snapper	1.4	0.3	0.3	0.3	38
Sole	1.2	0.3	0.4	0.2	50
Swordfish	2.6	1.1	1.0	0.3	39
Trout, Rainbow	3.4	0.7	1.2	0.6	60
Tuna Large	4.6	1.2	2.0	1.2	60
Whitefish	4.8	1	2	1.1	60

*The composition may vary depending on the habitat and the natural diet of the fish.

SFA=Saturated Fatty Acids; MUFA=Monounsaturated Fatty Acids; Omega-3 PUFA=Omega-3 Polyunsaturated Fatty Acids

benefits and safety of eating three to four seafood meals per week.

Other benefits of omega-3 polyunsaturated fat are summarized on the chart on page 121.

Several recent studies have shown that long term consumption of seafood, equivalent to even two seafood meals per week of mainly darker-flesh fish, significantly reduces cognitive

Shellfish	Fat	SFA	MUFA	Omega-3 PUFA	Cholesterol
Clams	1.2	0.2	0.2	0.4	36
Crab	1.1	0.2	0.3	0.6	60
Lobster	1	0.2	0.2	0.3	90
Mussels	2	0.2	0.2	0.4	67
Oysters	2.6	0.7	0.5	0.9	72
Scallops	0.9	0.3	0.2	0.3	35
Shrimp	1.7	0.4	0.5	0.5	157
Squid	1.8	0.7	0.4	0.6	280

FATTY ACID COMPOSITION OF SHELLFISH*
(Grams/3.5 oz)

*The composition may vary depending on the habitat and the natural diet of the fish.

SFA=Saturated Fatty Acids; MUFA=Monounsaturated Fatty Acids; Omega-3 PUFA=Omega-3 Polyunsaturated Fatty Acids

decline and dementia. Since our population is aging, the burden of dementia for those affected and their caregivers can be staggering. This is another reason for including at least two seafood meals per week in your diet.

A long-term prospective study followed up more than 41,000 Japanese men and women 40 to 59 years of age, for 10 years. During that time, there were 258 acute heart attacks and 37 sudden cardiac deaths.

For those with the highest fish intake (more than seven servings per week, a median intake of 180 gm/day, which equaled about 2.4 g/d omega-3 PUFA). The risk of a heart attack was reduced by 56% compared with those with the lowest fish intake (under one serving per/week, or a median of 0.3 gm omega-3 PUFA). Iso H; et al. Circulation 2006; 113: 195–202

Is plant omega-3 fat as good as omega-3 fat from seafood?

Certain plant-derived oils, such as avocado, flax seed, soybean, canola and walnut, contain an omega-3 fat called alpha-linolenic acid (ALA).

Contrary to much publicity, especially for flax seed and sesame seed oil, ALA *does not* have the same functions or benefits as seafood omega-3 PUFA. This is due to a different molecular structure. In fact, it is primarily the 24 carbon omega-3 PUFA, DHA (docosahexaenoic acid) that is responsible for most of seafood's benefits, especially its role in reducing the risk of dementia and Alzheimer's disease. (The 22-carbon seafood omega-3 is called EPA or eicosapentaenoic acid.)

Both EPA and DHA are essential fatty acids, meaning that we need them for our survival. Unfortunately, we can make our only a tiny amount of EPA and DHA. Fish don't make EPA or DHA either; they obtain theirs from plankton and algae and by feasting on other fish in the food chain.

If you don't eat seafood...

We can convert only about one percent to three percent of plant omega-3 fat (ALA) to EPA, and only a trivial amount to DHA, to provide the bare minimum of these two essential fatty acids. Human brain has the highest concentration of EPA

FISH CONSUMPTION AND RISK OF DEATH FROM CORONARY HEART DISEASE DEATHS*

Eleven studies with 222,364 individuals and an average follow-up of 12 years (relative risk compared with those eating fish less than once per/month) have shown the following risk reductions:

Fish Consumption	*% risk reduction*
1 to 3 times per /month	11%
1 per week	15%
2 to 4 per week	23%
5 or more per week	38%

Each 1 oz. per /day increase in fish intake reduces coronary deaths by 10%!

Five or more seafood meals per /week reduces the risk of sudden cardiac death by 70%!

*He K, et al (Northwestern and Harvard) *Circulation* 2004; 109: 2705–11

---

and DHA. Among people who do not eat an adequate amount of seafood, these essential fatty acid levels are reduced. During pregnancy, when estrogen is high, women are able to convert up to eight percent of plant omega-3 fat to EPA, a tiny fraction of which is then converted to DHA, enabling them to provide the fetus with the badly needed EPA and DHA for the brain's development. The importance of omega-PUFAs in the brain for neuro-cognitive development finally convinced baby food manufacturers to add EPA and DHA to their formulas.

Small amounts of plant omega-3 fat are quite safe and behave like monounsaturated fat. However, several recent studies have reported that high intake of ALA or supplements containing ALA, such as flaxseed oil, may increase the risk of prostate cancer, especially the advanced or aggressive type, by 30%. It is not yet clear why or how this happens. One plausible explanation is that when the plant-derived

ALA enters prostate cells, it prevents the entry of longer-chain omega-3 into these cells, depriving them of the robust anticarcinogenic benefits of seafood EPA and DHA.

Eating three to four seafood meals per week is one of the most important dietary changes you can make. By increasing your intake of omega-3 fatty acids, you can dramatically reduce your risk of a cardiovascular events and heart rate irregularities. Plus, each seafood meal replaces another meal that may be higher in calories, saturated fats or trans fatty acids.

Because the omega-3 fats are the healthiest nutrient in seafood, choose fish or shellfish with the highest (not the lowest) fat content. The boxes on page 118 and 119 provide a guide for choosing among many different types of seafood. In this instance, the fattier the fish, the better (nearly 25% to 30% of the fat in seafood is omega-3 polyunsaturated fat).

Most shellfish contain high concentrations of poorly absorbable cholesterol look-alikes. Much like their plant counterparts "phytosterols," they reduce the absorption of dietary cholesterol. The absorbed cholesterol from clams, shrimp or crab legs is actually much lower than 50%, making a shellfish meal (without butter or margarine, please) a guilt-free and enjoyable experience.

- Use olive oil, any vegetable oil (monounsaturated fat) instead of margarine, butter, cream or cooking fats in preparing your seafood.

- Grilling, barbecuing, baking, broiling and poaching or sauteeing in olive oil are reasonable preparation methods. I do not grill my seafood to avoid losing any omega-3 fat in the drippings.

- Eating several servings of vegetables with a shellfish dinner will also lower cholesterol absorption further (because of their phytosterol

WHAT DO SEAFOOD OMEGA-3 FATS DO?

They reduce...

- Triglycerides by 30%, but they raise the good HDL-cholesterol
- The number of small, more harmful LDL particles
- Activation and aggregation of platelets, and make them less likely to cause heart attack
- Activation of white blood cells, and the release of inflammation-causing compounds
- Coronary heart disease mortality by up to 38%[1]
- Sudden death from heart attack (due to extremely rapid heart rates) by more than 70%[2]
- Risk of atrial fibrillation (irregular heart rate) after coronary bypass surgery by more than 50%[3]
- Insulin resistance and risk of diabetes
- Progression of kidney failure, metabolic syndrome and fatty liver
- Symptoms of chronic lung disease (due to omega-3 PUFA's anti-inflammatory effects)[4]
- Risk of breast, colon and prostate cancer
- Risk of dementia by more than 40%, and Alzheimer's disease by over 50% (when three or more seafood meals per week are consumed)[5]

1-He K et al. Circulation 2004; 109: 2705–11
2-Albert CM et al. N Eng J Med 2002; 346: 1113–8
3-Calo L et al. J Am Coll Cardiology 2005; 45: 1723–28
4-Matsuyama W et al. Chest 2005; 128: 3817–27
5-Hashimoto M et al. J Nutr 2005; 135: 549–55

compounds), making the meal even more healthful.

On average we consume more than 20 to 30 grams of omega-6 fat per day in a typical Western diet compared with less than one gram seafood omega-3. Omega-6 PUFAs in vegetable oils, and trans fats in stick margarines, shortenings or cooking fats used for deep frying, compete with seafood's omega-3 PUFAs, and prevent them from entering tissues such as the heart muscle cells, white blood cells, platelets and brain or other cells. This defeats the purpose of eating the seafood in the first place.

Adding mayonnaise to your tuna fish sandwich does the same thing—it ruins your sandwich! A better choice is to add mild salsa, a touch of mustard, chopped celery or green onions to your sandwich to give it some zest and personality. Light or "lite" mayo is not much better than the regular kind. It has only about one-third less omega-6 fat. If you crave mayo on your sandwhich, choose a fat-free variety or fat-free whipped cream, or fat-free salad dressing.

Although most frozen or canned seafood loses a good deal of its taste and texture, its nutritional value will remain unchanged.

> *The three unforgivable "sins" with seafood are:* Buying stale fish (more than two or three days old, especially if it was not kept in the coldest part of the refrigerator), overcooking it (which releases unpleasant fishy odors and ruins the seafood's texture, flavor, delicacy and unique personality), and cooking or marinating it in vegetable oils with omega-6 PUFAs, such as corn, safflower, sunflower or soybean oil, adding mayonnaise or deep-frying.

Avoid frozen fried seafood. It's no better than deep-frying fresh fish yourself in cooking fat. It defeats the purpose of eating seafood. Fried fish sticks or deep-fried fish sandwiches from fast food places fall into the same category.

What about mercury and PCBs (polychlorinated biphenyls) in seafood?

Whenever I talk about the virtues of eating seafood, the questions follow: "What about mercury and the other compounds that cause cancer?" Do you also worry about these contaminants? Of course you do! But are the sound bites about mercury and PCBs in our seafood supported by fact? The answer is a resounding no! Mark Twain said, "I have known many problems in my life, most of which never happened." That sums up the fear of mercury and PCBs in our seafood!

Concern over mercury in seafood was centered on pregnant women. It was feared that mercury could cross the placenta and accumulate in the fetus' brain and create neuro-developmental defects. However, none of the US agencies—the US Environmental Protection Agency, the Food and Drug Administration, the US Department of Agriculture, the American Heart Association or the National Cancer Institute have cited mercury or PCBs in seafood as a major concern for non-pregnant adults. Even the cautionary note that pregnant women should limit their seafood intake to two meals per week was already dated and void by the time it was released to the public. But the media picked it up and the public now sees a hidden menace in every bite of every fish! The misinformation about "dangerous" levels of mercury and PCBs in our seafood gained a life of its own, uncorrected, and now it has become "a well-known fact," imprinted not only in the public mind but in the mind of healthcare providers as well.

So, what's the real story on mercury and PCBs in our seafood? Three studies have looked at the effects of prenatal exposure to mercury and child development.

First, there was an nine-year study of 779 mother infant pairs residing in Seychelles. Fish in Seychelles contain the same concentration of methyl mercury as fish available in the US. In Seychelles pregnant women eat an average of 12 seafood meals per week.

During the one-year follow-up, there was no evidence that even this extremely high fish intake in the prenatal period had any negative neurodevelopmental consequences in these women's offspring. (Myers GJ et al (US Natl Inst for Child Health) LANCET 2003; 361: 1686–92)

In the second study, among 7,421 British children, frequent fish consumption by mothers during pregnancy, and by children, was associated with higher neurodevelopmental scores. (Daniels JL et al. Epidemiol 2004; 15: 394–402)

The third study found that among 1,709 US women aged 16–49, less than four percent had blood mercury levels (slightly) above the EPA safe 5.8 microgram/l. (Schober SE et al. JAMA 2003; 289: 1667–74)

The FDA's safe level for PCBs is 2000 parts per billion (PPB). Even the most contaminated fish has less than 40–100 PPB.

How much fish should we eat?

Although seafood consumption in the US, Europe and other developed countries has slowly increased over the past 30 years (in Japan, it has slightly decreased due to higher consumption of beef and poultry), it is still relatively meager.

We often eat white-fleshed seafood with little omega-3 fat instead of darker-fleshed fish such as salmon, tuna or mackerel with higher omega-3 levels. Americans tend to eat deep-fried white fish or shrimp, a practice that essentially

MERCURY IN SEAFOOD: MUCH ADO ABOUT NOTHING!

In the past 40 years not a single case of (methyl) mercury poisoning from seafood has been reported in the US.

During the same 40 years, more than 30 million Americans, many in their 30s, 40s, or 50s, have died of cardiovascular diseases. About seven to 10 million of these people could have been saved by eating four to five seafood meals a week!

Traces of mercury (partly from volcanic activities at the seafloor) are present in some long-living, predatory ocean fish (king mackerel, shark, swordfish, tilefish and whale), and a few fresh-water fish, mostly from environmental mercury (large bass and pike).

FISH WITH METHYLMERCURY LEVELS UNDER THE FDA'S SAFE LIMIT

- Bass, sea or Chilean
- Black drum
- Butterfish
- Cod
- Clams and crabs
- Croaker
- Flounder
- Haddock
- Halibut
- Herring
- Lobster
- Mahi-mahi
- Mullet
- Oysters
- Perch
- Pollack
- Pompano
- Rockfish and salmon
- Scallops and shrimp
- Speckled (spotted) trout
- Skate and snappers
- Spot
- Whitefish

Farm-raised:

- Catfish
- Rainbow trout
- Red crayfish
- Salmon (fresh or canned)
- Shrimp
- Tilapia
- Trout

Note: Albacore tuna has 0.38 & yellow fin tuna 0.3 PPM, still below FDA's safe limit

defeats the purpose of eating seafood in the first place. (Remember, omega-6 and trans fats compete with omega-3.)

To obtain the vast benefits of seafood, have an average intake of 1½ to 2 grams of omega-3 PUFA per day, or 10 to 15 grams per week. This is especially important for people with major coronary risk factors and people with risk factors for cancers such as breast, colon or prostate (for this group, the higher their intake the better). This amount of omega-3 PUFAs can be obtained by eating at least three and preferably more than four seafood meals per week, particularly fish with darker flesh, which are fattier than white-fleshed fish or shellfish. Since approximately 25% to 30% of the fat in seafood is omega-3 PUFAs, as

a rule of thumb, the darker the flesh of the fish, the fattier it is, and the better it is for you.

The fat content of similar species of fish can vary as much as three-to fivefold, due to the habitat, water temperature, age and size (older and bigger tunas have a more enriched and fatty flesh than their younger and smaller counterparts). This is especially true of albacore tuna.

- A can of albacore tuna by the same canner may have as little as one gram fat per serving to as much as five grams.

- The omega-3 fat content of salmon also varies quite widely, ranging from two percent for Atlantic pink salmon to seven percent for Pacific coho, king or sockeye salmon.

The per capita seafood consumption in the US is about 16 pounds per year, compared with 51 pounds for chicken and 89 pounds for beef. About 86% of Americans eat less than three seafood meals per/ week, and more than 70% eat less than two seafood meals per week.

WHAT ABOUT PCB IN FARM-RAISED FISH?

There is no record of cancer death caused by eating PCB-contaminated fish.

Some (not all) farm-raised fish may have 1–5 parts per billion (ppb) PCBs, and a few samples have had up to 40 ppb PCBs.

Even assuming that *every* farm-raised fish has an extremely high concentration of 40 parts/billion PCBs, which is most improbable, one would have to eat *25,000 kg* (55,000 lb.) of such "extremely contaminated" seafood, or 0.7 kg (more than 1.5 lb.) *every day for 100 years* to receive 1 mg of PCBs.

There is no evidence that 1 mg of PCBs over 100 years of anyone's lifetime causes any cancer.

Farm-raised Atlantic salmon has actually higher concentration of omega-3 fat compared to wild salmon.

When you buy canned tuna and canned or fresh salmon, always choose the fish with the highest fat content, but do not buy any canned salmon or tuna in oil. Almost 30% of the fat in fish is omega-3 fat and the main reason for eating several seafood meals per week is to increase your omega-3 fat intake. The fattier the fish (except squid and shrimp), the better it is!

What about cholesterol content of shellfish?

Fish and shellfish have no more cholesterol (and in some instances even less) than chicken or turkey. Moreover, the fat content of most shellfish is about 10% less than chicken or turkey breast without skin, especially saturated fat, is so small that their cholesterol content is not a concern. If you sauté shrimp in olive oil, the monounsaturated fat in olive oil attaches to cholesterol in the shrimp's particles. What enters the liver does not satisfy liver cells' need for free (non-esterified) cholesterol, so the liver traps LDL-cholesterol from the bloodstream and extracts the needed free cholesterol from them. By doing so, the blood levels of LDL-cholesterol will actually drop!

Is raw fish and shellfish safe?

Eating raw oysters was commonplace in Europe as far back as Roman times. In Victorian times, pickled oysters were a favorite food of poor people. However, the tradition of eating raw oysters in the US, especially in the South, goes back more than 150 years. Only in the past 10 to 15 years have sushi and sashimi bars and restaurants sprouted everywhere in the US. Contrary to a common belief, raw seafood is not any more nutritious or healthful than the cooked variety. But are these raw seafood "delicacies" safe? With a few exceptions, the answer is yes!

Thanks to robust global economic, cultural, travel and migration patterns, we have had many culinary exchanges. We exported hamburgers, hot dogs, steaks and steak tartar (not an original American fare), and embraced sushi, sashimi and other raw seafood.

All raw fish (or meat), red, white or in-between, is perishable, and it may cause food-borne illnesses. Meat contains all the necessary nutrients for growth of bacteria, especially at room temperature, so it must be handled with care and kept at temperatures below 42°F (5°C) at all times to minimize the growth of bacteria. In fact, many top-notch restaurants serving sushi or sashimi use properly thawed (in the refrigerator, not on the countertop) *frozen seafood* to kill most of the bacteria, a safeguard against food-borne illnesses caused by raw fish.

☛ **WARNING:** Individuals with chronic debilitating or immune-suppressing disease should avoid eating raw oysters or any raw seafood.

Although properly handled oysters that are preserved at below 42°F are quite safe, never eat raw oysters from any vendor or restaurant if they are not chilled or kept and served on ice.

Although the risk of such illness is very low, safety depends upon the proper harvesting, handling and preserving the raw fish before it is served. There are *three different types of illnesses* associated with eating raw seafood...

Illnesses caused by bacteria

The primary culprit here is a bacterium called *Vibrio Vulnificus* that is associated with eating raw oysters. The contamination is worldwide and occurs in coastal waters or saltwater estuaries. Contaminated raw oysters, even if they have been harvested and consumed in cold places like Alaska, may cause nausea, vomiting and abdominal pain, and frequently blistering or necrotizing skin lesions, even in healthy individuals. This acute illness responds well if treated early with vigorous appropriate antibiotic therapy.

☞ **WARNING:** Although the risk of infection due to *Vibrio Vulnificus* is less than one per million persons eating raw oysters, it accounts for 95% of deaths associated with all seafood-related illnesses.

In persons who already have liver disease, diabetes or other chronic debilitating diseases, the risk of systemic infection and death is very high.

To illustrate how serious this illness can be, let me describe the aftermath of Hurricane Katrina. It hit Louisiana and Mississippi in late August 2005. Two weeks later, the US Centers for Disease Control and Prevention reported 14 cases of infection with *Vibrio Vulnificus* among residents of these two states. Because of the delays in diagnosis and treatment, three of them died.

✳ **CAUTION:** If you experience any acute illness, with or without skin lesions, following ingestion of raw oysters (or clams), inform your physician about what you ate.

Illnesses caused by parasites

Although rare, two kinds of parasitic infestations can result from eating certain raw fish. *Anisakiasis* (An-issa-ka-ya-sis) is a severe acute illness caused by ingestion of the larvae of tiny round worms present in some raw or undercooked fish such as cod, herring, mackerel and squid. It may cause severe abdominal pain, nausea, vomiting and allergic reactions like hives. In rare cases it may also cause intestinal inflammation and obstruction that requires surgery. Anisakiasis accounts for more than 90% of fish-caused parasitic infestations. There are some anti-parasitic drugs to treat this infestation, if they are started early. But being aware and avoiding infection from seafood is always preferable.

And, never eat any raw fish that's kept in cases or on counters without refrigeration or not kept on ice. Here, too, flash-frozen raw fish is much safer than unfrozen fish because freezing can kill the larvae of Anisakiasis.

Illnesses caused by toxins

The primary toxin associated with eating seafood (raw or cooked) is histamine produced by bacteria that causes spoilage of poorly handled or unrefrigerated seafood. The bacteria can break down seafood's protein and produce a large amount of histamine that is not destroyed by cooking. People who eat such spoiled fish, especially fin fish, such as bonito, mackerel or tuna, quickly experience severe allergic-type reactions. These reactions may include flushing, sweating, diffuse rash or hives, wheezing, abdominal pain, diarrhea and severe headache. Histamine-induced seafood poisoning accounts for 37% of all seafood-related illnesses, but fortunately it responds to commonly available antihistamines.

An uncommon but potentially serious illness from seafood is *ciguatera* poisoning from tropical reef fish such as barracuda, grouper, mullet, sea bass and snapper. Some saltwater planktons produce a toxin named *Ciguatoxin*. These planktons are eaten by smaller fish or shellfish, which in turn are eaten by larger fish. Although ciguatoxin is safe for the host fish, it is highly toxic when eaten by humans. Most outbreaks of poisoning by *ciguatoxin* in the US have occurred in Hawaii or Florida. Nausea, vomiting, abdominal cramps, diarrhea, neurological symptoms, including numbness and blurred vision, and irregular heart rhythm can occur as early as several minutes to more than 24 hours after eating contaminated fish.

Although there is no antidote for ciguatera poisoning, symptomatic treatment often prevents long-term, neurological complications. Since *ciguatera* toxin does not change the appearance, smell or taste of the fish, and has nothing to do with proper or improper handling of the fish, there is no specific way of preventing this disease unless you avoid eating these varieties of fish altogether.

✳ **CAUTION:** Ask what kind of fish is in the sushi or sashimi before you order it. If it contains cod, herring, mackerel or squid, do not order it unless you have confidence in food handling at the restaurant.

Can I take fish oil capsules instead of eating fish?

Not everyone likes seafood, especially many people who have been raised on a "meat and potatoes" diet. Replacing four to five less desirable foods every week with seafood is certainly preferable to taking fish oil capsules.

On the other hand, if you really dislike seafood, certain fish oil capsules can be reasonable alternatives. Be aware, however, that there may be confusion about the number of capsules you need to take each day and potential concerns about their purity, quality and cost.

Read the label. Misleading marketing and impractical dosage requirements occur with many brands of fish oil. Most over-the-counter brands have similar disadvantages. Only a few manufacturers make fish oil capsules that contain more than 600 mg of omega-3 PUFAs per capsule.

For example, the label of Nature's Bounty Salmon Oil 1000 mg gives the impression that each capsule contains 1000 mg of omega-3 PUFAs. On the back of the bottle, the fine print says something entirely different: The 1000 mg is per serving, but each serving is two capsules, not one. Furthermore, each capsule contains only 200 mg of omega-3 PUFAs, and the rest consists of other fish oil substances. Unsuspecting buyers may think that they are helping themselves with one or two fish oil capsules but, in fact, they are not. Worse, they may give themselves a false sense of security.

A seven-ounce (200 gm) serving of Atlantic salmon provides more than 1.5 gm of omega-3 fat, equal to eight Nature's Bounty Salmon Oil capsules. A similar serving of Alaska red salmon, fresh, flash-frozen or canned, equals 20 capsules! A can of Star Kist Solid White Tuna with 3 gm fat per serving (all six-or seven-ounce tuna cans contain 2½ servings per can) is equal to 10 capsules. You see my point? How many people are willing to take that many fish oil capsules every day, or even three to four times a week?

A purified omega-3 PUFA capsule containing more than 920 mg/capsule was approved by the US Food and Drug Administration, and is now available by prescription as Omacor. Omacor has the advantage of purity, consistency, high concentration and the assurance of getting a sufficient amount of omega-3 PUFAs in each capsule. But in my opinion, its high cost will continue to be an obstacle to wider use.

An over-the-counter fish oil capsule, Solgar Omega-3 100 is a reasonable choice since it contains about 640 mg of seafood omega-3 per capsule and is about half the price of Omacor.

Carbohydrates and Proteins: Fads vs. Facts

For most people, dietary carbohydrates (simple or complex) should constitute no more than 45% to 55% of daily calories. This means that about 30% to 35% of your calories come from dietary fats and 10% to 15% from proteins, allowing for an additional five percent from alcohol (in those who drink alcoholic beverages).

Eating too many dietary carbohydrates, especially sugar, high-fructose corn sweetener and starches can contribute to obesity, elevated blood glucose and insulin resistance (even among non-diabetics), elevated triglycerides, an increase in the level of coronary-unfriendly LDL-cholesterol and a significant decrease in the good HDL-cholesterol. The change from large LDL particles to small particles with long-term, high carbohydrate intake is coronary-unfriendly even if carbohydrates lower the LDL-cholesterol by five percent to 10%.

Dietary extremists on both sides argue about the benefits of very high- or very low-carbohydrate diets. On one side, the proponents of cholesterol-free and very low-fat diets extol the virtue of high dietary carbohydrate intake (in excess of 65% of calories). On the other side, "carbo busters" blame dietary carbohydrates for everything from tooth decay to early aging, chronic fatigue syndrome, cholesterol disorders and many other ailments. They are both wrong.

Numerous recent studies have shown that low-carbohydrate diets have no particular advantage over any other calorie-restricted diet for weight management. Any significant reduction in carbohydrate intake will restrict total caloric intake just as a low-fat diet would, with similar weight-reducing benefits. In other words, weight mismanagement and obesity problems are due to a long-term imbalance between calorie intake versus calorie output (burning of calories), but weight problems are not just carbohydrate-driven issues.

The current American diet has 55% to 60% carbohydrates, mostly high-glycemic carbs, such as sweets and starches.

The Glycemic Index: How Does it Affect Our Health?

There are three simple edible sugars: fructose, which is present in high concentrations in corn sweeteners and a small amount in fruits, galactose and glucose, which are breakdown by-products of table sugar. These simple sugars cause the blood sugar to rise quickly, and in response, the body produces a surge of insulin to help process them, and therefore lower the blood sugar.

The potential of these sugars and all other foods to raise blood sugar is referred to as glycemic index. Foods with greater potential to raise blood sugar levels have higher glycemic indices. Starches, such as bread, cereals, especially the frosted ones, pasta, potato and rice, break down quickly in the intestine into glucose molecules. They can raise the blood sugar within 30–45 minutes in the same way as a handful of table sugar. Starches also have high glycemic indices. (The glycemic index of all foods is compared with white bread, which is set at 100.) Generally, foods with glycemic indices below 70 are considered low glycemic; 70 to 100 are high glycemic; and foods over 100 are very high glycemic.

In healthy people, occasional high glycemic index foods have no serious adverse consequences. In those with cholesterol abnormalities, weight problems, or predisposition to diabetes, high glycemic index foods tend to make the underlying disorders worse. High glycemic index foods more readily convert to fat and accumulate

HIGH GLYCEMIC FOODS
WHAT DO THEY DO?

Long-term consumption of high glycemic foods can…

• Increase post-meal blood sugar and insulin levels, harmful to every organ

• Increase post-meal apoprotein B-100, the harmful protein that accompanies LDL-cholesterol

• Increase post-meal blood triglycerides for several hours

• Increase number of very harmful small LDL particles

• Increase the risk of weight gain and make weight loss more difficult

• Increase the risk of insulin resistance and diabetes

• Lower the good HDL-cholesterol level

• Increase the risk of cardiovascular events

• Increase the risk of colon cancer by more than twofold

GLYCEMIC INDEX OF GRAIN AND DAIRY PRODUCTS

Breads

Bagels	100
Bread, French, Italian, roll, white	100
Bread, hamburger or hotdog bun	100
Bread, multigrain, sourdough	80
Bread, pumpernickel, whole wheat	80
Bread, rye	90
Croissant	100
Kaiser roll	105
Melba toast	105
Potato bread	105
Waffles	110

Cakes

Angel food	105
Banana	80
Pound	85
Sponge	100
Most other cakes	110

Donuts, unglazed	105
Donuts, glazed	115

Cereals

All Bran	65
Bran Buds or Raisin Bran	90
Bran Chex	90
Cheerios, plain	90
Cheerios, frosted, honey	110
Coco Pops	110
Corn or Rice Chex, or flakes, unfrosted	105
Corn or Rice Chex, or flakes, frosted	130
Cream of Wheat	90
Crispex	125
Golden Grahams	110
Grape Nuts	105
Mini-wheats, unfrosted	80
Mini-wheats, frosted	105

GLYCEMIC INDEX OF GRAIN AND DAIRY PRODUCTS (*Continued*)

Nutri-grain or Product 19	90	Rice, low amylose	125
Oat bran	80	Rice cake	120
Puffed wheat	110	Wheat, whole	65
Quick oats	90	**Dairy**	
Rice Krispies	120	Cheese, cottage, goat, ricotta	45
Shredded Wheat	80	Cheese, processed	40
Shredded Wheat, frosted	105	Ice cream	95
Team	110	Milk, chocolate	50
Total	120	Milk, skim, 2% or whole	45
Grains		Yogurt, plain	20
		Yogurt, with fruit plus sugar or fructose	45
Corn	80	**Eggs**	
Rice, basmati	85	Eggs, hard or soft boiled, poached	40
Rice, brown	85	Eggs, omelets, scrambled	35
Rice, high amylose	90		

GLYCEMIC INDEX OF FRUITS, VEGETABLES AND MEATS

Fruit		Orange juice	75
Apples	50	Peach	40
Apple juice, unsweetened	55	Peach, canned in syrup	85
Apricot	45	Peach, canned in unsweetened juice	50
Blueberries, raspberries, strawberries	35	Pear	50
Banana	80	Pineapple	90
Cantaloupe	80	Plum	35
Cherries	35	Raisins	70
Fruit cocktail, unsweetened	70	Watermelon	95
Grapefruit	35	**Legumes**	
Grapes	70	Black-eyed peas	45
Kiwi	60	Butter beans	45
Oranges	65	Canned beans	55

GLYCEMIC INDEX OF FRUITS, VEGETABLES AND MEATS (*Continued*)

Chickpeas	50	Popcorn	80
Dried beans	40	Potato, baked	120
Green beans	45	Potato, french fries	110
Kidney beans	45	Potato, mashed	105
Lentils	40	Potato, sweet	85
Lima beans	50	Potato chips	105
Pinto beans	55	Tomato	45
Red or black beans	45	**Meats**	
Soy beans	40	Fish and shellfish	40
Split peas	45	Chicken and turkey	50
Vegetables		Beef, pork and lamb	50
Carrots	80	**Pastas**	
Celery	30	Various pastas and noodles	100
Corn	70	Pasta with tomato and meat or cheese	80
Corn chips	100	**Nuts**	
Green leafy vegetables	30	Almond, hazel nut, pistachios, walnut	40
Green herbs	30	Other nuts	45
Peas, dried	30		
Peas, green	50		

in fat cells; thus they are more *obesogenic*. Numerous studies have shown that high glycemic foods result in less satiety, more hunger and more total calorie consumption compared with the low glycemic foods.

A large body of evidence strongly suggests that long-term consumption of high glycemic index foods can contribute to insulin resistance or diabetes and significantly increase the risk of breast and colorectal cancers. (Long-term consumption of high glycemic index foods triggers the release of certain carcinogenic compounds such as insulin-like growth factors.)

Glycemic indices of foods are not etched in stone—they tend to vary depending on a number of factors. For example, the tiny amount of the weak acid added to sourdough bread *lowers* its glycemic index compared with white bread made with similar dough but without the acid. Physical characteristics, cooking method or added ingredients can also alter the glycemic index of a food. For example, bleached, low-fiber or finely ground flours have higher glycemic indices. Toasting the bread, adding jam or marmalades to bread or syrup to waffles, baking a potato or eating the potato without the skin all increase the glycemic indices. On the other hand, mixing a high glycemic food with vegetables, fruit or some fat lowers the glycemic index.

What About Dietary Fructose?

Fructose, mainly derived from corn, is a simple sugar increasingly used as a sweetener, mainly because it is the sweetest of all natural sugars and is less expensive than beet or cane sugar. Soda bottlers, for example, can save about a penny a bottle or can by substituting or replacing sugar in their products, saving millions of dollars each year. Most processed food that requires any sweetener—beverages, dairy products, canned, baked or other processed foods —contains high fructose corn sweetener.

Although small amounts of fructose are quite safe, regular high consumption may contribute to the risk of developing abdominal obesity, type 2 diabetes, lower levels of HDL-cholesterol and higher levels of triglycerides. It can also cause significant digestive symptoms such as gaseousness, bloating, cramps or diarrhea.

A recent study published in the *American Journal of Gastroenterology* showed that for people with irritable bowel syndrome, consuming even small amounts of fructose—including high fructose fruits, such as apples, bananas, cherries, dates, grapes, pears and plums—may aggravate their digestive symptoms.

The price of corn has doubled in the past few years, as huge amounts of corn are being diverted to produce ethanol and other "biofuels" for energy, making corn less appealing as a source of high-fructose sweetener. This shift might benefit the public by reducing the exposure to high-fructose sweetener and may encourage the food manufacturers to use less sweeteners of any kind in our food staple.

Dietary Proteins

In general, dietary proteins do not play a significant role in coronary artery disease. However, maternal protein malnutrition, which often results in low birth weight, is a major risk factor for developing coronary artery disease and diabetes in the future. On the other hand, excessive protein intake may increase blood levels of homocysteine, another major risk factor for coronary artery disease, or contribute to poor kidney function—especially among the elderly, diabetics or those with preexisting kidney disorders.

Adequate intake of high-quality proteins such as those in seafood, eggs, poultry and other lean meats provides a variety of essential amino acids for growth, development and normal function of nearly all humans cells.

Although elite athletes and bodybuilders need foods with more high-quality protein than most other people, their needs can usually be better met by eating more protein than by taking protein powders or supplements. Despite commercial hype and celebrity testimonials, there is scant evidence to show that these formulas have any advantage over dietary sources of protein for athletes. Elite athletes also need more complex carbohydrates to enhance their performance by providing adequate amounts of glucose to their muscles. Since glucose also has a protein-sparing effect, these athletes can actually benefit more by increasing dietary carbohydrates to about 55% to 60% of daily energy intake than by taking protein supplements.

Dietary proteins do not have any effects on heart health or cancer. Unlike dietary fat or carbohydrates, proteins do not contribute to obesity. High-quality proteins, such as seafood, poultry (without skin and not fried), legumes and low-fat dairy products, provide many choices for enjoyable eating. Since the rate of protein absorption is relatively slow, overeating at one meal loaded with dietary proteins may be a wasteful effort. You can utilize dietary proteins more effectively by spreading your intake over three or four meals instead of eating huge steaks at dinner followed by protein powder.

There is no scientific evidence to support the usefulness of high protein supplements, whether for weight loss, bodybuilding, enhancing "immune-power," menopausal symptoms, osteoporosis or anything else. Long-term use of very high-protein diets, especially those with very high-fat content, are counterproductive for individuals with cardiovascular disorders, kidney disease or diabetes.

What about soy protein and other soy products?

Soy products are promoted in the US as the cure-all nutrients that we have been missing. There has been endless hype and misinformation about the supposed benefits of soy products. In 1999 the US Food and Drug Administration allowed soy product manufacturers to make the claim that "25 grams of soy protein a day, as part of a diet low in saturated fat and cholesterol, may reduce the risk of heart disease." Their decision was based upon inadequate information available at the time. Soy product manufacturers have been running with that seal of approval ever since even though recent data provide no support for their claims.

In 2006, the American Heart Association Nutrition Committee reviewed 22 randomized studies of soy protein or its antioxidants (isoflavones). The AHA Nutrition Committee found no evidence that soy products have a significant impact on LDL-cholesterol, HDL-cholesterol, triglycerides or blood pressure and they provide no cardio-protective benefit. The AHA Nutrition Committee and many recent reports have not found any evidence to suggest that soy products have any beneficial impact on reducing menopausal symptoms or the risk of osteoporosis or any cancer.

It is now clear that soy milk, soy proteins and other soy products, especially as fermented and produced in the US, have no redeeming health value. A 2007 report from the US Department of Agriculture Human Nutrition Research Center on Aging (at Tufts University) showed that consumption of differently processed soy products had little or no effect on cardiovascular risk factors.

The impact of soy protein on blood pressure and cholesterol

- In 22 randomized studies with soy protein (about 50 gm, or nearly two-thirds of daily protein requirement), LDL-cholesterol was decreased by a trivial three percent.

- In 19 other similar studies, soy protein had no significant effect on blood pressure, LDL-cholesterol, HDL-cholesterol or triglycerides.

- A recent large study confirmed previous findings that high intake of fruits, vegetables and legumes (without soy products) lowered blood pressure by five to eight points.

- *A cautionary note:* There is a graded association between soy protein intake and bladder cancer (the higher the intake, the greater the risk).

Are soy products harmful?

Aside from the fact that most soy products have no taste or culinary "personality," even when disguised by various spices and sauces, an occasional serving is harmless. However, several reports strongly suggest that frequent consumption of soy protein may increase the risk of bladder cancer.

There are two major misunderstandings regarding soy products—and neither is discussed by soy promoters, nor understood by the public healthcare providers. First, soy products in the

US and most of Europe are distinctly different from soy products in the Far East. The Westernized versions are fermented in such a way that most of soy's flavonoids and antioxidants are stripped away. Second, people in the Far East start eating soy products and soy milk as infants and toddlers, so they are continuously exposed to soy's isoflavones for decades.

Americans tend to start eating soy products in their 30s and 40s, consuming a bit once or twice a week, believing that they are promoting their heath. A piece of tofu drowned in sugar or high-fructose corn sweetener or cubed as a cheese-imitation in salad offers no health (or culinary) benefit.

This is particularly true among meat and potato eaters who may not eat any dark fruits or vegetables.

Vitamin and Mineral Supplements: Which Ones And How Much?

Hundreds of biological actions happen constantly within each living cell. These programmed exchanges produce supercharged chemical compounds that are called "free radicals," or "oxygen free radicals," or simply "oxidants."

Sometimes free radicals cause havoc within a cell, interfere with its normal function or actually destroy it. One example of this is ultraviolet light that causes sunburn. In addition to causing physical damage, ultraviolet light triggers the release of free radicals inside the top layers of the skin, which in turn cause tissue damage, long after sunburn has healed.

Most cells readily defend themselves against the onslaught of oxidant charge; otherwise life would not exist. The defenders that fight off and neutralize the oxidants are called antioxidants. Some antioxidants are made within our own body, but many come from outside sources, such as foods and supplements. These two groups of antioxidants work in tandem and often in tiers, much like the deployment of military defensive forces; when one defensive line is exhausted or depleted, the other takes over.

Vitamin E

Vitamin E refers to a collection of eight different compounds. Alpha-tocopherol is the best known and most potent of these compounds. One main reason for the higher efficacy of alpha-tocopherol is that in humans and many mammals, vitamin E has a special "transfer agent," a protein that carries it from the intestine to and from the liver for distribution to various organs. Other forms of vitamin E are 50% to 70% less transportable. This makes these other compounds less effective. No matter how potent an antioxidant is in a test tube, it is worthless if it cannot be transported within the bloodstream to target organs.

Vitamin E is one of the most difficult nutrients to obtain through diet. This sounds surprising, doesn't it? In fact, only eight percent of US men and two percent of women have dietary vitamin E intake (from non-fortified oils and cereals) that meets the Estimated Average Requirement of 12 mg alpha-tocopherol per day.

Another issue is that we don't absorb every single milligram of vitamin E that we ingest. People who take supplements containing vitamin E often take them in the morning with fat-free or low-fat breakfast. But vitamin E, a fat-soluble vitamin, needs some accompanying at to be absorbed. On average only about 10% of vitamin E taken with a fat-free meal is absorbed compared to 20% with a low-fat and 33% with a high-fat meal. This low efficiency absorption of vitamin E may be one reason for conflicting data on the role of vitamin E in health and various diseases. The need for adequate fat intake to other fat soluble is similar vitamins, such as A, D and lycopene.

At present, research indicates that supplemental vitamin E has no significant heart health benefit among those who have already developed coronary artery disease. Although a large body of evidence suggests that dietary vitamin E may have a small role in the prevention of cardiovascular diseases, the studies are not compelling or convincing enough to justify recommending supplemental vitamin E for this purpose.

Does higher dietary or supplemental vitamin E have any health benefit?

Several studies have suggested that long-term use of vitamin E at high doses may slow down the progression of Alzheimer's disease. However, the Chicago Health and Aging Project report suggests that it's primarily dietary vitamin E (from food, oils, fruits and vegetables) that may have a protective effect against the cognitive decline of Alzheimer's disease, not supplemental vitamin E. In other words, it is the cooperation among various other nutrients and antioxidants with vitamin E that provides the protective effect.

A recent eight-year follow-up study of more than 29,000 men by the National Cancer Institute showed that among smokers, supplemental vitamin E in doses greater than 400 IU/day significantly reduced the risk of invasive prostate cancer. However, vitamin E showed no cancer protection for nonsmokers. These results suggest that smokers may have a relative deficiency of or higher requirement for vitamin E and vitamin C.

Consumers tend to expect too much from individual vitamins. This is particularly true for antioxidant vitamins such as beta-carotene, vitamin C and vitamin E. These vitamins, when taken alone, are not very effective because they cannot work in isolation. It is the synergy and cooperation among many vitamins, minerals and thousands of other compounds in a diet enriched with plenty of different fruits and vegetables over many years that collectively reduce the risk of various chronic diseases. Moreover, our bodies produce an endless number of oxidants. They differ from each other and they respond to specific antioxidants. In this way, oxidants are very much like bacteria and their sensitivity or resistance to different antibiotics. Vitamin C or E cannot be antioxidants to every single form of oxidant that the body produces or is exposed to. How this simple fact seems to escape antioxidant zealots is beyond comprehension! In fact, vitamins C and E can be oxidized themselves, making them turncoat oxidants! Nutritional isolationism and popping individual vitamins helps manufacturers of dietary supplements but they do nothing to enhance our health or promote positive, healthy aging.

VITAMIN E AND COGNITIVE DECLINE AND ALZHEIMER'S DISEASE

CHICAGO HEALTH AND AGING PROJECT, a four year-follow-up of 1,041 community residents over 65 years of age

- Each 5 mg/day increase in *dietary* a-tocopherol (from fruits/vegetables and olive oil) reduced the incidence of Alzheimer's disease by 26%.

- Each 5 mg/day increase in *dietary* a-tocopherol intake reduced the rate of cognitive decline by 20%.

- The protective effect of dietary vitamin E was observed only in those without Apoprotein E4. Apoprotein E4-E4 significantly increases the risk of Alzheimer's disease.#

- These findings explain in part the failure of high-dose a-tocopherol *supplements* to show a consistent benefit in the general population.

*Morris MC et al. Am J Clin Nutr 2005; 81: 508–14.
#Apoprotein E is a genetically inherited protein.

What's the dosage?

The biological potency (but not antioxidant potency) of all vitamin E preparations are standardized with international units (IU) instead of milligrams. The consumer should not be overly concerned about the natural versus the synthetic varieties. For those with severe cholesterol disorders or high triglyceride levels, and for diabetics, the high antioxidant potency of synthetic alpha-tocopherol is actually a desirable feature. In other cases, either the natural form or a mix of both natural and synthetic forms are reasonable alternatives. Except in cases of Alzheimer's disease, no valid scientific study suggests that doses higher than 400 IU per day provide any additional benefit.

What about a combination of multiple vitamins and minerals?

Many credible studies suggest that a combination of multivitamins and minerals may offer some health benefits. For example, age-related macular degeneration (AMD) is the most common cause of adult blindness in developed countries. The eye's retina is particularly sensitive to oxidant damage that occurs over many years, contributing to AMD. Thus an early preventive strategy might reduce the risk of this major disability.

A large, eight-year follow-up study of 4,170 men and women, 55 years or older, showed that high dietary intake of beta-carotene, vitamin C, vitamin E and zinc was associated with a 35% lower risk of developing macular degeneration. These results were reported in the *Journal of the American Medical Association*. Similarly, lutein lycopene and zeaxantine in dark fruits and vegetables provide significant protection against AMD.

Multiple vitamins with minerals have been shown in numerous well-conducted studies to improve immune functions.

A six-year, randomized study of women infected with HIV showed that a safe, inexpensive combination of vitamins and minerals delayed the progression and eventual death from HIV by nearly 30%, compared with those who took a placebo.

Since aging is frequently associated with decreased immune function and diabetics or those with chronic liver disease are all at higher risk for developing various infections or cancers, they, too, might benefit from taking one to two multivitamins with minerals tablets daily. Studies have also suggested a cancer-protecting benefit for a combination of multiple vitamins with minerals.

Vitamin C

Vitamin C is perhaps the most abused vitamin. More than 90% of Americans who take nutritional supplements take vitamin C, either alone or as a component of multivitamins.

Why take vitamin C?

Vitamin C can prevent (and cure) scurvy. That said, all other benefits attributed to vitamin C are vastly exaggerated. Smart consumers should view these claims with a healthy dose of skepticism. Taking 1,000 to 2,000 mg of vitamin C (approximately 10 to 20 times the recommended daily allowance) can shorten the course of a common cold by a day or a half-day. This trivial benefit can hardly justify taking such large doses on a daily basis.

The absorption of vitamin C from a 200 mg dose is almost complete. However, as you take more than 200 mg per day, its absorption from the intestine decreases sharply, and a large portion is essentially wasted in the stool. For example, of a 2,500 mg dose, only 10% to 20% (about 250 to 500 mg) will be absorbed. Also, as the blood level of vitamin C goes up, its excretion and elimination in the urine increases considerably.

Excessive doses of vitamin C increase urinary excretion of oxalate and uric acid and contribute to the formation of kidney stones. High doses of vitamin C can cause indigestion, heartburn, diarrhea or bloating. It can also increase the absorption of iron, which is not only an oxidant, but may accumulate in the heart, pancreas, liver, gonads and brain, at times causing severe complications in each of these organs. Vitamin C can also interfere with the absorption of chromium, and by doing so increase insulin resistance.

Does vitamin C provide any benefits?

Since vitamin C plays an important antioxidant role in the eyes. Moderate dietary or supplement intake can reduce the risk of cataracts. It may also reduce oxidation of LDL-cholesterol in the bloodstream, especially in diabetics who have a high oxidant load.

Recent studies have also shown that vitamin C reduces the oxidization of nitric oxide—a potent dilator and protector of coronary arteries. This role of vitamin C in preserving or promoting the function of nitric oxide may have a potentially beneficial impact for people with coronary artery disease or hypertension. A recent study, for example, showed that a 500 mg daily dose of vitamin C lowered the systolic blood pressure by 10 points.

How much do you need?

For optimal benefits from vitamin C supplements with minimal or no side effects, 200 to 500 mg per day is adequate.

Smokers should not think that taking 500 or 1,000 mg of vitamin C daily can protect against harmful effects of smoking. Nevertheless, for those who are unable to stop smoking, supplemental vitamin C may have some relevance.

For people who have diabetes, elevated blood cholesterol, abdominal obesity, or other coronary risk factors, and for those with chronic gastritis or pernicious anemia (which predisposes a person to a higher risk of stomach cancer), vitamin C at a dose of 200 to 500 mg per day is a reasonable addition to a diet high in fruits and vegetables.

Beta-carotene and the heart

Carotenoids are made up of a group of more than 1,200 compounds that are, more or less, close to vitamin A. Beta-carotene is the most publicized and perhaps one of the least useful commercially available carotenoids.

At current doses of 25 to 100 mg per day, beta-carotene has no significant cardiovascular benefit. Based on its biological activity, there is no plausible reason why larger doses would prove heart healthy. Although other carotenoids such as lutein, zeaxathine and lycopene have no significant cardio-protective role, they do have many other benefits. You can read more about them starting on page 147.

The B vitamins and vitamin B3

Despite side effects associated with niacin (vitamin B3), it is still the best drug for raising HDL-cholesterol, lowering lipoprotein(a) and reducing the number of small, coronary-unfriendly LDL particles. The minimum effective dose of niacin is about 1000 to 1500 mg per day.

At high doses, niacin has a number of undesirable side effects that cause nearly half the people who try it to stop taking it. It can cause flushing of the face and chest and a sunburn sensation that may last from minutes to an hour or so after each dose. It can also produce a generalized rash and itching. These skin side effects can be prevented by taking one regular aspirin (325 mg) or ibuprofen (200 mg). However,

IMPACT OF VARIOUS NUTRIENTS ON CANCERS				
Nutrient	**Breast**	**Colon**	**Lung**	**Prostate**
Saturated Fats	No effect	No effect	No effect	No effect
Omega-6 PUFA	Increases	Increases	No effect	No effect
Trans Fats	Increases	Increases	No effect	Increases
Omega-3 PUFA	Decreases	Decreases	No effect	No effect
Monounsaturates	Decreases	Decreases	No effect	Decreases
Fruits and Vegetables	Decreases	Decreases	No effect	Decreases
Folic Acid	Decreases	Decreases	No effect	Decreases
Selenium	Decreases	Decreases	No effect	Decreases
Lycopene	No effect	Decreases	Decreases	Decreases
Vitamins C and E	No effect	No effect	Unknown	Decreases
Calcium plus Vitamin D	No effect	Decreases	No effect	No effect
Dairy Products	No effect	Decreases	No effect	No effect
Alcohol*	Unknown	Decreases	No effect	No effect
Aspirin*	No effect	Decreases	No effect	Decreases

*Although alcohol and aspirin are not "nutrients," they are consumed widely by a large number of people, and so are inserted in this table.

frequent doses of aspirin or ibuprofen increase the risk of gastrointestinal side effects, including bleeding.

Niacin can also cause heartburn, nausea, elevation of blood sugar levels and abnormalities of liver tests. Liver test abnormalities are often innocent findings and are due to overproduction and leakage of certain enzymes into the bloodstream. In some rare cases, niacin can cause a drug-induced hepatitis.

Most niacin side effects can be avoided when it is used judiciously and under a physician's supervision.

Starting doses of niacin should not exceed 125 to 250 mg at mealtime. The dose can be increased slightly every week or two to allow for adaptation to higher doses. As the dose of niacin is increased, the side effects gradually subside and stop. But if the drug is missed for even a day or two, some of the side effects may return when it is restarted. This underscores the importance of daily compliance to your regimen.

 WARNING: More than 30 different formulations of niacin are commercially available. Unfortunately, some of them are not absorbed adequately when taken by mouth. Some brands claim to produce no flushing. They are essentially useless because they lack free nicotinic acid. Instead, these products may contain inositol, niacinamide, nicotinamide or other niacin derivatives that have no impact on HDL-cholesterol.

Delayed-release, sustained-action, long-acting or similar niacin products are somewhat more likely to cause liver injury than the short-acting varieties. However, they may also cause less flushing or stomach irritation. A prescription-only niacin (Niaspan) is designed to be taken at night. Unfortunately, as with all other brands at high doses (more than 1000 mg), many people may experience flushing and upper abdominal symptoms with Niaspan. And, the cost is several times higher than other brands.

Some drug companies are developing niacin-like drugs that are better tolerated and have fewer side effects. Some of these drugs should be available within the next few years and may prove to be extremely useful for raising HDL-cholesterol or lowering elevated levels of lipoprotein(a).

Vitamins B6, B9 (folic acid) and B12

The primary cardiovascular role of folic acid and vitamin B12 is in reducing blood level of homocysteine. Folic acid has many other benefits including lowering the risk of breast and prostate cancer, reducing the rate of cognitive decline and dementia and prevention of neurological defects.

Although vitamin B6 may have a small role in further lowering of homocysteine when added to folic acid and vitamin B12, it does not have any significant cardiovascular role.

✳ **CAUTION:** Large doses of vitamin B6 (pyridoxine) can cause sensory nerve damage. You should not take doses exceeding 100 mg per day. Since many individuals with elevated blood homocysteine levels do not show a good response to vitamin B6 alone, it should always be used with folic acid and vitamin B12.

Cardiovascular and health impact of minerals

Several minerals, including selenium, chromium, calcium, magnesium, iron, sodium and potassium, have significant impacts on the cardiovascular system.

Selenium

Selenium is a potent antioxidant in multiple tissues, including coronary artery wall and plaques therein. Selenium is also one of the most effective dietary anti-carcinogens (especially against prostate, colon and breast cancers). Any "healthy-heart" benefit is a bonus.

Decreased selenium intake can also contribute to age-relayed cognitive decline in older persons. A nine-year follow-up study of over 1300 people aged 60 to 71 showed that people whose blood selenium levels were low had greater cognitive decline than those with high levels.

At 200 mcg (0.2 mg) per day, selenium supplements are safe. At this dose, blood selenium levels will still be far below 1000 nanogram per millimeter of whole blood, the safe level set by the Environmental Protection Agency. Higher intake may be associated with diarrhea, irritability, hair loss and changes in the fingernail and toenail.

Seafood, kidney and liver (and to a lesser extent, other meats and grains) are good sources of selenium. Fruits and vegetables generally contain little selenium, especially if they were grown in selenium-poor soil.

Chromium

There have been many scientific studies of chromium. A recent US Department of Agriculture study showed that taking chromium supplements of 200 to 1000 mcg per day substantially improves blood sugar control in type 2 diabetics (those who do not require insulin). Higher doses showed proportionately better improvements, approaching the results obtained with oral anti-diabetes medications.

The average dietary intake of chromium in the US population is about 50 mcg per day. In another study, even adding 100 mcg of chromium picolinate—the most common form of over-the-counter chromium—to a daily diet significantly improved blood sugar control.

Some studies have suggested that extra chromium can reduce blood levels of LDL-cholesterol and triglycerides by as much as 10%

while raising the level of the good HDL-cholesterol by five percent. These beneficial cholesterol actions of chromium, combined with improved sugar metabolism, undoubtedly contribute to better cardiovascular health.

Another study suggested that chromium supplementation (200 to 400 mcg per day) can help overweight people lose body fat and improve their lean-to-fat ratio. This is an important distinction when compared to other weight loss medications that usually cause loss of lean muscle tissues as well as body fat.

How much chromium do you need?

Because chromium can decrease insulin resistance and improve the metabolism of carbohydrates, it is a reasonable and safe supplement, especially for sedentary or obese individuals and diabetics. For these uses, 200 mcg taken two times a day should be sufficient.

Foods containing high levels of chromium include: Processed cheeses (such as American or cheddar), wheat germ, brewer's yeast, organ meats (liver and kidney) and seafood. Since vitamin C interferes with the absorption of chromium, the two should not be taken together, especially with vitamin C doses exceeding 100 to 200 mg.

Iron

Numerous studies over the past two decades have strongly suggested that excessive iron increases the risk of heart attacks, while iron depletion has a "healthy-heart" role. It is thought that iron, especially at high concentrations, may act like an oxidant, promoting the oxidization of LDL-cholesterol, and it may increase tissue damage within the heart muscle.

The consensus of recent studies is that excessive body iron does not play a role in the initiation of coronary plaques, but it does increase the risk of a heart attack and other cardiovascular events.

Although excessive body iron can increase the risk of a heart attack, iron deficiency can be harmful, too. It is associated with anemia, tiredness and the reduced capacity of the heart and other muscles to perform at optimum levels or to provide enough oxygen to vital organs.

Nearly one out of 400 Americans has a genetic disorder that predisposes him or her to absorb a very high percentage of dietary or supplemental iron. This condition is called "hemochromatosis," and it causes severe heart, liver, pancreas and brain damage. Recent studies have shown that in people with hemochromatosis, even in its mild form, the risk of heart attack is increased more than twofold. The combination of high body iron with smoking and high blood pressure is even more dangerous—it raises the risk of a heart attack.

 CAUTION: Routine use of iron supplements for "energy," "pep," "stress," or other falsely advertised reasons—especially when combined with vitamin C, which increases iron absorption—is quite harmful especially in people with hemochromatosis.

Excessive body iron is one of the "unknown" risk factors for coronary artery disease.

Should you take iron?

Supplemental iron, invariably present in "multivitamins with minerals," is completely unnecessary for men and post-menopausal women who do not have iron deficiency. Further, iron products do not boost or provide energy and they cannot help tiredness or fatigue if you are not iron-deficient. The potential harmful effect of iron supplements is even larger among people with elevated blood cholesterol or homocysteine and in hypertensives and smokers.

Avoid iron pills unless you have a diagnosis of iron-deficiency anemia.

Women in their childbearing years who lose blood with their monthly menstrual flow may benefit from small amounts of iron added to their daily diet. Others who wish to take multivitamin or mineral supplements should choose one without iron.

Dietary sources of iron include red meats, poultry, seafood, eggs, vegetables, and fortified cereals. Absorption of iron from various meats (red or white) is far more efficient than from vegetables, fruits or cereal, because they contain different kinds of iron, with different degrees of bioavailability.

Calcium

Calcium is essential for the proper function of many cells, including muscle cells of the heart and arteries throughout the body. Calcium's impact on coronary arteries, however, is relatively minor.

Although calcium may be present in many coronary and other arterial plaques, it does not play a roll in producing these plaques. Along with other compounds in the bloodstream such as copper, iron and magnesium, calcium is trapped in pre-existing and usually advanced plaques. This passive entry of calcium into plaques has spawned marketing gimmicks by manufacturers of CAT scanners and clinics that promote "coronary calcium scan" as a lifesaving test. I find the coronary calcium scan a nearly useless test.

Data from 22 randomized studies showed that calcium supplementation decreases systolic blood pressure by an average of only two points. For most hypertensives, this is a trivial drop.

Since there may be a threshold of calcium intake below which the blood pressure may rise, calcium supplementation may still be useful for some hypertensive persons. Some hypertensive people, for example, tend to eat fewer dairy products (a rich source of calcium), either on their own or on the advice of a health provider to "cut down fat and cholesterol."

Pregnant women are also at risk for developing hypertension. Recent studies have shown that calcium supplementation reduces pregnancy-induced hypertension by 70%, and toxemia of pregnancy—a serious disease—by nearly 60%. Certainly, in this group, extra calcium can be beneficial in helping to keep the mother and fetus healthy.

Calcium and osteoporosis

Most consumers assume that taking one or two calcium tablets can improve bone mineral density and reduce the risk of osteoporosis bone fractures. These assumptions are not exactly justified.

Many studies have suggested that any benefit of calcium and vitamin D supplements, especially at low doses (under 1200 mg/day for calcium, and under 800 IU for vitamin D), on bone mineral density and osteoporosis at best is very small. This is particularly true among post-menopausal women who are not on estrogen replacement therapy or other anti-osteoporosis drugs.

The Women's Health Initiative Clinical Trials recruited more than 36,000 post-menopausal women, from 50 to 79 years of age, and followed them for seven years. The women who took an average of 1000 mg calcium carbonate along with 400 IU of vitamin D daily, showed no significant reduction in the risk of hip or spinal fractures compared with those who took the placebo.

Unfortunately, this study was somewhat flawed in that the recommended doses of both calcium and vitamin D were too low. It was designed in early 1990s, when the requirement for higher doses of calcium and vitamin D were not fully understood. Even at these low doses, less than 60% of women took them for the duration of the study. Thus it is possible, as suggested by other studies, that higher doses taken for many years could have some protective effect. Optimal total calcium and vitamin D intake should be higher than 1500 mg/day and 1500 IU/day respectively. This requires supplementation of 1200 mg and 1200 IU of calcium and vitamin D.

Remember that other measures are needed to improve bone mineral density and decrease the risk of fractures in both women and men. These measures include better nutrition, higher protein, fruit and vegetable intake, regular physical activities; estrogen replacement therapy for younger menopausal women when appropriate, and anti-osteoporosis drugs for those who have already developed osteoporosis.

Does supplemental calcium have any cancer protective role?

Colorectal cancer is the only cancer for which calcium supplementation may have a protective role. Many studies have shown that supplemental calcium and vitamin D in doses greater than 1200 mg/day and 800 IU/day, respectively, can reduce the risk of developing colon polyps. That's significant because polyps may have the potential to become cancerous.

A Swedish study of 45,306 men, from 45 to 79 years of age, who were followed up for more than 6½ years showed a 30% risk reduction for those with the highest calcium intake. Thus, the findings of this and other studies support the potential benefit of calcium and vitamin D supplements of more than 1200 mg/day and more than 800 IU/day, respectively, for protection against osteoporosis and colorectal cancer.

Vitamin D has been the subject of many recent studies, which have shown that at high doses (more than 1200 IU), it can reduce the risk of some cancers, including breast, colon, prostate and pancreas.

Can calcium supplements cause kidney stones?

More than 90% of kidney stones are made up of a mixture of calcium and oxalate. Doctors and other healthcare providers, including nutritionists, often tell people who have had a history of kidney stones to avoid taking calcium or vitamin D. This is a common mistake based on inadequate understanding of how kidney stones are formed.

Oxalate is present in many foods and is readily absorbed from the intestine. The kidneys eliminate oxalate in the urine. However, some calcium is also eliminated, and once the two of them meet in urinary tubes inside the kidneys they bind together, forming the core of a kidney stone. As this tiny piece grows, eventually it becomes a jagged and often irregular-shaped stone, which may vary in size from a grain of sand to a pea or larger.

When calcium is taken with meals, it binds with dietary oxalate in the intestine and will help dramatically reduce the absorption of oxalate. The oxalate-colon combination is then eliminated in the stools. Hence, there is none or very little oxalate in the bloodstream to be filtered out by the kidneys and cause kidney stones. When calcium supplements are taken with meals, on a daily basis, approximately 200 to 300 mg of calcium is used up to bind oxalate in the intestine and dispose of it. The absorbed calcium is then utilized for other body needs, including bone formation and prevention of osteoporosis, without increasing the risk of kidney stones.

The amount of calcium "wasted" in binding with oxalate in the intestine does not reduce the available calcium. That's because we never absorb all the calcium we put in our stomach. In fact, we don't absorb more than 30% to 50% of the calcium. The rest is eliminated in the stools anyway, but when it binds with oxalate, at least it serves a useful purpose.

Bioavailability of different calcium products may vary by formulation by as much as 200% to 300%. Calcium citrate seems to be more efficiently absorbed than calcium carbonate. The fractional absorption of calcium decreases further with high doses so taking too much calcium at one time is counterproductive. For this reason, divide the dose between breakfast and dinner to improve the absorption efficiency instead of taking all of it once a day.

Calcium from dairy products and fortified orange juice is more bioavailable than other types of calcium such as Oscal, oyster shell pills, Tums or Rolaids. However, bones need calcium and phosphorus, both of which are preserved in a balanced ratio in milk and non-processed dairy products (milk, yogurt, cottage cheese). Calcium fortified juices or soy milk do not have the balanced calcium and phosphorus.

Good dietary sources of calcium and phosphorous are…

- All low-fat dairy products. Processed cheeses not only have too much saturated fat, but a large amount of salt.
- Leafy and green vegetables, such as kale, spinach and broccoli.
- Calcium-fortified foods and beverages (including orange juice).
- Drinking water, which surprisingly, contains some calcium and phosphorous. However, home water filters or water purifiers remove a substantial amount not only of calcium and phosphorous but other minerals as well. Most bottled waters have practically no calcium, phosphorous, fluoride or other minerals.
- Some sun exposure (but not sunburn). This helps our own body produce far more vitamin D than we could ever obtain from dietary sources or supplements. In fact, your skin can

synthesize as much as 10,000 IU of vitamin D, equal to 25 vitamin D pills or several gallons of milk.

The common warning to stay out of the sun, or the recommendation to cover your body, wear hats, and use plenty of sunscreen lotion before you step outside is an irrational approach to protect people against skin cancers. Skin cancers, including the dreaded melanoma, may be triggered by repeated sunburn, an issue distinctly different from sun exposure for an hour or so daily.

As noted earlier, high blood levels of vitamin D can dramatically reduce the risk of many catastrophic cancers, including breast, colon, pancreas, prostate and even melanoma by as much as 45% (Giovannucci, E et al. J Natl Cancer Inst 2005, 98: 451–59).

Approximately 200,000 people die each year from these few cancers, and another 85,000 die from osteoporosis. Basal cell skin cancers are nuisances that are readily cured by removing them.

A more balanced and rational approach is to encourage people of all ages, especially those over 50, to get out as often as they can during the non-peak hours of ultraviolet light (1pm to 3pm). Strolling in shorts and tee-shirts, or stretching out prone and supine for 30 to 60 minutes daily when possible (*without suntan lotion*) are reasonable means of synthesizing your own vitamin D. For those with a previous history of facial skin cancer or repeated sunburn, the use of sunscreen on the face or wearing a hat should enable them to have sun exposure to other parts of their bodies.

Magnesium

After potassium, magnesium is the second most abundant mineral in human tissues, except in bones. National survey data have shown that dietary magnesium intake is inadequate in the US population, especially among women and elderly. Magnesium has numerous functions, but within the cardiovascular system, its main role is to relax the arteries and prevent irritability of the heart muscle that contributes to irregular heart rhythm. Intravenous infusion of magnesium in people who suffer an acute heart attack has been shown to significantly reduce the risk of life-threatening cardiac arrhythmias.

A recent study examined the relation of blood magnesium levels to coronary artery disease. Nearly 14,000 middle-aged adults from four communities (who were free of cardiovascular diseases at the beginning of the study) were followed up for four to seven years. The results showed that women with the highest blood magnesium levels had about 50% less risk of developing coronary artery disease compared to women with the lowest blood levels. Men who had the highest blood magnesium levels had 27% less risk than men with the lowest levels. The study also showed that mortality from coronary artery disease is significantly lower among men and women who live in hard water areas (containing higher calcium and magnesium levels) than among those living in soft-water areas.

It is unclear how or why low blood levels of magnesium contribute to coronary artery disease. In animal studies, magnesium deficiency can cause swelling and distortion of endothelial cells (lining the inner wall of the arteries), thereby allowing LDL-cholesterol and white blood cells to cross through this barrier. Several studies have suggested that low intake of magnesium can raise the triglycerides and lower the good HDL-cholesterol, and increase the risk of diabetes, which itself is the most potent risk factor for cardiovascular diseases. A recent Harvard University study showed that dietary magnesium also has a modest anti-inflammatory effect, which may improve the

---

CHELATION THERAPY: FAITH, HOPE AND HOAX

Advertisers promote chelation therapy as a method to remove calcium and other mineral deposits from the arterial wall, thereby "reversing atherosclerosis." However, chelation therapy is no more than modern-day snake oil. Chelation therapy involves intravenous infusion of a compound called EDTA, usually in combination with vitamins and minerals, once or twice weekly for four to six months. The total cost may be thousands of dollars, and few, if any, health insurers cover it.

Recent studies have clearly established that chelation therapy with EDTA is a useless practice and cannot reduce the size of coronary artery plaques, improve blood circulation or remove much of anything from the atherosclerotic arteries.

EDTA cannot penetrate the plaque core, nor can it dissolve, separate or remove the calcium from the pile of debris in the plaque. Calcium, iron, copper, fibrous tissues, overgrown muscle cells, oxidized cholesterol and other deposits within coronary artery plaques have contributed to a tough, cement-like structure that does not permit EDTA to penetrate it. Even if some deposits could be removed by EDTA, the plaques will not shrink or disappear, and the underlying processes that caused hardening of the arteries in the first place will continue during and after chelation therapy.

---

function of endothelial cells (the inner lining of the arteries) and reduce the risk of cardiovascular events. (Song Y et al. *Am J Clin Nutr 2007*; 85: 1068–74).

Since kidneys have a dominant role in eliminating magnesium, daily variations in dietary magnesium intake do not play a critical role, but long-term low magnesium intake or frequent bouts of diarrhea, which contribute to magnesium loss in the stools, may result in magnesium deficiency.

In general, magnesium supplementation is unnecessary and, at best, it is of doubtful benefit. But in people who have chronic recurrent diarrhea, vomiting, profuse sweating (during sustained rigorous exercises or outdoor activities on hot days), short-term supplementation may be helpful.

Rich dietary sources of magnesium include whole seeds such as nuts, legumes and various grains. Unfortunately, processing removes more than 80% of the magnesium in cereal grains. Green vegetables are also rich in magnesium, but fruits (except bananas), meats, dairy products and seafood are poor sources of magnesium.

Potassium

The role of potassium in cardiovascular health, like calcium, is to regulate heart rhythm, smooth muscle tone in the arterial system and lower blood pressure. Normally, dietary potassium deficiency does not occur. However, a good deal of potassium can be lost through the kidneys (especially when diuretics are used on a regular basis), the gastrointestinal tract (in people with protracted vomiting, diarrhea or laxative abuse) or by profuse sweating. Excessive potassium loss can cause tiredness, weakness, poor appetite, nausea, listlessness or irrational behavior. It can also cause severe (and, rarely, fatal) irregularities of the heart rhythm.

Three recent studies showed that higher potassium intake is associated with a modest drop in systolic (by three points) and diastolic (by two points) blood pressure. African-Americans and older persons are especially responsive to increased potassium intake.

Potassium is abundant in all living cells and can be found in a wide variety of foods. Rich sources of potassium include most fruits (such as figs, oranges, bananas and cantaloupe), fruit juices and vegetables (including root vegetables such as potatoes, carrots and radishes) and various meats, red and white. The average daily intake of potassium in the United States is about 3500 mg per day. However, studies show that among African-Americans, the average daily intake is only half that amount. This lower intake of potassium may be a factor in the high incidence of hypertension in this segment of the population.

One of the easiest ways to increase your dietary potassium and at the same time reduce sodium intake is to use salt substitutes instead of regular salt. Many salt substitutes contain mainly potassium chloride instead of sodium chloride. There are also different "light" or "lite" salts that, depending on the manufacturer, may contain various combinations of sodium chloride, potassium chloride or magnesium chloride. The net result is that they all have less table salt (sodium chloride) than regular salt. These are all perfectly safe and reasonable alternatives to regular salt for all your cooking needs as well as in the salt shaker on your table.

Potassium supplements are available by prescription, but they have side effects, especially in the pill form. Many are not readily dissolved and may cause irritation of the esophagus and the stomach, causing indigestion and, in rare instances, ulcers. But for those who are on diuretics for various indications, taking potassium supplements under supervision is reasonably safe.

Salt: Sodium chloride

Salt is the most intensively studied mineral in medicine, yet it is still the most controversial. It seems like everyone feels obligated to point out the evils of salt when they spot someone looking at a salt shaker. The proponents of salt restriction have manipulated the public opinion and many healthcare providers into believing that dietary salt intake should be restricted for everyone. The currently recommended allowance is less than 4 grams per day. That's equal to one teaspoon of salt and its meant to include the salt in all foods and snacks, and what you add at the table. Do you think you could limit your salt intake every day? I certainly can't.

On the other hand, the salt lobby has stubbornly resisted a sensible response to the compelling scientific data showing that the present high level of salt consumption (more than 12 grams/day) is unnecessary and may be harmful. The anti-salt evangelists have countered by accusing the salt lobby of collusion with the soft drink industry. They supposedly conspire with food processors to maintain the high salt content of processed foods that increase thirst, thus contributing to greater intake of soft drinks. Here is another case in which science, emotion and commercial interests all clash in a storm of controversy. Consumers are left confused by the conflicting messages.

What's right for you?

Salt restriction is helpful to some people, harmful to a few others and of very little value to most people. Recently, researchers have discovered two versions of the "anti-angiotensinogen gene," which determine the salt-responsiveness of an individual. Those who have inherited the AA version of the gene are sensitive to fluctuations in salt intake, whereas people with the other version, BB, are not salt-responsive.

Among African-Americans, 65% to 80% have the AA version, and as a result, their, hypertension responds much better to decreased dietary salt intake. In contrast, only 10% to 15% of white Americans and 35% to 50% of Hispanics have this gene. Approximately 85% to 90% of white Americans do not respond to dietary salt

restriction. Older persons and people with significant abdominal obesity are usually salt-sensitive.

The test for salt-responsiveness is not widely available and is still being used as a research tool. I suggest to my hypertension patients of every ethnicity and age to reduce the total salt intake to about 6 grams per day by avoiding salty crackers, pretzels, chips, sausages, bacon, all canned soups and processed cheeses. However, the world won't end if you occasionally consume more.

A rigorous analysis of 23 scientific studies (on mostly Caucasian people) showed that even a drastic reduction in salt intake produced only a minor reduction in blood pressure. On average, systolic blood pressure dropped six points and diastolic pressure dropped three points. For a person with blood pressure of 180/105 (systolic over diastolic), this would mean a small reduction in pressure to 174/102—numbers just as dangerous as the prior ones and numbers that would still require vigorous medical treatment.

Most people who develop stroke or heart attack do no necessarily have very high blood pressure. Most have moderate hypertension—that is systolic blood pressure of about to 130 to 150, or diastolic pressure of 85–95. Regrettably, many healthcare providers still don't use effective antihypertension drugs for these patients, but rely on self-restriction that's often unsuccessful.

Salt restriction may have some harmful side effects. A significant decrease in salt intake to below 4,000 mg per day may be associated with higher blood triglycerides, lower HDL-cholesterol and increased vascular tone (stiffness of the arteries), which paradoxically, can raise the blood pressure. This is of particular importance to white hypertensive persons under 45 to 50 for whom the potentially adverse metabolic effects of salt restriction may be further compounded by increasing the blood pressure rather than lowering it.

The average salt intake of an adult in the United States and other developed countries is relatively high at about 10,000 to 12,000 mg per day. (About half is sodium and the rest is chloride.) Most dietary salt (70% to 80%) comes from processed foods, while only 20% to 30% is from salt added to foods during cooking or at the table. As I noted earlier, any effort at reducing salt intake should be directed at processed foods such as cold cuts, sausages, bacon, canned soups, pickled products, vegetable juices, chips, pretzels and fast foods.

High dietary salt intake results in high urinary output of sodium, the major route for eliminating sodium. Along with sodium, calcium is also excreted through the kidneys. This process may contribute to osteoporosis, particularly in postmenopausal women and in older men. In fact, a modest reduction (not restriction) of dietary salt may have the same effect on bone mineral density as an increase in calcium intake of nearly 900 mg per day. This is an important consideration, especially among young girls whose calcium intake is habitually low and who may consume salty processed foods and snacks.

Numerous studies have shown that you can maintain a salt reduction diet for the long term. There is good evidence that when people cut down salt intake, their taste preference changes rather quickly. This is because salt taste receptors on the tongue become more sensitive, and salt-reduced foods give them the same taste as salty ones. After several weeks on a lower salt diet, most people prefer less salty foods, which helps them stay with their salt-reduced diet.

On the basis of the available scientific research, here are recommendations for dietary salt intake...

- Older persons, African-Americans and obese persons of any age who have high blood pressure tend to be salt-responsive and therefore

The test for salt-responsiveness is not widely available. But I suggest that you consider taking it before going on an extreme restricted salt diet (under 4 grams daily), especially if you are a hypertensive white American and do not have severe heart, kidney or liver failure. On the other hand, because up to 80 percent of African-Americans have the salt-sensitive gene, those who have even mild hypertension should restrict salt intake.

should lower their salt intake to less than 4,000 mg per day (sodium intake of less than 2,000 mg). This is equivalent to just under one teaspoon of salt for the entire day.

- If you are in this group, avoid nearly all salt-laden processed foods. Using salt substitutes or sodium-reduced products for cooking or in the salt shaker is another way of cutting down salt intake. Many salt substitutes (sodium-free or reduced-sodium salts) have the added advantage of providing potassium which helps lower the blood pressure.

- Other people with high blood pressure and postmenopausal women with or without risk factors for osteoporosis, should cut their salt intake to less than 6,000 mg per day. This can be achieved by cutting down on salty processed foods, fast food, chips and canned soups and switching to a potassium-containing salt substitute.

- Even if you do not have hypertension, avoid salty processed foods and lower your salt intake to less than 8,000 mg per day (less than two teaspoons for all foods and drinks).

Cafeterias at schools and military bases are notorious for serving salt-laden fatty meals to children and young adults. These young people often adapt to a salty diet and eat that way for life.

It is scandalous that that no one has taken the initiative to change these practices. At fast food chains, some entrees contain more than 1,500 mg of sodium (or 3,000 mg of salt). When side dishes are added, the sodium content of the meal may exceed 2,000 mg (or 4,000 mg of salt).

Although food processing companies and fast food eateries can voluntarily cut back the amount of sodium in their products, which makes good public health sense and good business sense, they won't until they are forced. Salt-lowering will follow the slow demise of trans fats in our food staple.

Fruits, Vegetables, Herbs And Nuts: Proven Heart Protectors

Fruits and vegetables are irreplaceable in human nutrition. They contain minute quantities of many compounds that contribute to balanced nutrition. Multivitamin pills and other supplements offer only a limited number of compounds, often with unbalanced quantities and qualities.

Numerous studies have shown an inverse relation between cardiovascular diseases and the consumption of fruits, vegetables, herbs and nuts. These "heart-healthy" benefits have been observed across many populations—among those who have high and low rates of cardiovascular diseases.

Of course, not all fruits, vegetables, herbs and nuts provide the same amount of cardioprotective or anticancer benefits. There are profound differences in the types and quantities of produce consumed. Regional and seasonal availability of different fruits and vegetables will change the type of ingredients we consume.

In addition to many healthful ingredients, consuming fruits, vegetables, herbs and nuts may mean eating less saturated fat, trans fatty acids and total calories. The shift in dietary fat to more monounsaturates, primarily derived from olive oil, or to more omega-3 fatty acids from seafood, also provides additional health benefits to people who consume large amounts of fruits and vegetables.

Recent studies suggest that consumption of blueberries and dark purple grape juice can help decrease the risk of coronary artery disease. In laboratory experiments (US Department of Agriculture and Tufts University), researchers gave rats daily doses of blueberry extracts (equivalent to one cup of blueberries for humans). These animals showed considerable improvement in age-related loss of balance and lack of coordination when compared with rats who were not given the extract. Strawberry and spinach extracts showed similar but more modest benefits.

In a study from Finland (which has had one of the highest rates of coronary artery disease in the world), people who ate apples and onions frequently (both rich sources of antioxidant compounds) had a nearly 30% reduction in the rate of heart attacks or death from coronary events.

Two recent Harvard University studies also showed that high consumption (more than five servings per day) of vegetables and fruits reduced the five-year risk of coronary events by 30%.

Various nutrients in fruits, vegetables, herbs and nuts such as potassium, antioxidants, vitamins, flavonoid compounds and blood "thinners" may account for a substantial part of these benefits. However, the role of healthy eating habits and healthy lifestyles, such as regular exercise, not smoking and controlling other coronary risk factors are all relevant.

Although several recent studies have suggested that eating five or more servings of fruits and vegetables can lower the blood pressure, this effect is rather small and no more than three to five points. However, an analysis of eight recent studies that included more than 257,000 individuals followed-up for an average of 13 years

BIOLOGICAL POTENCIES OF SOME COMPOUNDS IN VEGETABLES AND FRUITS				
Compound	**Source**	**Anti-Oxidant**	**Cardio-Protection**	**Anti-Cancer**
Carotenoids:				
Beta-carotene	Yellow Fruits and Vegetables	++	0	0
Zeaxanthin	Fruits, Dark Leafy Vegetables	+++	++	+++
Lutein	Green Leafy Vegetables	++	++	++
Lycopene	Tomato and Tomato Products	+++	++	++++
Alpha Tocopherol	Green Leafy Vegetables	++++	++++	+
Flavonoids	Berries, Apples, Onions, Tea	++++	+++	++++

+ to ++++=Low to High Level of Effectiveness
0=No Effect

showed that those eating five or more servings of fruit and vegetables daily had a 26% lower risk of stroke.

Frequent consumption of fruits and vegetables significantly reduces the risk of osteoporosis. Among older women, this protective effect is as much as or even greater than what is achieved with anti-osteoporosis drugs (Prynne, CJ et al. Am J Clin Nutr 2006; 83: 1420–28). Some of this benefit is due to the role of fruits and vegetables in reducing the body's "acid environment" which contributes to loss of calcium and phosphorus through the urine. However, fruits and vegetables also contain folic acid, vitamin K and plenty of potassium and magnesium, which have active roles in improving the "mineral density" of bones or new bone formation. The role of vitamin K (in dark fruits and leafy vegetables) is especially notable because osteocalcin, an abundant protein in the bones and cartilage needs vitamin K for their action. So here is another reason for eating your five or more servings of fruits and vegetables.

What you should do

Include a variety of deeply colored fruits with their skins, vegetables and herbs in your diet. Their healthful nutrients, including vitamins, antioxidants, flavonoids and plant chemicals, vary from one fruit, vegetable or herb to the next. Plus, some of these compounds may be more, or less, digestible depending on the source. Recent data from the US Centers for Disease Control and Prevention show, regrettably, that overall fewer than 15% of American engage in regular physical activity and eat five or more servings of fruits and vegetables daily.

Remember, you need a variety of fruits and vegetables. Eating too much of a single nutrient, even a fruit or vegetable, is not balanced enough to provide a fighting tool against cardiovascular diseases, diabetes, cancers, osteoporosis or other chronic diseases. The nutritional benefits of fruits and vegetables are distinctly different from each other. Although dark-colored fruits (such as berries, black grapes, plums, nectarines and peaches) and vegetables (such as spinach, broccoli, and

RANKING OF FRUITS AND VEGETABLES WITH HIGH CONCENTRATIONS OF CAROTENOIDS			
Ranking	**Beta Carotene**	**Lutein**	**Lycopene**
1	Apricots	Kale	Tomato Catsup
2	Carrots	Spinach	Tomato Paste
3	Sweet Potatoes	Mustard Greens	Tomato Sauce
4	Collards	Dill	Tomato Juice
5	Kale	Celery	Raw Tomatoes
6	Spinach	Broccoli	Watermelon
7	Parsley	Romaine Lettuce	Guava, Raw
8	Swiss Chard	Green Peas	Guava Juice
9	Mustard Greens	Green Peppers	Pink Grapefruit
10	Chicory	Pumpkin	Apricots

outer leaves of lettuce, watercress, parsley and herbs) are the most helpful, eating a cucumber, some mushrooms or zucchini is not exactly sinful. The lighter-colored vegetables don't have the same heavy concentration of antioxidants or anticarcinogens, but if you like them, so be it—mix and match.

Many dark, tart fruits, in addition to numerous vitamins, minerals and antioxidants, also have an abundant amount of procyanidins, which improve the endothelial functions (inner lining of the arteries) and are potent antioxidants. Nearly all darker-colored and tart fruits (all berries, black or dark red grapes and their juices or wines made from them, pomegranates, black plums, figs, apples) are rich sources of procyanidins. Dark chocolate is also an excellent source, but not milk chocolate, which is often made with shortening containing trans fats.

A recent study from Johns Hopkins University showed that a diet rich in fruits and vegetables without the use of vitamin supplements resulted in sufficient blood antioxidant levels to reduce oxidation of LDL-cholesterol. This and other studies have clearly established that habitual intake of sufficient fruits, vegetables, herbs, and nuts provide a genuine and effective increase in the concentration of antioxidants in the blood.

Many children and adolescents do not learn to eat sufficient amounts of fruits and vegetables and maintain their poor dietary habits into adulthood. Ideally, prevention of cardiovascular diseases and cancers requires an early start and almost a lifetime of healthy dietary and lifestyle practices. But, it is never too late to start.

In the United States and most developed countries, fresh fruits and vegetables are available year-round. Fresh-frozen fruits or vegetables are just as nutritious, but not as tasty as their fresh counterparts. Canned fruits in juices (but not in heavy syrup) are another alternative in winter months, provided you discard the "juice," which has plenty of undesirable high fructose corn sweeteners. In fact, I wash canned fruits under cold water to remove as much of the fructose-tainted juice as possible.

Because of high salt content, avoid canned vegetables and choose the fresh-frozen (or preferably fresh) variety. Dried fruits such as raisins,

TOTAL FIBER CONTENT OF FRUITS AND VEGETABLES
(Per 100 gm)

Fruits	Grams	Fruits	Grams
Apples, with Skin	2.2	Nectarines	1.6
Apples, without Skin	1.8	Olives, Black	3
Applesauce	1.5	Olives, Green	2.8
Apricots, Dried	8	Oranges	2.5
Apricots, Fresh	2	Orange Juice	0.2
Avocados	2	Peaches, Dried	1.6
Bananas	2	Pears, Dried	8
Blackberries	7	Pears, Fresh	2.6
Blueberries	2.2	Pineapples, Canned	1.3
Cantaloupe or Honeydew	1	Pineapples, Fresh	1.2
Cherries	1.5	Plums, Dried	7
Figs, Dried	9.2	Plums, Fresh	2
Fruit Cocktail	1.5	Prunes, Stewed	6
Grapefruit	1	Raisins	5
Grapes, Seedless	1	Raspberries	5
Kiwi Fruit	3.4	Raspberries	2.6
Mangoes	1.5	Watermelons	0.4

apricots, peaches, figs, black cherries and various berries are wonderful for snacking. Even a few dark chocolate-covered (but not milk chocolate-covered, since milk chocolate is commonly made with shortening and contains unhealthy trans fats) almonds or raisins are far better than candy bars.

Some people take multivitamins or other "nutritional" supplements every day with the explanation, "I don't eat enough fruits or vegetables." In my view, pills are not a logical substitute for the real thing. Fruits and vegetables contain thousands of healthful nutrients that can never be put in a pill or capsule.

 CAUTION: As a reminder, rinse all fruits, vegetables and herbs thoroughly before eating. Many outbreaks of food-borne illnesses from imported raspberries or domestic green onions, spinach, alfalfa sprouts and other produce have occurred in the past several years. It is always prudent to wash all your fruits and vegetables.

People with abnormal immune systems (diabetics, those with chronic liver or kidney disorders, people who use immune-suppressant drugs or who have a transplanted organ, AIDS or other immune-deficiency disorders) must be even more vigilant. They should consider washing all their fruits and vegetables with permanganate to kill many organisms and parasites.

TOTAL FIBER CONTENT OF NUTS, SEEDS AND BREADS
(Per 100 gm)

Nuts and Seeds	Grams	Breads	Grams
Almonds, Roasted	11.2	Cornbread	2.4
Cashews, Roasted	6	Cracked Wheat	5.3
Chickpeas, Canned	5.8	French	2.7
Filberts (Hazelnuts)	6.9	Italian	3.1
Mixed Nuts, Roasted	8	Mixed Grain	7.1
Peanuts, Roasted	8	Oatmeal	3.9
Peanut Butter, Chunky, Roasted	6.8	Pita, White	1.6
Peanut Butter, Creamy	6	Pita, Whole Wheat	7.6
Pecans, Roasted	6.5	Pumpernickel	5.9
Pistachios, Roasted	10.8	Rye	6.2
Sunflower Seeds, Roasted	6.8	Wheat	4.3
Walnuts, Roasted	5	White	2.3
		Whole Wheat	6.9

Garlic: No magic bullet

Every week, there's a headline or a sound bite praising one fruit or vegetable for its potent, life-saving virtues. These claims are usually exaggerated and sometimes nonsensical. Nevertheless, many fruits and vegetables may contain distinct ingredients with heart-friendly or cancer-fighting effects.

Garlic promoters tout it as an effective cholesterol-lowering, "natural" alternative to drugs. Unfortunately, most of the studies reporting positive results (five percent to seven percent cholesterol-lowering) with garlic are flawed because they have ignored the role of simultaneous dietary changes. In these studies, the cholesterol-lowering is primarily due to changes in dietary practices, not garlic pills.

The findings of four diet-controlled, double-blind studies (from the United States, Great Britain and Germany) using garlic powder pills (Kwai) or steam-distilled garlic oil capsules were recently published. All the studies showed that garlic had no effect on any blood lipids, LDL, HDL or tri-glyceride levels. Results were no different in those who took garlic preparations compared with those who took placebos. Even at much higher doses of garlic (fresh, powder or oil), the effect of lowering blood cholesterol by five percent to seven percent is too meager to have a positive result on your heart.

The most recent report was a six-month study of three garlic preparations—fresh garlic, powdered garlic supplement or garlic extract supplement—conducted by researchers at Stanford University. None of the garlic forms, when given at an approximate dose of a four-gram clove (one average sized clove), six days a week for six months, had any significant effect on LDL, HDL

151

or triglyceride concentration (Gardner CD et al. Arch Intern Med 2007; 167: 346–53).

Collectively, those well conducted studies have fully documented that garlic in any form has no impact on blood cholesterol levels. Still, garlic may have some other minor cardioprotective benefits. For example, garlic reduces the clumping of blood platelets and thus reduces the stickiness of platelets and the risk of clot formation and perhaps heart attacks. This particular benefit of one or two cloves of garlic per day is nearly similar to taking one low-dose aspirin tablet daily. Since not all garlic products have a similar antiplatelet effect, the choice of garlic products is important. For example, fresh garlic and freeze-dried garlic powder are similar in potency, while steam-distilled oils are 35% as effective, and oil macerates only about 10% as effective. Aged garlic preparations have no such anticlotting effects.

Garlic products are not always harmless. In some individuals, especially those with irritable bowel or esophageal acid reflux, garlic preparations can aggravate symptoms of belching, heartburn, gaseousness and bloating. Garlic can also cause allergic reactions including contact dermatitis. A strong garlic breath or garlic body odor also has an antisocial effect that you should consider before starting a garlic regimen.

The bottom line on garlic is that a small amount of garlic adds a distinct flavor and taste to many meals, and you should enjoy it for that reason. As a bonus, garlic is also a rich source of many nutrients, antioxidants and anticlotting compounds that can provide some minor heart health protection. No amount of advertising and testimonials by well paid celebrities makes garlic supplements an effective tool in lowering blood cholesterol levels.

A high blood cholesterol level and coronary artery disease are not trivial matters, and you should never trivialize them by taking one or two garlic pills daily instead of a more proactive approach to control any of the 20 major coronary risk factors you might have.

Onions

Like garlic, onion is also extremely versatile and a rich source of many nutrients. It has a high concentration of quercetin, a flavonoid with very potent antioxidant effects. A recent European study suggests that people who consume onions frequently (or apples and tea, also high in flavonoids) have significantly lower rates of cardiovascular disease, especially heart attacks.

Quercetin is often bound to some other compounds. For example, the quercetin in onions is mainly quercetin glucoside, which makes it more absorbable; approximately 50% of it is absorbed. (Calcium also has a variable rate of absorption. The bioavailability—or absorbability—of calcium gluconate or calcium citrate is 30% to 50% higher than calcium carbonate.) Black tea is mainly in the form of quercetin rutinoside, which lowers its bioavailability to less than 20%. However, the high concentration of quercetin in a strong cup of tea compensates for its reduced bioavailability.

Onion has far less sulfides than garlic, especially allicin, which is responsible for garlic's odor. As a result, fewer volatile compounds come out in your breath. This makes onion more user-friendly and avoids the stale garlic odor that appears in the air we exhale for 12 to 24 hours. However, if you have certain digestive disorders such as acid reflex or irritable bowel syndrome, you may not be able to tolerate too much onion, especially if it is raw.

Fortunately, makers of nutritional supplements haven't exploited onions yet! Enjoy the real thing; both raw and cooked versions provide the same benefits.

Tomatoes

Tomato is a rich source of the antioxidant "lycopene" and other nutrients. But the available studies suggest that the role of lycopene in heart health is relatively small. Because lycopene (like vitamin E) is a fat-soluble antioxidant, it is carried by various lipoproteins into the arterial wall, where it backs up vitamin E to fight the oxidization of LDL-cholesterol.

Since lycopene (like vitamins A, D, E and K) is fat soluble, it requires some fat to facilitate its absorption. So, tomato juice with a fat-free breakfast does not suffice. Instead, have your tomato juice or mixed vegetable juices with lunch or dinner, which usually contain some fat.

Heating releases more lycopene from tomato and tomato products, which is not destroyed by cooking. Since tomato sauces or pastes are used in foods with some fat (preferably olive oil), they are excellent sources of lycopene—even better than tomato juice or raw tomato.

Some studies suggest that high blood levels of lycopene reduce the risk of prostate cancer by 30%. For those who are concerned about (or have) prostate cancer, a diet rich in tomato products, along with a lycopene supplement, 10 to 25 mg once a day, is a practical way of reducing your risk.

Cruciferous vegetables

Broccoli, broccoli sprouts, cauliflower, cabbage and brussels sprouts reduce the risk of cardiovascular diseases and they significantly lower the rates of many cancers, especially esophagus, stomach, colon, pancreas, prostate and ovarian. Aside from a vast number of antioxidants, cruciferous vegetables also provide a good deal of dietary fiber that can prevent blood sugar surges in diabetics or obese persons.

Since cruciferous vegetables are available year-round in the United States, make every effort to eat several servings per week. These vegetables are not very popular, and overcooking them—a rather common mistake—can give them an unpleasant odor, color or texture. Adding salt, pepper, olive oil, a touch of lemon juice or other herbs and spices during a three- to five-minute steaming (in the microwave or on the stovetop) may make them more appealing.

Green, leafy vegetables

Dark, green, leafy vegetables are rich sources of many vitamins including A, C and E, many healthful minerals and flavonoids. Numerous studies have shown that, like cruciferous vegetables, green, leafy vegetables are both cardioprotective and anticarcinogenic.

Kale, spinach and watercress have the highest concentrations of antioxidants of all vegetables. (Their fruit counterparts with the highest concentrations of antioxidants are blueberries, blackberries, raspberries, strawberries and concord grapes.) Eating green, leafy vegetables regularly provides you with many cardioprotective antioxidants. It's also the most effective dietary means to reduce your risk of many cancers. Using kale, spinach and watercress (instead of lettuce) and broccoli florets provides a healthful and tasty alternative to regular salads.

Some physicians warn their patients who are on "blood thinners" (anticoagulants like warfarin) to cut down on or avoid green leafy, vegetables, but this is based on misunderstanding, not fact. Their concern is that vitamin K in these products may counteract the effect of anticoagulants. This would require you to eat several pounds of kale or spinach every day—which is unlikely to happen, Green, leafy vegetables also contain vitamin E and tiny amounts of aspirin-like substances (salicylates) that negate the impact of their vitamin K.

Herbs and spices

Is there a food whose personality, character and delectability cannot be enhanced or brought to life by herbs and spices? Happily, herbs and spices contain many vitamins, trace minerals, antioxidants and other compounds that are heart healthy, cancer protective, or provide other health benefits. Some herbs and spices also contain low levels of salicylates (close relatives of aspirin), which enhance their heart protective properties. These include oregano, mint, rosemary, paprika, pepper, curry and cumin.

A recent joint study by Swedish and Greek investigators showed that extracts of thyme and sage reduced oxidization of fats in various cells to the same extent as vitamin E. This study and other studies suggest that frequent use of herbs may also provide many health benefits beyond pleasurable eating. Habitual consumption of hot peppers (containing capsaicin) improves insulin resistance and may lower the blood sugar and triglycerides. Unlike fruits and vegetables, herbs and spices cannot be consumed in large quantities, limiting their overall contribution to a cardioprotective or healthful diet. Nevertheless, because of higher concentration of health-promoting compounds in herbs and spices, even at a low level of consumption they can still make your foods delicious and at the same time, healthy.

Grapefruit

Grapefruit is another food that has been touted to have cardioprotective, anticancer and weight-control benefits and other exaggerated health claims. Although grapefruit is a rich source of vitamin C, potassium and some antioxidants, it is not a miracle fruit. If grapefruit has any anti-obesity effect (which is highly improbable), it is due to its filling effect, similar to cantaloupe, watermelon or other melons. This is true for every fruit, vegetable and even drinking water. Grapefruit does not possess any magical or mysterious weight reducing or disease-modifying properties.

Grapefruit and grapefruit juice deactivates a special enzyme in the wall of the intestine called "cytochrome P3A4." This enzyme is responsible for the partial breakdown of many drugs taken orally, making them less available for absorption. When a certain drug is taken with grapefruit or grapefruit juice, the amount of drug that is absorbable is increased by one-third compared with taking the same drug with water or other juices. For most drugs, this is not a major problem. In fact, for some drugs it improves their bioavailability efficacy. But for many cardiovascular drugs, anticoagulants, diabetes drugs, this may cause undesirably higher blood levels with some complications.

Researchers from the University of North Carolina at Chapel Hill recently identified the compound in grapefruit responsible for deactivating the CYP-3A4 enzyme furanocoumarin. It's actually a close relative of the anticoagulant drug Coumadin. When volunteers were given regular grapefruit juice, it nearly doubled the absorption and blood level of the blood pressure-lowering drug felodipine that was taken along with grapefruit juice. The absorption and blood level of felodipine taken with a grapefruit juice out of which its furanocoumarin was removed was about 50% lower than levels found with regular grapefruit juice.

 CAUTION: Always avoid grapefruit or grapefruit juice for at least two hours after taking various heart, blood pressure, diabetes, anticoagulant or anti-AIDS drugs and all oral chemotherapy (anti-cancer) agents.

Some recent studies suggest that a daily glass of grapefruit juice might increase the risk of kidney stones by more than 40%. Although it's not clear how grapefruit juice contributes to kidney stones, one possibility is that an ingredient in grapefruit combines with dietary oxalate, a main component of most kidney stones, and makes it form sediment when it is excreted by the kidneys.

Grapefruit provides no significant advantage over other citrus fruits. Except for precautions and reservations, grapefruit and its juice should be enjoyed for what it is.

Oranges and orange juice

Oranges and their juice are rich sources of antioxidants as well as vitamin C, folic acid and potassium. In a recent study, Canadian researchers gave a group of volunteers three glasses of orange juice daily (more than 1.5 pints) for several weeks. On average, HDL-cholesterol levels rose by about 20% with no change in LDL-cholesterol. Three glasses of orange juice add an additional 80 grams of carbohydrates (or about 320 calories) to the diet, so this is an impractical way of raising HDL levels, especially for diabetics or people with weight mismanagement.

Still, even one or two glasses of orange juice with pulp and fortified with calcium is far superior to soda and caffeinated "power" drinks.

Cranberries and cranberry juice

Cranberries are a rich source of antioxidants, but cranberry juice is one of the most acidic juices, far more than tomato, grapefruit or orange juice. This property of cranberry juice has made it a very safe and highly effective way of making the urine more acidic, which helps reduce the risk of urinary tract infection (in people with frequent attacks of bladder and kidney infections). Most people eat cranberries or cranberry juice sparingly because of their tartness. An occasional glass of cranberry juice is unlikely to have significant cardioprotective benefit.

Taste for fruits and vegetables

Everyone knows that eating plenty of fruits and vegetables is good and healthful. So why it is that so few Americans eat adequate servings?

Clearly, what we feed our children can set a lifetime pattern. Recent data also suggest that genetic makeup can affect distaste for certain fruits and vegetables. Nearly a third of the population of the United States is genetically very sensitive to certain tastes such as bitter and tart —tastes that, in most fruits and vegetables are due to flavonoid compounds. These individuals are called "super tasters." Unless they retrain their taste buds or make a conscious effort, they shy away from broccoli, cruciferous vegetables and certain tart fruits such as various berries— which are the best plant sources for many healthful flavonoids. Unfortunately, super tasters (like former President George Bush, who made "I hate broccoli!" one of his lasting legacies) have a hard time with their fruit and vegetable selections. They often eat few vegetables other than the occasional salad. The rest of the population is made up of "normal tasters" and "nontasters."

PROP (propylthiouracil) is the main chemical substance that gives taste to many fruits and vegetables. In a recent study, researchers at Rutgers University examined vegetable intake among preschool children. When given the choice of different vegetables, only eight percent of children who could not taste the PROP, the nontasters, did not eat any vegetables compared to 32% of tasters. For most of these children, this behavior tracks into adulthood.

By and large, nontasters are thinner, more physically active, and have higher HDL-cholesterol, but lower LDL-cholesterol and triglycerides. They also eat and enjoy all kinds of fruit and vegetables, which, in part, may explain their lower risk profile for cardiovascular diseases and cancers. Normal tasters east some fruits and vegetables, but are a bit finicky. Still, they will eat various greens from time to time without too much fuss.

Nuts

Most nuts are rich sources of vitamins, minerals, proteins, monounsaturated or polyunsaturated fats, dietary fiber. They also are versatile and have a long shelf life. Numerous studies have suggested that frequent consumption of certain nuts (about 10%, several times per week) can reduce the risk of cardiovascular events by more than 20%. This is even more so if these desirable nuts (almonds, hazelnut, pecans, pistachios and walnuts) displace other foods or snacks, many of which may be overburdened with saturated or trans fats, and sugar or high fructose corn sweeteners.

Peanuts have a high concentration of saturated fat (18% in peanut oil) and a small amount of two coronary-unfriendly longer chain saturated fats—arachidonic acid, which has 20 carbons in its chain, and behenic acid, which has 22 carbons. Still, a handful of peanuts or an occasional peanut butter sandwich will not cause a heart attack or derail your efforts to have a happy and healthy heart.

Brazil nuts, pine nuts and pumpkin, sesame and sunflower seeds also have high concentrations of saturated fats and omega-6, which make them less desirable than other nuts.

Enjoy nuts but avoid Brazil nuts, pine nuts, cashews and peanuts. And, beware of the calories. Nuts have far more calories per 100 gm weight than fruits. For example, 100 gm (3.5 oz)

of dry-roasted sunflower seeds provides more than 600 calories. On the other hand, fresh fruits (except avocado) are fat-free and have less than 100 calories per each 100 gm serving. A handful of tasty almonds, filberts, pistachios or walnuts are superior to sweet snacks or ice cream.

Whole grains

Whole grains are important sources of many nutrients including fiber, starch, proteins, trace minerals, vitamins, plant chemicals and antioxidants. They provide a balanced blend of ingredients that are cardioprotective and reduce the risk of developing hypertension, diabetes and stomach and colon cancers. Unfortunately, most healthful nutrients (except for the starch and protein) are removed in the milling process, making many grain products (white breads, rice, pastas and most cereals) no more than ghosts of the real things. They have no significant cardioprotective or anticarcinogenic benefits, and may contribute to insulin resistance, obesity, and diabetes, higher levels of bad LDL-cholesterol and triglycerides, but lower levels of the good HDL-cholesterol.

Several recent studies in both men and women have shown that long-term use of whole grains on a regular basis can reduce the risk of coronary artery disease by about 30%. Although some of this benefit may be attributable to healthier dietary and lifestyle behavior of people who eat whole grain products, the ingredients in whole grains contribute to their cardioprotective benefit. Excessive amounts of wheat bran or bran cereals may produce gas, bloating or cramps due to fermentation of bran in the colon by intestinal bacteria. This is especially true if you have diverticulosis or irritable bowel. Oat products and wild rice are healthful alternatives for such individuals.

Herbal Supplements: A Marketing Hoax?

Herbal and "nutritional" supplements have become increasingly popular in the United States. The allure of "natural" products is rooted in the belief that natural products are benevolent, safe and—with the help of misleading advertising—also "effective" against a wide variety of diseases.

Consumers tend to think that natural products are inherently better or healthier than synthetic ones. The truth is that "natural" does not mean they are safe, healthful or harmonious with nature. After all, poisonous mushrooms, snake venom, pneumonia, malaria, hurricanes and earthquakes are all natural phenomena but they are hardly good for you. Many Europeans, and now Americans, take herbal supplements, for their perceived health benefits or for therapeutic purposes. This is especially common among people with chronic diseases.

In most instances, herbal products are no more than very weak chemical compounds or drugs that lack the scrutiny of the Food and Drug Administration. How can it be that untested, unproven, often contaminated and ineffective "natural" drugs flourish in a technologically advanced and well-informed society? The answer is advertisements, blogs, misinformation and outright bogus claims on internet sites.

Since there is no standard for many herbal products, both their ingredients and their biological activity vary from manufacturer to manufacturer and from batch to batch. Soil, storage, handling, manufacturing and shelf life of the finished product and the scruples of supplement producers all affect their potency. The potency of different brands of a given herbal supplement may vary by 5,000- to 10,000-fold. While a particular herbal supplement may claim 500 mg

of a certain herb, it may actually contain only 5 to 10 mg. Often, the product is manufactured incorrectly or inadvertently contaminated with toxic or nontoxic material.

In brief: You can never be sure that an herbal supplement is safe or even genuine. I can bottle the grass from my front yard and claim it can help reduce pounds without dieting, hair loss, erectile dysfunction, stress, and improve cardiovascular health, stamina, osteoporosis, insomnia, and whatever else I want. No one, the FDA, or any other watchdog agency can stop me! A law passed in 1994 by heavy lobbying and campaign contributions removed the FDA's jurisdiction over supplement manufacturers, so a supplement can be whatever the manufacturer claims it to be. In the United States, herbal supplements that claim to benefit heart health include ginseng, ginkgo biloba, garlic products, hawthorn and evening primrose.

Ginseng

Ginseng is among the most heavily hyped and controversial supplements, with the status of cure-all miracle supplement. Ginseng comes from the roots of some plants grown in the Far East (Korea, China and Japan), Canada, the United States and Brazil. And therein lies the problem.

Almost all fruits, vegetables, herbs and spices are more or less similar all over the world. More than 50 different plants are called ginseng, but with the exception of a few, they have nothing in common with the genuine Asian or American ginseng. The ginseng in Korea is not the same as that found in Russia, Brazil or the United States. Moreover, despite of claims of purity by manufacturers and retailers, there is no product standardization guarantee of its purity.

People who buy aspirin are assured that 500 mg of aspirin manufactured by different companies is the same almost anywhere in the world. By contrast, 100 mg of ginseng may contain different ingredients according to different manufacturers, in different regions of a country—not to mention different countries.

More than 25% of the products sold as ginseng have no detectable ginseng. Another 60% contain very little (far less than half) of what is advertised or printed on the bottle. Some types of ginseng, like the Brazilian or the Russian (Siberian) varieties, are not even true ginseng, but they are still marketed as such.

In the United States, about 90% of the ginseng crop is grown in Wisconsin by more than 1,500 ginseng growers. Although ginseng

THE BOTTOM LINE ON GREEN TEA

Although green tea has received a lot of publicity for its heart health benefit, these claims are mostly hollow. One of the world's largest green tea companies petitioned the US Food and Drug Administration for permission to claim that green tea reduces the risk of cardiovascular diseases. The FDA rejected the petition, after a careful review of the documents and studies the petitioner submitted. The FDA found, "There is no credible evidence to support qualified health claims for green tea or green tea extract and a reduction of a number of risk factors associated with cardiovascular diseases."

AMOUNTS OF FIBER IN VEGETABLES
(Per 100 gm)

Vegetables	Grams	Vegetables	Grams
Artichokes	5.2	Lettuce, Iceberg	1
Asparagus, Green or White	2	Lettuce, Romaine	1.7
Beans, Black or Kidney	7	Mushrooms	1.3
Beans, Lima	7	Onions	1.6
Beets	1.7	Peas, Sweet	2.6
Broccoli	2.8	Peas, Black Eyed	9.6
Brussels Sprouts	4.3	Peppers, Sweet	1.6
Cabbage	1	Popcorn	4
Cabbage, Red	2	Potatoes, with Skin	4
Carrots	3.2	Potatoes without Skin	1.5
Cauliflower	2.4	Spinach, Raw	2.2
Celery	1.6	Squash	2
Corn, Sweet	3.7	Sweet Potatoes	3
Cucumbers, with Skin	1	Tomatoes, Raw	1.3
Cucumbers, without Skin	0.5	Turnip, Greens	2.4
Eggplant	2.5	Watercress	2.3
Kale	2	Zucchini	2

is supposed to be cultivated without pesticides, Wisconsin's Department of Agriculture recently uncovered widespread and illegal use of the pesticides Lindane and PCMB by ginseng growers.

There are endless, exaggerated claims for what ginseng can do. Depending on the zeal of the promoter and the gullibility of the target audience, ginseng "can do anything." These claims include: the ability to improve cardiovascular health, lower cholesterol and blood pressure, protect against cancers, reduce stress, increase sexual potency and improve athletic performance. All of these claims are either trivial or nonexistent.

Because Oriental ginseng is expensive, producers often cut and dilute it with fillers. Some merchants do not even put any ginseng at all in their products! But they label and promote their non-ginseng as a "pure" and "potent" ginseng.

✳ **CAUTION:** For people with chronic heart failure who are taking digitalis, Siberian "ginseng" can raise digitalis blood levels to toxic and even fatal levels. If you have cardiovascular disease for which your doctor has prescribed digoxin or other digitalis derivatives, do not take any ginseng products.

Ginkgo biloba

Unlike ginseng, which comes from the plant's roots, ginkgo biloba is extracted from dried leaves of ginkgo trees. Ginkgo preparations have been used since 2800 B.C., but it has become very popular lately and is one of the best-selling herbal medicines in Europe. Ginkgo is among the few herbs for which standardized extracts are available.

A number of European studies have suggested that the regular use of ginkgo biloba over two to four months might improve cognitive functions, memory and stress tolerance. Since ginkgo has a slight antiplatelet effect, it might also have some relevance to reducing the risk of heart attack or stroke. Because of this antiplatelet activity, it may enhance the effect of aspirin or other anticlotting drugs slightly, but it does not contribute to bleeding tendencies.

Ginkgosan

Ginkgosan is a combination of ginkgo biloba (60 mg) and ginseng (100 mg). At the dose of two tablets per day, the combination may have a mild blood pressure-lowering effect.

For most users, ginkosan provides no more than a placebo effect. Since it is nearly impossible to obtain genuine ginseng or ginkgosan at a reasonable price, the meager benefits of most commercially available products do not justify the trouble and expense. Although one to three pills per day have no major side effects, it is unlikely that you will receive sustainable health benefit from either ginseng or ginkgo biloba. The concern is that some users rely too much on these supplements and delay modern, safe and effective interventions to correct their risk factors.

Hawthorn

The flowers, fruits and leaves of hawthorn were popular 100 years ago for palliating various cardiovascular ailments, at a time when we had no safe or effective drugs. Hawthorn has been shown to increase blood flow through coronary arteries and improve the heart's performance in people with mild heart failure. It has also shown a very mild antihypertensive effect. These effects, however, are minor at best and pale in comparison with today's highly effective and safe cardiovascular drugs. In the 21st century, it's not sensible to rely on hawthorn to treat deadly diseases. At the commonly used dosage, hawthorn is relatively free of major side effects, but it has very little clinical usefulness.

> ✳ **CAUTION:** On occasion, hawthorn can cause digitalis toxicity in people with chronic heart failure who take digoxin (or Lanoxin), very much like the effects of Siberian ginseng.

Evening Primrose

The seeds of this native North American weed contain about 14% oil. A small portion of this oil, amounting to less than two percent overall, is made up of gamma-linolenic acid, a plant omega-3 fatty acid, for which various outlandish claims are common.

Exaggerated claims for primrose oil include its ability to help with weight loss, lowering cholesterol, hypertension and rheumatism, as well as relieving menstrual cramps, premenstrual syndrome and cardioprotective benefits. To obtain this questionable cardiovascular benefit would require taking 10 or more capsules per day (a few dollars daily), and the accompanying moderate digestive symptoms.

Adulterated products may include impurities and dilution with other oils. An important concern is that a portion of the oil in evening primrose may be oxidized during its shelf life in the capsules. These oxidized fatty acids may potentially cause liver damage and could possibly be carcinogenic.

The unproven benefit of evening primrose oil certainly cannot justify spending $50 to $100 a month on this supplement. And, at lower doses, which is what most users take, it is practically useless.

Herbal supplements have no magical cardiovascular or other benefits. More importantly, cardiovascular diseases should not be treated with old-fashioned remedies. In developed countries, the average life span has gone up from 47 to nearly 80 years since the mid-nineteenth century, almost entirely due to advances in medicine, public health and food technology. Relying on or regressing to herbal supplements may enrich their manufacturers and purveyors but offers close to no benefit to consumers.

Coenzyme Q10

Coenzyme Q10 is a fat-soluble compound produced inside most human cells and is present in high concentrations in the heart, liver and kidneys. It participates along with other compounds and enzymes in regulating energy production within the cells and maintaining cellular health.

Companies who promote coenzyme Q10 as a miracle drug are misinterpreting its synergistic function. For example, coenzyme Q10 has been extensively promoted for treatment of heart failure or to "improve heart muscle function". It does neither.

Recent studies among patients with heart failure have shown that even at high doses, coenzyme Q10 was not any more effective than placebo. A possible use for coenzyme Q10 is for patients who develop muscle pain from taking cholesterol-lowering statins. Statins may reduce the production of cellular coenzyme Q10, and the assumption is that supplements might replenish it and thereby reduce the aches and pains. Unfortunately, here too, its effect may be no better than a placebo. Overall, coenzyme Q10 is an expensive but practically worthless supplement.

Dietary Fiber

"Dietary fiber" refers to certain components of plants that are not broken down or digested in the small intestine. Horses, cattle and other herbivore animals have enzymes such as cellulase and hemicellulase to digest plant fiber, while humans do not have them. That's why a cow can graze on green pasture and grow in size while humans would starve to death eating grass, even though it is mainly complex carbohydrates.

How humans lost these enzymes is a question that dates back at least two million years to our distant ancestors. Over the past 10,000 years, we have been mainly carnivorous, also eating fruits, vegetables and seeds. Although humans cannot digest or absorb plant fiber (it is mostly eliminated in the stool), we can process many other ingredients in fruits and vegetables.

There is a big difference between a high-fiber diet and a diet that contains plenty of fruits and vegetables. Nutrients like bran cereals contain very high concentrations of dietary fiber, along with added vitamins and minerals, but also plenty of high fructose corn sweeteners or sugar. Fruits and vegetables have between one percent to 10% dietary fiber and a vast number of healthful ingredients, the majority of which are not present in "fortified" bran products (or vitamin/mineral tablets). The physical form of dietary fiber (for example, coarse grains compared with finely milled flour products) can also alter the impact of dietary fiber.

Researchers studied more than 34,500 postmenopausal women for an average of nine years. Women with the highest intake of whole grains (an average of three servings per day) had a 30% lower risk of developing coronary artery disease when compared with those who had less than three servings per week. Although dietary fiber accounted for some of the benefit, most of the benefits were due to the antioxidants, plant chemicals, folic acid and other (as yet unidentified) ingredients in whole grains. Plus, people who eat whole grains are usually more health conscious and have other healthy habits and lifestyles (being physically active, nonsmokers and weighing less).

Soluble vs. insoluble fiber

All plant fibers hold water and swell. Fibers that have a high water-holding capacity are soluble fibers and those with very low capacity are insoluble. Soluble fibers include psyllium (such as Metamucil and Bran Bud), pectins and gums from plants, fruits and some vegetables.

Most plant fibers are a mix of soluble and insoluble.

- Oat bran has approximately 16 grams of fiber in each 100 grams (3½ oz.) of which 40% fraction is soluble. More importantly, oat bran contains 10% beta-glucan, a compound that is responsible for oat bran's cholesterol-lowering effect, even though it is minimal.

- In contrast, wheat bran has nearly 42 grams of fiber in each 100 grams, most of which is insoluble. Wheat bran has only two percent beta-glucan, which explains why wheat bran products do not lower blood cholesterol levels.

The cholesterol-lowering effect of soluble fiber depends on the dose.

- An effective dose of oat bran, for example, is approximately three to five servings per day, equal to three to five cups, to lower cholesterol by five percent. Lower doses, such as an occasional breakfast of oatmeal or oat cereals, have no cholesterol-lowering impact. Eat them if you enjoy them, but not for any health claims, no matter what the box says!

- Higher doses of oat bran, phyllium, guar gum, pectin or other soluble fibers—along with other dietary modifications—can reduce blood cholesterol level by an average of seven percent to 10%.

- Higher doses, however, amounting to 50 to 60 grams per day, usually have unpleasant side effects, including excessive gas, bloating, fullness, diarrhea and abdominal pain. On rare occasions, they may cause intestinal obstruction, especially in older persons.

✻ **CAUTION:** Most people should avoid fiber pills, particularly older persons or those with a history of digestive problems. Occasionally these pills can swell and cause small bowel obstruction, especially in people who have abdominal adhesions from previous surgeries.

There are many well-promoted fiber products on the market, all geared toward cholesterol reduction. Some of them are very expensive (up to $6 to $8 a day to lower blood cholesterol by approximately five percent). And some would require taking as many as 12 tablets daily. I can't imagine anyone falling into this trap and not thinking, "There must be better ways to lower my cholesterol." There are!

Despite advertisers' claims, these products, even if they do lower blood cholesterol by five to seven percent, have no relevance to cardiovascular health. Low doses are utterly ineffective and may create a false sense of security, and prevent consumers from seeking proper medical care. It's even worse for women, who require even more fiber to lower their cholesterol by a few percentage points.

What you should do

In general, try to eat several servings of fruits and vegetables (fresh, canned, frozen or dried) along with legumes or nuts (excluding Brazil nuts, peanuts, pine nuts and pumpkin or sunflower seeds) and eat cereals containing soluble fiber such as oat and barley. Remember canned fruits have a high concentration of fructose corn sweeteners. So you should drain and wash under cold water your canned fruits, such as apricots, peaches, and pears, even when it is in "fruit juice," to which they add corn sweeteners.

People often assume that they have enough fiber in their diet from an occasional serving of salad or fruit, but ingredients of a typical garden salad have very little fiber. If one medium-sized cucumber has one gram of fiber, how much fiber can there be in two or three slices? Or in two or three small wedges of a tomato? Similarly, many common summer fruits (such as cantaloupe or melons) do not have much fiber; more than 95% of the volume of these melons is water.

Some simple ways to increase dietary fiber: Switch to rye or dark bread from white bread, to oat-based cereals or whole wheat from sweetened or frosted brands; and to baked potato with skin from french fries. Eat fresh or dried figs, prunes, apricots, peaches and various berries, beans, peas, corn and carrots. Eat fruits (oranges, apples and prunes) instead of drinking their juices, which have little or no fiber. To avoid gas and bloating, be sure to increase your dietary fiber slowly to reach desirable levels of 10 to 20 gm per day.

Beverages: Tea, Cocoa, Coffee, Alcohol, Water, Soft Drinks and Fruit Juices

Tea

After water, people drink more tea than any beverage in the world, especially in Asia and Europe. Black tea is the fermentation by-product of green tea leaves. The tea master's expertise and creativity in combination with the soil condition, region, weather, rainfall and growing conditions account for the tea's taste, flavor, aroma and other characteristics, very much like wine.

Tea is a rich source of many antioxidants. Within 30 to 50 minutes after drinking a cup of brewed tea, blood levels of tea's antioxidants rise by 40% to 50% and may last for up to 80 minutes. Green tea, but not black tea, has certain polyphenolic compounds that can block the action of an enzyme called "urokinase" in some cancer cells. Some of tea's antioxidants include quercetin and catechins that can reduce the risk of coronary artery disease and stroke with high intake. A substantial portion of these antioxidants are readily absorbed from the intestine and go to work soon after arrival in the bloodstream. But despite unbridled enthusiasm for tea as an antioxidant, cardioprotective and anticarcinogen, keep in mind that all these benefits are quite small compared to controlling the 20 major risk factors (smoking, dietary miscues, obesity, sedentary lifestyle, failure to screen for breast, colon and prostate cancer).

Tea also lowers the blood level of homocysteine, a protein compound that is damaging to the cardiovascular system. Recent data from the Boston Area Health Study showed that among men and women with no previous history of coronary artery disease, those who habitually drank one or more cups of tea per day had 45% less risk of developing a heart attack compared with people who didn't drink tea. In a 15-year study from the Netherlands, the risk of suffering a stroke was 70% less in men who drank an average of four-and-a-half cups of tea per day compared with those who drank less than two-and-a-half cups. However, tea drinkers frequently have other healthy lifestyle and dietary practices, and have fewer major coronary risk factors, all of which can contribute to their lower risk of cardiovascular events.

Tea and cancer

Both black and green teas have an abundance of antioxidant *polyphenols* with potential cancer-fighting benefits that have been demonstrated in both animal and human studies. A recent 15-year follow-up study of 61,057 Swedish women, ages 40 to 76, showed a significant reduction in the risk of ovarian cancer among women who drank more than two to three cups of tea daily. Another study among Japanese (who have a high

prevalence of stomach cancer) did not show a significant protection against stomach cancer even among green tea drinkers. Whether these results reflect the difference between heavy green and black tea or the existence of predisposing risk factors that overcome the benefits of tea drinking is not clear at this time.

Contrary to the incessant hype, the overall benefits of individual nutrients, including tea, are relatively small. We need a basket of healthful nutrients to provide us with significant health benefits. So let's enjoy our tea, black or green, but let's tame our boundless expectations about its benefits.

✳ **CAUTION:** The cardiovascular and anti-cancer benefits of tea are substantially reduced when milk is added to the brew, a practice common in England, Canada, Australia and New Zealand. This is because some ingredients in milk may bind to tea's antioxidants and phenolic compounds and reduce their absorption from the digestive tract. In other words, these compounds become less bioavailable when milk is added to a cup of hot tea.

However, this reaction does not occur when you take tea without milk, following a meal with milk or dairy products. That's because gastric acidity and lower temperature of the stomach content (98° to 99° as compared with more than 200° in a cup of hot tea) prevents this kind of binding. As a result, food does not interfere with the absorption of tea's ingredients.

The evidence strongly suggests that drinking a few cups of tea daily is a healthful practice that can reduce your risk of heart attack, stroke and perhaps cancers such as esophagus, stomach or bladder. (Since tea has other ingredients that act like diuretics, it may reduce the risk of bladder cancer by increasing the volume of the urine and diluting any carcinogens in the bladder.) Tea can also reduce the risk of forming kidney stones by diluting the urine. Coffee offers none of these benefits, so it's prudent to consider tea as an alternative to coffee. Note that iced tea is too diluted to have a significant amount of phenolic compounds or other antioxidants compared with brewed hot tea. But a glass of iced tea is still preferable to carbonated beverages.

To fully extract the qualities of tea from tea leaves, boil water in excess of 210°. You should allow your tea leaves (or bag) to simmer at high temperature for at least three to five minutes to allow most of the phenolic compounds to seep through.

 CAUTION: Don't brew tea in the microwave! Microwave-heated water is not as hot as kettle- or pot-boiled water. In the microwave, the bubbles rise from the outer layers of water while the center is not fully heated. When you pour the water over a tea bag, the temperature is usually much less than 210 degrees. The result is a cup of tea with not much personality or healthfulness. A slight foaming over the surface of the cup indicates that the water was not adequately hot.

Brewing tea the old-fashioned way is still the best way to have a healthful and enjoyable cup of tea. Remember, adding milk turns a delightful cup of brew into an unappealing and muddy-looking drink, and strips it of its heart-healthy and cancer preventative properties. Instead of sugar, you may add a teaspoon of dark honey to your cup of tea. Dark honey (more so than light honey) is a rich source of healthy phenolic compounds.

Cocoa

Cocoa (and dark chocolate) is a paradox. Despite its relatively high sugar and saturated fat content, chocolate is a rich source of antioxidants. These antioxidants prevent the fat in chocolate from turning rancid and reduce the need for preservatives to extend the chocolate's shelf life. They can also reduce oxidization of LDL-cholesterol.

A cup of hot chocolate, for example, contains approximately 150mg of phenolic compounds, and a piece of dark chocolate (1.5 oz or 41 gm) provides almost 200 mg. In comparison, a 5 oz (140 ml) glass of red wine contains approximately 210 mg of phenolic compounds. The most active phenolic compounds in dark chocolate are procyanadins, similar to dark fruits and red wine.

Chocolate is also a rich source of many vitamins, including A and B vitamins, as well as a number of minerals, such as calcium, phosphorous, potassium, copper and iron. Moreover, it contains phenylethylamine, which stimulates the brain and produces euphoria and pleasure. In addition, good, dark chocolate (unlike the milk chocolate varieties) does not contain added shortening or a big dose of butter. Nearly one-third of dark chocolate's fat content is stearic acid, a saturated fat that behaves like monounsaturates.

So, an occasional piece of dark chocolate or a cup of hot chocolate offers pleasure and perhaps some minor cardioprotection. If you are a chocolate lover, do not overdose. Over time, the cholesterol-raising potential of excessive chocolate intake may prove more harmful than the sum of its antioxidants or pleasurable benefits.

Coffee

Moderate amounts of coffee (less than four cups a day) are neither cardioprotective or harmful. On the other hand, high consumption (more than four cups per day) of either regular or decaffeinated coffee may raise the blood level of LDL-cholesterol slightly.

The cholesterol-raising compound in coffee is not caffeine, but a special oily substance in ground coffee that seeps out during brewing. The active compounds of this oily substance are mainly cafestol and kahweol, which are usually filtered out by paper coffee filters and to a lesser extent by metal filters. Relatively high levels of these compounds are present in boiled coffee (Scandinavian style) and in unfiltered and espresso coffee.

Large coffee consumption (six to eight cups a day or more) can also increase the blood level of homocysteine, a harmful protein compound that damages coronary arteries. It is unclear whether cafestol, kahweol or other compounds in coffee are responsible for this harmful effect.

Frequently, heavy coffee drinkers are also heavy smokers, especially among Europeans and Latin Americans. For these people, smoking plays a far more important role in increasing the risk of cardiovascular diseases than does drinking coffee.

What is the impact of coffee on blood pressure?

A cup of coffee on average contains about 120 mg caffeine compared to 30 mg to 40 mg for tea. Coffee is also a rich source of many phenolic and flavonoid antioxidants, potassium and magnesium. Although caffeine pills and caffeine-containing sodas can raise the blood pressure by about 5 mmHg, moderate coffee consumption (less than four cups per day) reduces the blood pressure.

This is because at low to moderate coffee consumption, antioxidants in coffee counterbalance the blood pressure-raising action of caffeine. However, excessive coffee drinking can raise the blood pressure because the antioxidants may not be adequate to balance large doses of caffeine.

✳ **CAUTION:** Colas and other sodas and power drinks contain caffeine but have no antioxidants to blunt the blood pressure-raising effect of caffeine. If you have high blood pressure, switch to caffeine-free varieties.

Does coffee increase or decrease the risk of a heart attack?

There is a near unanimity in recent studies that moderate coffee consumption decreases the risk of cardiovascular disease, and specifically of heart attack. In a 15-year study of 27,312 women, consumption of up to three cups of coffee per day was associated with a 24% lower risk of death from cardiovascular diseases. However, the benefits decreased as the consumption levels rose.

The heart-healthy benefit of coffee at low doses is attributed to its plentiful antioxidants, which reduce the inflammation within the coronary artery wall. In fact, among Norwegians, coffee accounts for more than 60% of their dietary antioxidants.

In the combined 14-year follow-up of the Male Health Professional Study (with 44,005 men) and the Nurse's Health Study (84,488 women), coffee consumption had no cardiovascular impact, either beneficial or harmful. One reason for this discrepancy may well be the relatively younger age of the two groups in the later study.

Other recent studies suggest that more than four to five cups of coffee daily may increase the risk of heart attack, especially among people younger than 50 years of age. High intake of caffeine has been identified as the most likely compound responsible for this increased risk. Caffeine raises the heart rate, blood pressure and the levels of stress hormones (such as adrenaline compounds) in the bloodstream. Caffeine also reduces the concentration of a potent blood vessel dilator (vasodilator) called adenosine in the wall of coronary and other arteries. Reduction of adenosine contributes to spasm and constriction of the arteries. So blood flow to heart muscle and brain may be reduced for a few hours while blood caffeine levels are high. This time-dependent effect of caffeine explains why the impact of coffee on the risk of heart attack is acute and is not accumulative.

Caffeine is metabolized and broken down in the body by a specific enzyme system. Some people have a mutation in this enzyme system that reduces its effectiveness and keeps blood caffeine levels high. People who have this mutant enzyme system are "slow caffeine metabolizers." On the other hand, people with the normal enzyme system are able to rapidly break down caffeine and lower its blood level. They are "rapid caffeine metabolizers."

In a collaborative study, researchers from the University of Toronto, Harvard and Costa Rica evaluated more than 2,000 Costa Rican men and women who had experienced a first nonfatal heart attack and a similar number of people with no history of heart attack. The researchers were interested to see whether caffeine metabolism has any relevance to the risk of heart attacks. Results showed that among slow caffeine metabolizers who habitually drank more than four cups of coffee per day, the risk of nonfatal heart attack was 60% higher than in rapid caffeine metabolizers who also drank more than four cups per day. The risk of heart attack among men and women younger than 50 years of age was greater than in older persons. This suggests that the high prevalence of other coronary risk factors in an older population may dilute or reduce the impact of caffeine.

In this study, approximately 55% of subjects were slow caffeine metabolizers, but this number may vary among different populations. These findings, especially the age factor, may in part explain inconsistencies in some previous studies, which had not shown a significant increase in the risk of heart attack with up to six cups of coffee per day.

 NOTE: Although we estimate coffee consumption by measuring "cups," many Americans use coffee mugs or large cups from coffee bars that may be equal to or larger than two cups.

Does coffee have any impact on diabetes?

Although two or three cups of coffee may not have a positive or negative impact on diabetes, larger intake of decaffeinated coffee may reduce the risk of diabetes. For a detailed discussion of regular and decaffeinated coffee, please see, Diabetes.

Does coffee have any impact on the liver?

In a study by the US National Institute of Diabetes and Digestive and Kidney Diseases, nearly 10,000 people were followed up for an average of 19 years. In this long-term study, people who drank two to three cups of coffee per day had a 40% lower risk of chronic liver disease than those who drank less than one cup per day. The impact of drinking several cups of tea was similar but less striking, likely because tea has about one-quarter of the caffeine in coffee.

The findings of this report were confirmed in a much larger study of 125,580 members of a comprehensive prepaid health care plan. However, in this later study, the protective effect of coffee was only against alcohol-induced liver disease, especially cirrhosis. The liver-protective effect of coffee is primarily attributed to caffeine and, to a minor degree, to coffee's various antioxidants.

The bottom line on coffee

Aside from the pleasure, taste and minor physical and emotional lift, coffee lacks any cardioprotective, anticancer benefit. However, among people with weight issues, insulin resistance or diabetes, and possibly in those who have more than two alcoholic drinks daily, a few cups of coffee may have some benefits. So if you enjoy a few cups of coffee each day, there is no compelling reason to change. However, mixing coffee with smoking, or abusing alcohol will offer no protection against the consequences of these destructive behaviors.

Alcohol

Alcohol is not a nutrient, but a large percent of people in the world (except in Muslim countries) drink it frequently. In the past decade, more than 100 long-term studies have consistently shown that a small amount of alcohol (less than two drinks per day) is associated with a 30% to 50% reduction in the risk of developing coronary artery disease. Mortality data from 21 developed and relatively affluent countries have also shown cardioprotective benefits from all alcoholic beverages, not just red wine. To date, the weight of the evidence supporting the heart-health of light drinking is so strong that it can no longer be considered controversial.

How do alcoholic beverages help the heart?

Alcoholic beverages (wine, beer or spirits) reduce cardiovascular deaths in three ways.

(1) Alcohol (not other ingredients of alcoholic beverages) raises blood levels of (good) HDL-cholesterol by approximately seven percent to 10% depending on one's initial HDL level. If your HDL level is 35 mg/dl, raising it by 3 mg/may not appear significant, but it is. On the other hand, those who have higher HDL, such as 70 or 80 mg/dl can raise theirs by twice as much (7 to 8 mg/dl) as individuals with low levels. This effect accounts for approximately half of alcohol's cardioprotective benefit.

(2) Alcohol reduces the tendency of blood to form a clot inside the arteries and therefore significantly decreases the risk of coronary thrombosis. This is especially helpful when alcohol is consumed with meals. The blood's tendency to clot inside the arteries increases for several hours after eating. So the alcohol's anticoagulant effect is at work while the risk of heart attack or stroke is raised. This anticlotting effect represents about 30% of alcohol's heart-health benefits.

(3) Some, not all, alcoholic beverages contain flavonoid antioxidants (such as catechin, quercetin, and especially procyanidins) that can potentially reduce the oxidation of both HDL and LDL-cholesterol by more than 75%. These antioxidants in both red and white wine seep through the grape's skin during the wine-making process and account for approximately 10% to 20% of the cardioprotective benefits of alcoholic beverages.

Red or white wine?

We've seen a torrent of publicity about the wonders of red wine. It is true that certain red wines contain more procyanidins than others, red or white. These procyanidins are present in black and dark red grapes, mainly in the skin. During wine making, various compounds, including procyanidins seep through the grape's skin giving wines their distinct color, aroma, flavor and other characteristics. The same compound is also present in grape juice, grapes and raisins —provided that you chew them well to crush the skin.

The concentration of compounds in wines vary from batch to batch, year to year based on geographic location, soil, sun, rainfall, harvesting time, wine making technique, and the wine-maker's selection of what kind of grapes go into a given wine. Overall, the concentration of red wine flavonoids is greater than white wine. As noted before, the absorption rate of all flavonoids is not the same; for example, it is greater for onion flavonoids than it is for tea, but teas have a much higher concentration. Similarly, the red wine and its white counterpart have different flavonoids at different concentrations.

In a recent study, chardonnay (white) wine reduced oxidation of LDL-cholesterol by 30% compared to 15% for cabernet (red) wine. The clotting of blood was also reduced twice as much by white wine versus red wine (29% and 12%, respectively). The reason for these unexpected findings is that the flavonoids in white wine, even though they are present at lower concentration than in red wine, are more readily absorbed, achieving a higher blood concentration. However, the red wine enthusiasts need not despair.

The effects of tannin were recently studied in rats that were given alcohol containing tannins. Usually, after the anticlotting effects of alcohol wear off in a few hours, the blood's tendency to clot reverts back to what it was before the drink.

The rats given red wine had far less clotting rebound than the animals given other forms of alcohol. A similar phenomenon also occurs in humans. This is understandable since the benefit of nearly all drugs for diabetes, blood pressure, etc., are short-term as well. The tannins, however, have a much longer effect than alcohol itself.

Young red wines with tannins have a high concentration of procyanidins that can improve the endothelial function (the inner lining of the artery), so it can more effectively repel the invasion of LDL-cholesterol while blood cells and reduce the risk of plaque formation. So if you like red wine, enjoy one or two glasses with meals. Dark grapes or their juices (Concord and others) provide about 20% of wine's benefits. This is because they have similar (but at a slightly lower concentration) flavonoids and antioxidants as wine (the 20% benefit), but no alcohol (the other 80% benefit of wine).

Red wine (and the skin or juices of all dark grapes) contains a special antioxidant called "resveratrol" that can significantly reduce oxidation of LDL-cholesterol in a test tube. Unfortunately, its concentration in blood is far too low to protect LDL-cholesterol oxidation. Two or three glasses of red wine may still have significant cardioprotective benefits. Again, this result only happens when you have the wine or the purple grape juice (12 to 16 oz) right after eating.

What about other benefits of alcoholic beverages?

Low doses of alcohol (two drinks or less per day) reduce the risk of a stroke by 50%. But for heavy drinkers, the stroke risk is increased threefold.

Light drinking can make insulin's action more efficient so the breakdown or metabolism of carbohydrates becomes easier. In diabetics, especially those who are treated with oral medications, one or two drinks with the evening meal might help control diabetes more efficiently.

Contrary to what's commonly thought, sautéing with wine or beer does not totally evaporate the alcohol content or denature alcohol's other ingredients. In fact, as much as 70% to 80% of alcohol may be retained. But, since very little alcohol is used for cooking, it has virtually no health impact.

Alcohol's side effects

Alcohol is an additive drug that has a narrow safety margin. Beyond one or two drinks daily, alcohol has no medical benefit and is associated with serious or fatal side effects. Nearly all of alcohol's cardioprotection is achieved with the first drink. After the second drink, it's downhill. Some negative health effects of alcohol include…

- Excessive drinking increases the risk of irregular heart rate, hypertension, heart attacks and stroke.

- Among heavy drinkers, men are twice and women are seven times as likely to suffer a stroke as nondrinkers.

- A recent study of sudden deaths in women without a history of heart disease showed that nearly 40% of the deaths were alcohol-related. A number of studies have shown similar data in men. In nearly all of these fatalities, the cause is sudden irregularities of the heart rate and eventual cardiac arrest.

- Heavy alcohol consumption is a known risk factor for premature death. A recent long-term study of 1,600 middle-aged men revealed that the risk of death from all causes was substantially increased in people who regularly drank six or more beers at a time. The association was even stronger with deaths from external causes (such as accidents) and heart attacks. Many heavy drinkers are also often heavy

smokers. The combined burden of excessive alcohol intake and smoking contribute to increased cardiovascular mortality among heavy drinkers.

How much should you drink?

If you have no personal objection to drinking alcohol, one or two drinks with your main meal may provide cardioprotective and other healthful benefits.

So what kind of alcoholic beverage is best? With a few minor differences, they are essentially the same. One interesting distinction is that beverages produced by fermentation (beer, wine, cognac and champagne) cause a 50% to 90% increase in stomach acid secretion. Distilled beverages such as gin, vodka and whisky have no measurable impact on gastric acid secretion.

In experiments, distillation of wines removes the compounds that increase acid secretion. Distilled beverages generally are from various grains, which lack the compounds in grapes and would be filtered out anyway. So, if you have acid reflux or stomach problems, you may be better off with distilled beverages, preferably diluted.

Given all the evidence favoring low-dose alcohol intake, one or two drinks with the main meal for those at high risk of cardiovascular disease may be helpful.

But remember, it's not essential to drink alcoholic beverages to reduce your risk of heart attack. Alcohol can be a deadly drug when abused. For heavy drinkers, William Shakespeare was correct when he wrote "'First the man takes a drink, then the drink takes a drink, then the drink takes the man!"

> Data from 22 recent studies of alcoholic beverages offers inconsistent conclusions. These conclusions often suit the intentions of their sponsors.
>
> Depending on the study's design, the beverage, population and the gender studied, red wine, white wine, beer and liquor each came out on top.
>
> For example, in a study from California, white wine appeared to be more cardioprotective than red wine, red wine was more protective than beer, and beer more so than liquor.
>
> In the Female Nurses Study, beer was associated with the lowest risk of coronary artery disease, while in the Male Health Professionals Study, liquor was the most cardioprotective alcoholic beverage.
>
> And in France, red wine won the honors!

Water

Over the past decade, sales of bottled water in the United States have increased by more than 400%. The annual per capita consumption of bottled water has risen to more than 15 gallons. In California, the annual per capita consumption exceeds 20 gallons. Amazingly, people pay far more for bottled water than they pay for gasoline, and they don't even complain!

Because bottled water is a highly profitable enterprise, there are more than 100 national and regional brands of bottled water in the United States. Even Donald Trump has come up with his own "luxury" brand of expensive bottled water. Contrary to their claims, some brands are nothing more than bottled city water with no relation to "pure spring water." Nearly one-third of bottled water is filtered tap water to which some mineral has been added. Some bottlers add oxygen to bottled water and make outlandish claims that the product improves athletic performance. People are not fish—adding oxygen to drinking water has no effect.

The growth of the bottled water industry is mainly due to the power of advertising, exploiting consumers' concern about the taste and safety of tap water, even though the safety of US (and nearly all developed countries) drinking water is excellent.

IS THERE A "FRENCH PARADOX"?

For centuries the French diet has included relatively high levels of fat. Yet, except for the Japanese, certain regions of France have the lowest rates of coronary artery disease of all developed nations. This "paradox" is attributed to the traditional French habit of drinking red wine with meals, but it ignores many other heart-healthy factors. For example...

- The French (from the regions with low rates of coronary artery disease) consume much monounsaturated fat, especially olive oil. They eat very little margarine or shortening. Most poultry and red meats come from free-range and grazing animals whose flesh has less saturated fat and more monounsaturated than feed-lot fed animals. Free-range meat and eggs also contain some omega-3 polyunsaturated fats.

- The French diet often includes plenty of seafood with all of its benefits.

- The French tend to eat more fruits and vegetables (several times more) than people in northern Europe.

- The French eat 58% of their total daily calories by 2 PM, Americans eat 38% of daily calories by 2 PM. The French are also physically more active, and tend to have much lower rates of abdominal obesity.

- The French drink wine with their meals, which reduces the risk of coronary artery disease during the vulnerable post-meal hours.

- In many regions of France, the population has remained homogeneous for centuries. Thus some of these "heart-healthy" genes track through generations.

- The "French paradox" is not a paradox at all. It is a readily explainable consequence of long-term healthy diet and lifestyles.

The composition of bottled water differs from one bottler to the next.

- Some bottled waters, such as Lithia Springs, Montclair and Vichy Springs, have higher sodium content than others (but still at very low levels).

- Many brands contain little or no sodium. *Some of these include:* Canadian Glacier, Carolina Mountain, Deer Park, Evian, Great Bear, Mountain Valley Spring, Poland Spring, Pure Hawaiian, Sierra, Talking Rain and Zephyrhills.

- Most bottled waters have little or no magnesium or calcium, minerals that reduce the risk of cardiac rhythm irregularities in dehydrated individuals. In fact, among the more than 30 brands recently tested only Mendocino has an adequate and balanced amount of these two minerals without going overboard with sodium. Evian is a distant second to Mendocino.

- All bottled waters lack fluoride, zinc, selenium, iodine and other trace minerals.

HARMFUL EFFECTS OF HEAVY ALCOHOL INTAKE (3 OR MORE DRINKS DAILY)

Increases the risk of:
- Heart attack, stroke and irregular heart rate
- Sudden death, especially among women
- Dementia by over 20%
- Depression (70% of heavy drinkers have depression)
- Pancreatitis, alcohol-induced hepatitis, fatty liver and cirrhosis of the liver
- Testicular atrophy and impotence in men and reduced libido in women
- Breast cancer by 40%
- Violence and accidents (accounts for 25,000 traffic deaths each year)

And:
- It is an addictive drug (more than 20 million Americans are alcoholics)
- Tears families and friends apart
- Costs more than $150 billion annually

Is bottled water a fad?

Water, strange as it sounds, is actually quite "heart-healthy" and can significantly reduce the risk of heart attack. In a six-year study of more than 34,000 Seventh-Day Adventists, men who drank five or more glasses of water a day had a 51% lower risk of fatal heart attacks than those who drank less than two glasses per day. Women who drank more than five glasses of water daily had a 35% lower risk of fatal coronary events. Even after adjusting for other risk factors, these remarkable differences persisted. Equally important, the study found that men and women who drank more than five glasses of water a day had a 44% lower risk of fatal strokes.

In a Swedish study, women 50 to 69 years of age, who had lived in counties with hard water (high levels of calcium and magnesium), had a 30% lower risk of dying from a heart attack. Among Swedish men, high-magnesium water conferred similar protection against fatal heart attacks.

Why should water lower the risk of fatal heart attacks?

- One plausible explanation is that water dilutes the blood, making it less viscous, and therefore less likely to cause clot formation.

- An untested explanation is that platelets in a well-hydrated bloodstream do not stick together or to the endothelial cells of coronary and cerebral arteries to initiate clot formation.

- A well-hydrated person also passes a lot of urine. A high urine output makes the blood even less prone to clotting, because small amounts of some clotting factors in the blood are filtered out in the urine.

- Both calcium and magnesium in hard water have been found to lower death rates from coronary artery disease and decrease the risk of fatal arrhythmias after a heart attack.

Bottle or tap?

Aside from taste and portability, bottled water offers no advantage over city water in areas with high standards for water purification and safety. Because most city water contains healthful minerals such as magnesium, calcium, fluoride, potassium, iodine, selenium and zinc, city water is preferable to heavily filtered and mineral-stripped bottled waters.

This is especially important for athletes who exercise vigorously and might deplete their potassium and magnesium. Similarly, individuals exercising strenuously may have a higher risk of cardiac rhythm irregularities. Children, too, need calcium and fluoride for healthy teeth and bones and should be discouraged from drinking bottled waters and colas.

However, if the taste or smell of your city water is unpleasant, bottled waters are certainly preferable to dehydration.

Most faucet-mounted home water filters (with solid block carbon filters) remove more than 90% of water-borne germs, parasites, and "impurities" from tap water and provide a tasty and safe source of drinking water. Depending on usage, you should change the filter frequently, at least once every two to three months. Some newer models of granular activated charcoal filters can also remove water-borne parasites, but this varies from manufacturer to manufacturer.

For those whose immune systems are severely compromised, more expensive and effective under-the-sink filters should not only remove the parasitic contaminants but other microorganisms as well.

Bottled waters generally provide convenience and a false sense of safety. Since the majority of bottled waters are neither pasteurized nor sterilized (they are usually filtered), they may still have some bacterial contaminants. You will deprive yourself of healthful benefits of tap water if you exclusively rely on bottled water.

Soft drinks

An occasional soft drink with or without caffeine or sugar has no effect on heart health, cancer or other health issue. But, I stress "occasional." Although soft drinks have no direct impact on cardiovascular health, they do have significant side effects...Nearly all colas contain phosphoric acid, which increases loss of calcium through the kidneys into the urine, and may contribute to the epidemic of osteoporosis among people in their 40s and 50s. The sugar and high fructose corn sweeteners in soda are also contributing to obesity and type 2 diabetes. In addition, soda can aggravate symptoms of acid reflux disease and irritable bowel syndrome, two disorders that afflict more than 50 million Americans of all age groups.

What about sugar-free, caffeine-free sodas?

Isn't it incredible that we happily pay to drink something that is nothing? We are a consumers driven society. Advertising makes us believe that although caffeine-free diet sodas have no redeeming value and are actually harmful, we should still pay for the privilege of drinking them!

Fruit juices

All unsweetened fruit juices (with or without calcium fortification) are excellent alternatives to colas and soft drinks. Unpasteurized juices (such as apple juice) may pose a health risk due to bacterial contamination. Several recent outbreaks of E. coli infection in the United States and Canada have been traced to these unpasteurized products, even though the manufacturers used standard procedures. (Most of these outbreaks of E. coli infection have been traced to the farm or orchard from which the produce came, and not to the factories themselves.) For this reason, choose only pasteurized fruit juices, especially those who have compromised immune systems. 🍎

4

THE TWENTY RISK FACTOR DIET

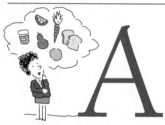

Any nutritional approach to cardiovascular health must take into account almost all risk factors. Most popular diets designed to lower cholesterol or to aid weight loss often take a simplistic, sometimes harmful, approach. Before I introduce my nutritional approach to cardiovascular health, let's see why current dietary programs are obsolete, ineffective or even unsafe.

Low-fat, Low-cholesterol Diets: Ineffective and Possibly Harmful

Low-fat, low-cholesterol diets became popular over 40 years ago, when it was believed that coronary artery disease was a direct consequence of an elevated blood cholesterol level. Today, we know that this was a flawed assumption. Another flawed assumption was that a low-fat, low-cholesterol diet would significantly lower blood cholesterol and consequently lower the risk of coronary artery disease. These diets did not live up to their high expectations, because even if they lowered the LDL-cholesterol, they did not address the other major coronary risk factors.

For approximately 30% of people, low-fat, low-cholesterol diets may lower LDL-cholesterol by an average of 7 to 10 mg/dl, and in about one out of six diet responders, the blood cholesterol might fall by even more than 20 mg/dl. However, this modest reduction in LDL-cholesterol is unlikely to have a significant cardiovascular impact, especially in people who have very high blood cholesterol levels, or have already developed coronary artery disease. Moreover, the 70% of the population who do not respond to dietary cholesterol and saturated fat benefit even less from low-fat, low-cholesterol diets.

Since a low-fat, low-cholesterol diet usually has a much higher level of carbohydrates, it may lower the cardioprotective HDL-cholesterol, raise triglycerides, and actually counteract any benefit from lowering the LDL-cholesterol.

Is total dietary fat relevant to coronary artery disease?

Eskimos obtain more than 60% of their energy supply from fat, but they have the lowest risk of coronary artery disease in the world. Similarly, many low-risk populations—Mediterraneans, many ovo-lacto-vegetarians, or the majority of Americans who do not have coronary artery disease—have a dietary fat intake that ranges from 33% to more than 40%.

Dietary fat intake among various populations is not correlated with their rates of coronary artery disease. A recent 14-year study of more than 80,000 healthy American women between 34 and 59 years of age showed that the total amount of dietary fat intake had no relation to coronary artery disease. The investigators, however, estimated that replacing five percent of calories from saturated fat with unsaturated fats (monounsaturates or nonhydrogenated vegetable oils) would reduce the risk of coronary artery disease by 42%. Replacing two percent of calories from trans fatty acids (present in margarines, shortenings, cooking fats and other foods) with unsaturated fats would reduce the risk by 53%.

The Multiple Risk Factor Intervention Trial followed nearly 13,000 healthy, low-risk men with no previous history of coronary artery disease for 16 years. One group followed the American Heart Association Phase II diet, which has less than 20% fat and less than 200 mg of cholesterol per day. They took medications to lower their high blood pressure, stopped smoking and lost some weight. During the 16-year follow-up, deaths from coronary artery disease in the treated group dropped by only 11% compared to the control group (which was not so treated).

In contrast, a recent study from Lyon, France, showed that in a group of high-risk individuals (i.e., people who have already developed coronary artery disease and had at least one heart attack), those who followed a Mediterranean diet experienced 70% fewer heart attacks, 56% fewer overall deaths, and, surprisingly, 61% fewer cancers. These dramatic effects occurred even though the fat content of the diet was more than 30%, mostly from monounsaturates and omega-3 polyunsaturates from seafood.

Can low-fat diets reduce the risk of cardiovascular diseases?

More than a thousand studies have failed to provide any evidence that reducing total dietary fat has any significant impact on either prevention or treatment of coronary artery disease.

In the long-anticipated Women's Health-Initiative Trial, 48,835 women aged 50 to 79 years, were enrolled in a randomized controlled study of a low-fat versus regular-fat diet to see the impact on cardiovascular events. After an eight-year follow-up, the low-fat diet had no significant impact on the risk of coronary artery disease, stroke or other vascular events. However, in women who had lower intake of saturated fat or trans fat there was a trend toward lower risk for various cardiovascular diseases. These studies demonstrate that it is not the total fat but the type of fat that is relevant to heart health.

Can low-fat diets help in weight management or prevention of various cancers?

Numerous trials of low-fat diets for weight loss over the past two decades have not shown any significant benefit. For example, in the Women's Health Initiative Trial, described above, the women on the low-fat diet had lost slightly over one pound more than women who were not on the low-fat diet.

In the most recent study, Stanford University researchers placed four groups of women with weight problems on one of the following four diets for a year: an extremely rigid, very low-fat, very little to no cholesterol, vegetarian diet (Ornish diet); Zone diet (low-glycemic index); LEARN diet (Similar to American Heart Association, Phase II diet), and Atkins diet (very low-carb, very high-fat, high cholesterol). After 12 months, the group on the most rigid

Ornish diet lowered their LDL-cholesterol by only 4 mg/dl! (Gardner, CD et al., *JAMA* 2007; 297: 969–77).

In a previous study, researchers for Tufts University in Boston compared Ornish (very low-fat, cholesterol-free), Atkins (very high-fat, low-carb), the Zone (low-glycemic index) and Weight Watchers (small portions and low-calorie) diets. After one year, there was no difference among the four diet groups in terms of weight loss or cardio-vascular risk reduction. However, the dropout rates were higher among the Atkins and Ornish dieters than for the two other groups (Dansinger, ML et al., *JAMA* 2005; 293: 45–53).

For over two decades the notion that reducing total dietary fats lowers the risk of breast cancer in women has been vigorously promoted without scientific evidence to back it up. From the very beginning this was a sound bite "low-fat diet," instead of a sound dietary recommendation to reduce trans fatty acids and hydrogenated fats and increase monounsaturated fat and omega-3 fat from seafood. Several studies have shown that a low-fat diet does not reduce the risk of breast cancer, colorectal cancer or any other malignancies.

Aside from depriving people of the joy of eating, and imposing inflexible restrictions on their food choices, low-fat, low-cholesterol diets may even be harmful.

In a 20-year study of 832 men between 45 and 65 years of age, a low-fat, low-cholesterol diet increased risk of a stroke by more than 50% compared to those who were not on cholesterol- and fat-restricted diets. That is because the smaller brain arteries need fat, cholesterol and lecithin to maintain their integrity and not crack or rupture and bleed into the brain, or clog up and prevent blood flow to brain tissue. Is this an effective, practical, or safe diet to prevent a heart attack?

Very low-fat, very low-cholesterol diets

Let's look at very low-fat, very low-cholesterol diets. Pritikin's Longevity Program contains less than 10% of calories from fat (less than three percent from saturated fat) and about 25 mg of cholesterol per day, whereas Ornish's Lifestyle Heart Trial provides seven percent of calories from fat and no cholesterol. Further the Lifestyle Heart Trial forbids all oils, meats, poultry, seafood, nuts, dairy (except a small amount of skimmed milk), eggs, alcohol, tea, coffee and chocolate. What's left to eat?

Unlike many studies that are based on hundreds or thousands of cases, Dean Ornish's Lifestyle Heart Trial diet evolved from the study of only 22 men with severe coronary artery disease, obesity and sedentary lifestyles. These individuals were enrolled in a supervised program of regular exercise (one died while exercising), stress management, weight reduction, smoking cessation, antihypertensive therapy, aspirin and various vitamins, along with repeated follow-up visits. In addition, they closely followed the strict vegan diet described above.

After five years on this rigid program—impossible to follow for most people—the researchers reported a 50% lower relative risk of new coronary events compared to another small control group. They touted this 50% response rate as proof that a rigid vegan diet might be the answer to the epidemic of coronary artery disease.

But does a 50% reduction in the relative risk of coronary events in five years support the efficacy of a rigid vegan diet? These individuals also received comprehensive treatment for numerous other risk factors. Why do these researchers attribute the 50% improvement (as meager as it is) to their punitive and next-to-impossible diet? A rigid vegan diet has no relevance to prevention or treatment of coronary artery disease (and may be counterproductive).

Since patients in the Ornish Lifestyle Diet took aspirin (with a 30% expected risk reduction), lowered their LDL-cholesterol (30%) and blood pressure (30%), exercised regularly (50%), lost weight (40%), stopped smoking (30%) and participated in regularly scheduled, twice-a-week stress management therapy (at least an expected 50% risk reduction), they should have earned a risk reduction close to 260%. Yet their relative risk reduction was only 50%. Moreover, such rigid diets, outside of research settings, have even fewer benefits, as the Stanford University study described on p. 175, demonstrated. I don't think an extreme approach is a rational, safe, or practical way to deal with a deadly epidemic.

Some vegetarian zealots and proponents of very low-fat, no-cholesterol diets argue that the human digestive tract is generally unsuitable to eat meat. Our distant ancestors, Homo erectus, made tools and chased animals for food at least 2½ million years ago. Thus any genetic mutation would have favored a meat-eating diet, not the other way around. With a few exceptions, even rodents, insects, birds and fish are avid carnivores when they have the opportunity. Monkeys and other primates often supplement their protein-deficient diet by devising ingenious tricks to catch ants and other insects. They also resort to occasional cannibalism.

Extremely low-fat, low-cholesterol diets (or the newer cholesterol-free versions) became popular some 20 years ago when there were no effective or safe cholesterol-lowering drugs. These diets were the counterparts of salt-free diets (for hypertensives and people with heart or kidney failure) and sugar-free diets (for diabetics). Fortunately, salt-free and sugar-free diets

had their "fifteen minutes of fame" and faded into oblivion as effective drugs became available. Very low-fat, cholesterol-free diets are punitive, ineffective and may even be harmful. They have no place in preventing or treating coronary artery disease.

The 10 dietary commandments

Now that low-fat, low-cholesterol diets are ruled out, the key question is: What are the aims of dietary interventions is? An ideal dietary intervention should prevent, slow down or stop the coronary quartet. To achieve these goals such a diet should be consistent with all or most of my "10 commandments." See page 184.

The Twenty Risk Factor (TRF) diet presented here fulfills all of these dietary "commandments," while low-fat, low-cholesterol and vegetarian diets do not. The TRF diet is not based on personal beliefs, a bias for or against any particular nutrient or food group, or my own unsupported opinions. In science, and especially in medicine, opinion must be supported by facts.

The TRF diet is based on a modified and contemporary Mediterranean diet, analyzed and computed for use by people of all ages, whether or not they have any risk factors for coronary artery disease. It is backed by several thousand scientific works published in the past 10 years and a 3,000-year-old history of healthfulness and safety.

In addition to its heart-healthy role, the TRF diet also reduces the risk of many cancers (such as breast, colon and prostate), diabetes, hypertension, obesity, kidney stones and osteoporosis. It provides endless choices without the boredom of a fixed, rigid menu. In essence, the Twenty Risk Factor diet is designed to replace almost all other diets.

One Diet for All Coronary Risk Factors: The TRF Rating System

Food is not the enemy. Foods have many heart healthy and cancer-fighting ingredients. They also can promote health in numerous other ways. On the other hand, over-consuming some nutrients, such as saturated fats, trans fatty acids or high glycemic carbohydrates, can have a negative health impact. So it's a dual role—foods can be credited for their health-promoting role and blamed for their disease-causing potential. We need to choose healthy foods for healthy hearts.

Eating should be a pleasurable activity not an exercise in algebra or biochemistry. Judging food solely on the basis of its fat and cholesterol content is not valid, because it ignores the exceedingly diverse roles of different nutrients in foods. Rigid and punitive dietary practices have no relevance to preventive medicine. Fad diets with emphasis on single nutrients such as broccoli, grapefruit, oat bran or garlic, or components such as carbohydrates, fat and cholesterol, are unbalanced and may be harmful.

Furthermore, short bursts of dieting have no long-term benefits. You can't bank benefits of short-term dietary or lifestyle changes somewhere in the human body.

The TRF diet is the result of more than a decade of research in the area of food technology, nutrition, medicine and health. The TRF diet is broad-based and takes into account all the important nutrient groups.

For example, in the TRF diet, the overall health impact of a piece of chicken is distinctly different from that of fish, even though they may have the same amount of fat and cholesterol content. Similarly, olive oil or canola oil is different from corn oil or margarine, even though they have the same amount of fat and calories, and no cholesterol.

For most consumers, it is impractical to be constantly figuring out what is in their foods. The TRF diet eliminates all these concerns. Most important, the TRF diet is designed to meet dietary requirements for the management of *all* 20 major coronary risk factors. There is no need for a separate diet if you have heart disease, hypertension or diabetes, or obesity, if you're young or elderly. Moreover, the TRF diet has drawn from a huge database of research on various cancers to provide a rational dietary approach to reduce the risk of the most common cancers dramatically, including breast, colon and prostate. The TRF diet is the lifetime diet for all people—for those who are healthy and those who want to be.

The formula for the TRF scoring system is presented for information only. Readers will not have to do the math themselves because I have already computed the scores for many common foods and snacks. The formula should be a helpful tool for other researchers, nutritionists and government or private agencies involved in public health and nutrition policies.

Tips, tricks and practical guidelines for using TRF scores

TRF scores provide a liberating tool to help you choose healthy foods. As long as the 24-hour TRF scores are kept under 30, the choice of foods is limited only by your creativity and personal preferences.

Although the TRF scoring system allows plenty of room for flexibility and choice, it is qualitative. You cannot offset an unhealthy choice by adding a healthy one.

The purpose of the TRF scoring system is to provide a valid and worry-free tool to choose healthful meals, not to provide loopholes for "cheating" or "outsmarting" the system. Although a single meal, or a single day, of dietary indiscretion will not have a lasting impact, to minimize your risk of a cardiovascular event, diabetes, or various cancers, you should not make a U-turn.

Here are some questions you might ask about the TRF diet.

Should you eat red meat?

More than 70% of Americans think that red meat is a contributing factor to heart attack and more than 50% think or have heard that red meat may cause colon or breast cancer. Even healthcare providers routinely advise their patients to cut down on red meat without valid evidence to back up such recommendations. They include unprocessed lean red meats such as beef, veal, pork and venison with processed red meats such as hot dogs, bologna, sausages, etc. The second group has very high concentrations of saturated fats and TRF scores, and they increase the risk of cardiovascular diseases, whereas lean red meats have no impact on cardiovascular health and similarly have no role in diabetes, obesity, or various cancers.

Most studies of red meat consumption have created more confusion than clarity. For example, a Finnish study showed that high consumption of red meat increased the risk of colorectal cancer in men, but not in women; a Swedish study showed no increased risk in either men or women. Other studies have shown no association between fresh red meat and any cancer, but have shown an increased risk with heavy consumption of processed red meat.

A recent European study has provided a new perspective and a plausible explanation for the association between processed red meats and colorectal cancers. Heavy meat eaters often eat very little fish, and so deprive themselves of the significant cancer-fighting benefits of seafood. It is not the consumption of the red meat that may increase the risk of colorectal cancer, but the lack of adequate seafood in the diet.

Several studies have shown that moderate amounts of lean red meats do not raise LDL-cholesterol any more than chicken or turkey. For example, extra-lean ground beef has four to seven percent total fat, about one-half of that is saturated. However, about 50% of this saturated fat is stearic acid which acts like monounsaturates and does not raise the LDL-cholesterol. Therefore, a quarter pound of uncooked, extra-lean ground beef has a mere one to two grams of undesirable saturated fat, which should not affect blood cholesterol level.

You should, however, avoid greasy red meats—regular hamburger, ribs, meat loaf, steak, hot dogs, sausages, bacon and processed cold cuts such as bologna. The problem is not the red meat, but the white fat. Extra lean ground beef (four to seven percent fat) for hamburgers, meat loaf and kabobs, or lean London broil, sirloin, and tenderloin, or lean pork products, veal, venison, or buffalo meat all provide delicious and healthful meals, provided they are small servings of less than six ounces.

Since grilling can make hamburgers made with lean ground beef dry, you can always mix one tablespoon of olive oil with it to make it as juicy as regular hamburger, but without the undesirable saturated fats. Chops, whether lamb, veal or pork, are too greasy and have very high TRF scores, unless they are trimmed thoroughly after cooking.

Should you eat poultry?

Although chicken and turkey can provide many delicious and healthy meals, they should not become the "alternative" to lean red meats. Chicken and turkey are neutral; they neither prevent nor promote coronary artery disease. But if you have a high risk of developing coronary artery disease, or already have it, neutrality is not productive. By doing "no harm" (remaining neutral and relying on chicken and turkey), you miss the opportunity to reduce your risk of a coronary event.

When you grill, bake or broil chicken, you can leave the skin on to prevent the meat from drying and making it tough and inedible. In these instances, the fat of the skin does not transfer to the meat; but always remove the skin before eating it. When you cook chicken with other ingredients in a pot or pan, however, these ingredients can absorb some of the melted fat, especially potatoes, carrots and other vegetables. Remove the skin before cooking it.

Should you eat seafood?

As you have seen, seafood provides a vast number of cardioprotective benefits, unmatched by any other food. Since seafood's cardioprotective role is directly related to its omega-3 polyunsaturated fat content and not to its protein or other nutrients, the fattier the fish, the better it is. Approximately 30% of the fat in seafood is omega-3 polyunsaturated fat, and another 20% to 30% is monounsaturates. A big chunk of saturated fat in seafood is stearic acid, which acts very much like monounsaturates, leaving little coronary-unfriendly saturated fat to worry about. As a rule, the fat content of white fish is substantially less than that in fish with pink or dark meats.

To achieve the full benefits of omega-3 polyunsaturated fat, eat three to four seafood meals per week. For example, two days a week, eat some seafood for lunch (such as tuna fish sandwiches without mayonnaise). Then, two nights of the week, you can eat seafood of your choice for dinner.

You should not prepare seafood with vegetable oils or fats (which contain a very high concentration of omega-6 polyunsaturated fat), because it defeats the purpose of eating seafood in the first place. Sautéing with olive oil, canola oil or hazelnut oil (all predominately monounsaturated)

THE COMPOSITION OF THE TWENTY RISK FACTOR DIET

Dietary Nutrient	Grams (or mg) per day #
Saturated fat, from foods and snacks	less than 14
Omega-6 fat, from vegetable oils, margarines, cooking fats	less than 20
Omega-3 fat, from seafood (or fish oil supplements)	more than 2
Monounsaturated fat, from olive oil, nuts (and canola oil)*	more than 40
Total fat, from all foods and snacks	more than 70
Cholesterol, from foods and snacks	300–400 mg
Total carbohydrates, from starches, sugars, grains, produce	more than 200
Protein, from animal and plant sources	more than 70
Fruits and vegetables, mostly darker varieties and less starchy	5 or more servings

#Grams or milligrams of nutrients are based on 2000 calories per day. These amounts change with higher or lower calories per day.

*Although canola oil has about 52%–54% monounsaturates and another 6%–8% plant omega-3, with only 5% saturated fat, which are desirable, it also has more than 30% omega-6 fat, which is not so desirable. Canola oil is preferable to all other vegetable oils. (Olive oil is a fruit oil, not vegetable oil.)

is the better alternative. Shrimp and many other shellfish have very low-fat content, about one percent total fat, compared to 30% for a choice grade T-bone steak. On the other hand, fish with pink or red flesh contains more fat (usually less than five to seven percent), about 25%–30% of which is the cardioprotective omega-3 polyunsaturated fat. For this reason, try to choose fattier fish, such as salmon and tuna, instead of tilapia, flounder or perch.

The cholesterol content of all fish is comparable to, or even lower than, chicken or turkey. Among shellfish, only squid has moderately high cholesterol content, but most people do not eat squid frequently. Shrimp, while its cholesterol content is slightly higher than chicken or turkey, can still provide a heart friendly meal because of its very low saturated fat. In other shellfish, such as clams, a large portion of "cholesterol" content is not actually cholesterol, as we know it, but cholesterol look-alikes or sterols that are poorly absorbed from the intestine. These cholesterol look-alikes, moreover, actually prevent the absorption of cholesterol from the intestine, making them quite healthful.

Should you eat dairy products and eggs?

All low-fat dairy products (such as milk, yogurt or cottage cheese) are excellent nutrients for people of all ages, except for people who are lactose intolerant. Approximately half of adult Hispanics, 60% of African-Americans, 70% of Asians and 50% of Middle Easterners are lactose intolerant, as well as 10% of the Caucasian population of the United States. For these groups, products containing lactose can cause gas, bloating, diarrhea or abdominal cramps.

Combining lactose-free milk, such as Lact-Aid, or combining one or two Lact-Aid tablets with milk and cottage cheese, are reasonable options for lactose intolerant people.

In processed cheeses, such as American, cheddar, mozzarella, provolone, parmesan and Swiss, lactose is fermented and broken down. Therefore, processed cheeses do not cause any symptoms in lactose intolerant individuals. Unfortunately, processed cheeses have very high TRF scores. Meals containing cheese as the main ingredient, such as pizza, ravioli and grilled-cheese sandwiches, are not coronary-friendly. Still, an occasional piece of cheese should not be viewed as poisonous or a trigger for a coronary event.

People often say, "I get my calcium from cheeses," or, "Cheeses have a lot of calcium." Processed cheeses do have some calcium but not much. What they have a lot of is sodium, which in healthy people is mostly eliminated, in the urine. Unfortunately, as sodium is eliminated, it also drags calcium along with it. The net effect is loss of calcium, and eventually low mineral density of bones and osteoporosis. Therefore, processed cheeses are not good sources of calcium.

Eggs have been mistakenly and arbitrarily eliminated from our diet because of the unwarranted fear of raising blood cholesterol level. This misconception is due to the cholesterol content of each yolk (an average of 220 mg per egg). But total fat content of eggs is about four percent—the same as the dark meat of chicken or turkey. And the yolk and the egg white provide wonderfully nutritious meals for people of all ages, especially the young and the elderly.

Numerous studies have shown that eating seven to 10 eggs per week (without butter or shortenings) does not raise cholesterol levels. In fact, making your omelette or sunny-side-up eggs with olive oil causes the olive oil's monounsaturated fat to attach to cholesterol (or esterify the cholesterol). Esterized cholesterol does not raise the blood cholesterol level. The TRF scores of an omelet with two medium-sized eggs cooked with olive oil or canola oil is about 7. An omelet or other egg dish (without added cheese) is

OIL ABSORBED PER 100 GRAM PORTION DURING STIR-FRYING

	Grams
Shredded low-fat pork	4
Fresh soybean	5
Cubed chicken	7
Green peppers	8
Kidney beans	9
Onions	11
Pea pods	12
Cauliflower	13
Cabbage	13
Spinach	13
Mushroom	14
Carrot	14
Eggplant	14
Bamboo shoot	15
Broccoli	15

a reasonable choice, two to three times per week, and provides a good deal of flexibility in your diet.

What's the right amount of fruits and vegetables?

During the past 25 years in the United States, consumption of fruits and vegetables has increased by 22% and 19% respectively. Unfortunately, more than half of the vegetables Americans eat are potatoes, half of them fried, containing a big dose of undesirable trans fatty acids. Dark leafy vegetables and deeply colored fruits (such as all berries, plums, nectarines and grapes) are rich sources of cardioprotective antioxidants/flavonoids. For this reason, the TRF diet encourages at least five to seven servings per day of vegetables and fruits.

What types of dietary fat should be avoided?

Avoid butter, creams, stick margarine, shortening, cooking fats, lard and mayonnaise. All of these fats have very high TRF scores. Stick margarines and shortenings not only have a high concentration of saturated fats, but they also contain 15% to 25% trans fatty acids, which makes them quite coronary-unfriendly. Given the choice between butter and stick margarine, the best choice is olive oil!

Olive oil, canola oil or hazelnut oil can be used for all cooking needs, but a small amount of soft, trans fatty acid-free margarine (such as Benecol, Brummel & Brown, Smart Balance, or Take Control) or a low-fat variety can be used sparingly. (The TRF score of two tablespoons of Benecol spread is 1, and for Brummel & Brown spread, it is 4, compared to an average of more than 16 for many stick margarines.)

Foods and snacks prepared with margarines, shortenings or cooking fats are coronary-unfriendly. For example, having a Danish pastry for breakfast is no better than eating two fried eggs, with bacon and buttered bread. Donuts, muffins and croissants also have relatively high concentrations of saturated and trans fatty acids, which raise their TRF scores. The same is true for cakes, cookies, pastries and pies.

All deep-fried food—deep-fried chicken, seafood, onion rings, french-fried potatoes or donuts—has a high concentration of trans fatty acids and omega-6 polyunsaturated fat and unacceptably high TRF scores. On the other hand, you can sauté various foods in a nonstick pan using a small amount of olive oil, canola oil or hazelnut oil.

High intake of omega-6 polyunsaturates present in all vegetable oils, such as corn, sunflower, safflower, sesame and soybean oils— contrary to decades of misleading advertising —is also unhealthy. The three major concerns with these vegetable fats are that they: (1) lower HDL-cholesterol; (2) increase oxidation of LDL-cholesterol— a major disadvantage, since oxidized LDL particles are quite coronary unfriendly; and (3) spark a lingering concern that omega-6 polyunsaturated fat might increase the risk of certain cancers, such as breast, colon and prostate.

Current recommendations to increase consumption of polyunsaturated fat to 10% of dietary energy intake were based on the knowledge available 30 years ago. Such recommendations are now obsolete and have no relevance to cardiovascular health, especially since virgin olive oils are healthful alternatives and are readily available at prices comparable to or slightly higher than vegetable oils. Substituting olive oil (which is fruit oil, not a vegetable oil) for all other oils and fats in the diet raises the HDL-cholesterol and lowers the LDL-cholesterol. But more importantly, this simple change in the type (but not necessarily the amount) of dietary fat inhibits the oxidation of LDL-cholesterol.

Palm oil, palm kernel or cottonseed oil, often used in baked products, have very high concentrations of saturated fats and, proportionately, very high TRF scores. Although the amount of these oils in a daily diet is relatively small, when added to other saturated and trans fatty acids in a typical Western diet, you cannot ignore them. On the other hand, an occasional slice of pie or cake would not clog your coronary artery overnight.

Should you avoid eating out?

Dining out need not be a "coronary trap." Dishes prepared with creams, butter, margarine or cooking fat may be appetizing, but they have quite

---

FAST FOOD OR HAZARDOUS MATERIAL?

Some examples of Denny's breakfast menu…

- *Farmer's Slam* has 80 gm of fat (24 gm saturated), 704 mg cholesterol, and 3,200 mg sodium and a TRF score of +48!

- *French Slam 2* has 82 gm fat (26 gm saturated), 825 mg cholesterol, and 2,900 mg sodium and a TRF score of 59!

- *Breakfast Dagwood* has 90 gm fats (38 gm saturated), more than 800 mg cholesterol and 3,600 mg sodium and a TRF score of 84!

WHAT IS WRONG WITH DEEP-FRIED FOOD?

Long-term consumption of repeatedly heated fats…

- **Impairs** the ability of the arteries to properly dilate when needed.

- **Increases** the blood pressure.

- **Increases** the LDL-cholesterol and **lowers** the HDL-cholesterol.

- **Increases** oxidation of LDL- and HDL-cholesterol (makes LDL-cholesterol more harmful and HDL-cholesterol less cardioprotective).

- **Increases** the risk of heart attack, stroke, insulin resistance, diabetes and dementia.

- **Increases** the risk of breast, colon and prostate cancer.

- **And carries all other misdeeds of trans fats.**

How does deep-frying make foods unhealthy?

- Repeatedly heated fats contain more than **400% oxidized** fat by-products than fresh oils/fats.

- Oxidized and unhealthy fat by-products enter the foods that are deep-fried.

- These fats also contain high concentrations of omega-6, trans and saturated fats.

THE DIETARY COMMANDMENTS

A rational diet...

- Should *lower* the bad LDL-cholesterol and *raise* the good HDL-cholesterol
- Should *lower* triglycerides
- Should *lower* the number of very harmful small LDL particles
- Should *lower* the oxidant load and oxidization of LDL- and HDL-cholesterol
- Should *lower* insulin resistance and risk of metabolic syndrome and diabetes
- Should *lower* platelet and white blood cell activation, which reduces the risk of plaque rupture and heart attack or stroke
- Should *lower* inflammation within the wall of the arteries and plaques
- Should *lower* the risk of cancers such as breast, colon, prostate and pancreas
- Should *not be* energy dense (highly caloric) or have a high glycemic index to help with weight management and diabetes control
- Should *not be* rigid or boring

high TRF scores. This is particularly true with cream, butter and Alfredo or most French sauces, such as béarnaise and hollandaise. The sensible approach is to ask your server if a particular dish can be prepared with olive oil instead of butter, cream or margarine. At good restaurants, this request is usually honored. In fact, choosing a seafood entree, especially if it is grilled, lightly sautéed, baked, poached or broiled (preferably using olive oil), minimizes any concern about hidden and unwanted fats.

In fast food restaurants, grilled chicken or roast beef sandwiches without added butter or margarine or greasy sauces are reasonable options. The TRF scores of various sizes of french fries are high, so choose the smaller sized portion. Similarly, salads with cheese and sauce are no better than hamburgers at these restaurants. Breakfast at fast food restaurants is even worse in terms of its fat content. However an occasional meal with eggs, bacon or even sausages is permissible.

You should also avoid large portions of any meal—anywhere, anytime—because invariably they have too many calories and too-high TRF scores. "All you can eat" buffets, smorgasbords, two-for-one specials and extra-large sizes are notoriously coronary-unfriendly, have too many calories, very high TRF scores and are often conducive to overeating everything but the "right stuff."

French, Italian and even Chinese restaurants in the United States often prepare meals with an inordinate amount of hidden fat. Many Chinese restaurants use peanut oil so excessively that it covers every piece of vegetable and meat in the dish, turning it into a most unhealthy meal. The box on pg. 182 shows how much fat is absorbed by various foods during stir-frying. When eating out, choose a simple entree that is not disguised with, or swimming in, various ingredients.

What about fast foods?

The fast food industry is an American creation that has mushroomed all over the world. In the United States, nearly everyone, especially families with young children, visits a fast food establishment at least once a week. Although over two-thirds of the people consider fast foods "junk food," this does not seem to deter them from eating them.

Whether we like it or not, the fast food industry is here to stay. The Tables showing TRF scores of fast food start on p. 225. With a few exceptions, similar foods at other fast food eateries have the same TRF scores with minor variations.

Among the reasons so many people eat at fast food establishments are that they are convenient and informal, the service is fast and the food is predictable and reasonably tasty (especially for youngsters). But, of equal importance, these foods are affordable, and some actually have nutritional value!

After pressure by citizen groups in the early 1990s, a few fast food chains in the United States began a public relations campaign and lowered the fat content of a few of their entrees. Some even introduced low-fat items to provide consumers with so-called "heart healthy" choices. But by the late 1990s, regrettably, most of the lean items had disappeared from the menus of nearly all fast food eateries. In 2005–2007, fast food chains intensified the race to make their sandwiches bigger or meatier, and by adding various sauces or garnishes, even more calorie- and fat-laden. Many recent items added to menus at fast food eateries are far worse than previous items.

Puzzling to me is the silence of public health officials, citizen advocacy groups, and the public in general, who seem to have given up and have even embraced them with enthusiasm. Could the fast food eateries opt for healthy food, when the public is telling them they like the unhealthful ones?

The TRF scores of some fast food entrees are so unhealthful that, like alcohol or tobacco products, they should be forced to carry a health warning. For example, one Double Whopper with Cheese at Burger King has 67 grams of fat (100% of total daily requirement), 26 grams of saturated fat (more than 100%), and nearly 3,000 mg of salt (60%). Overall, the TRF score of this atrocious concoction, not counting any french fries or desserts, is 57. A king-size french fries portion adds another 26 points, and a medium milk

shake, another 12 points, giving that meal a total TRF score of 95! This is more than the allowed TRF score of all meals for three whole days.

McDonald's and Taco Bell's offerings have also become fattier, and pack much higher TRF scores than they did a few years ago. Among the big fast food chains, only Wendy's resisted the trend for a while, but they, too, have succumbed to the notion that "bigger is better." For example, they have introduced "Cheddar Lovers Bacon Cheeseburger," a dreadful combination with about 50 gm of fat, of which nearly half is saturated, and more than 3,000 mg of salt. Just as disheartening are the TRF scores of Wendy's Taco Salad and Greek Salad which are 21 and 15, respectively. In contrast, the scores of their Deluxe Garden Salad and Grilled Chicken Salad are quite reasonable at 3 and 5, respectively.

At Taco Bell, very few entrees have TRF scores below 10. A Taco Salad with Salsa scores 29, and a Chicken Club Burrito scores 21. These chains could lower the fat content, especially saturated and trans fatty acids, but like the rest of the fast food industry, they choose not to.

Kentucky Fried Chicken has managed to turn the harmless chicken into a coronary-unfriendly meal by deep-frying it in cooking fat loaded with saturated fat and trans fatty acids. For example, their Tender Roast Breast without skin has a healthful TRF score of 4. In sharp contrast, Extra Crispy Breast has a coronary-unfriendly score of 15, and Chunky Chicken Pot Pie's score is nearly twice as bad at 26.

Subway sandwiches are another example of good and bad all mixed up. For example, the average consumer may not suspect that a Subway Tuna Sub has a TRF score of 20 and a Seafood and Crab Sub a score of 19—five times higher than a TRF score of Roast Beef or Ham (with TRF scores of 4), and more than six times higher than a Turkey Breast or Chicken Breast Sub (with TRF scores of 3).

Pizza Hut and nearly all other pizzerias, national and regional, are no better. For example, most people think "vegetarian" means nutritious and healthy foods. At pizzerias, vegetarian no longer means what it implies. Instead, it means a greasy, cheese- or margarine-laden concoction with a few slivers of onions, green peppers, mushrooms or black olives. TRF scores of all of these pizzas are very high, especially since most people tend to eat more than one piece. For example, the TRF score of four pieces of Pizza Hut's Veggie Lovers Stuffed Crust Pizza is a disheartening 50, equal to the allowed TRF scores of all foods and snacks for two days.

Recent studies have shown that consumption of fat that has been used for deep-frying in fast food restaurants impairs artery wall function, and the ability of the arteries to dilate properly. This is because repeatedly heated cooking fats have a concentration of oxidized fatty products 400% higher than that of previously unused fat. Thus, fried items at fast food restaurants put consumers in a double jeopardy—too much fat with very high TRF scores, and far too many oxidized fat by-products.

Although McDonald's executives had pledged to stop using cooking fats containing trans fats by mid 2005, two years later they still had failed to deliver on that public relations promise. On June 8, 2006, Wendy's announced that they found a mixture of cooking fats that contains no trans fats, and would begin to use it for french fries and chicken nuggets in their more than 6,500 restaurants in the US later that year but they, too, have not done what they had pledged. Even if fast food restaurants stop using toxic trans fats in their menus, the problem of repeatedly heated cooking oils and the partial conversion of cooking fats to oxidized by-products remains a health threat. Furthermore, if they use "interesterified" fat in place of cooking fat, as they have used in the past, we may be jumping from the frying pan into the fire.

The contribution of fast foods to our epidemics of obesity and diabetes is not just the excess fat or "empty calories." Soft drinks, potato chips or french fries, and nearly all desserts have practically no dietary fiber, but have very high glycemic index, so they provoke insulin surge and a reduced sense of satiety. Thus they contribute to further eating or snacking. The almost obligatory soft drinks also help to wash the food down and encourage buying (and eating) the big-portion, extra large or super sized sandwiches with added garnishes, which have far more saturated and trans fats than smaller fare. In particular, baked potatoes, and french fries have a large amount of rapidly absorbed starch with very high glycemic index.

A recent 20-year follow-up study of 84,555 female nurses in the U.S. showed that frequent consumption of potatoes or french fries was associated with a 20% increase in the risk of type 2 diabetes (Halton TL et al. Am J Clin Nutr 2006; 83:284–90). This association was stronger for french fries than baked potatoes, a finding explained almost entirely by the high concentration of trans fatty acids in french fries.

In addition, people who often eat fast foods tend to eat far less seafood and fruits or vegetables, but they often claim that "I eat my vegetables," referring to the one or two thin slices of tomato, pickles or lettuce on their sandwiches. Fast food eaters also tend to be sedentary people, further contributing to an energy (calorie) surplus that they simply cannot burn.

It is helpful to know in advance which items among fast food menus have low TRF. To reduce TRF scores and caloric content of any item, choose those without (or ask the server to leave out) sauces, mayonnaise, margarine, fried onions, mushrooms, bacon, melted cheese or "double" portions. Grilled chicken, roast beef or turkey sandwiches without these items are usually reasonable choices. Baked potato instead of french fries is also another way of cutting down on the unnecessary trans fatty acids. Still, an occasional small serving of french fried potatoes will not cause irreparable harm to your coronary artery. But when in doubt, use the TRF scores.

What about desserts and snacks?

Desserts are often very calorie-rich and contain hidden margarine, shortening or butter, which makes them far more unhealthful than most main dishes. Cakes (especially cheesecakes), cookies, pies, tarts and other pastries all have high TRF scores and should be avoided whenever possible.

Even "light" ice creams often are not what "light" implies. They are still loaded with undesirable saturated fat and unneeded calories. But small servings of sorbet, sherbet or frozen yogurt, garnished with or added to a bowl of berries or a fruit cocktail, are reasonable choices. Even a few pieces of dark chocolate-covered almonds or raisins are better than other milk chocolate-rich snacks or desserts containing high levels of margarine, shortening or coconut.

Should I skip meals?

A recent joint study by the US Food and Drug Administration and the National Heart, Lungs and Blood Institute showed that in the United States, 20% of adults, 51% of female high school students, and 18% of male students skip breakfast on a regular basis.

People skip breakfast because they get up too late for work or school, or to take care of children or the elderly. A large number of people skip breakfast intentionally, and think they are helping themselves by cutting down on their calories. But numerous studies in both laboratory animals and humans have consistently shown that fewer meals lead to weight gain. To lose weight and keep the lost weight off, have three to four separate, but small meals. Often, people who skip breakfast or lunch eat a huge dinner, followed by frequent snacks until bedtime. For many, total calories consumed with dinner and snacks equal or exceed that which they would have eaten in three or four small meals. The large calorie load at dinner, the usual sedentary state after evening meals, and the frequent nibbling or snacking until bedtime, all contribute to more calories.

Skipping meals means we burn fewer calories than we would have during the day and store more calories as fat at night. Meal skipping also increases the level of certain enzymes within fat cells which will enhance the storage of fat. In addition, skipping meals will reduce the ability of the liver to produce LDL receptors, and can contribute to higher blood cholesterol levels. When the stomach and the small intestine have not received food for several hours, the abundant amount of unused digestive enzymes will increase the efficacy with which the next meal is digested and absorbed, thus increasing the total calories that enter our bloodstream. Eating breakfast helps one have to a better attitude toward work, school and self, more stamina and less tiredness during the day, better maintenance of blood sugar level, less hunger and less subsequent snacking.

I can't remember whether a certain food is coronary-friendly or not!!

When in doubt about how much or which ingredients are in your food, or when you are simply wondering, "What can I eat?" always use the

TRF scores as your guide. Remember that the lower the TRF score of a food or meal, the better it is. Try to keep the TRF scores of breakfast and lunch to less than 5 each. This way, there are far more choices available for dinner (or the main meal).

One of my primary goals for developing the TRF system is to provide you with a flexible and practical guide for cardiovascular health. Do *not* turn this flexibility into a rigid or fanatical scorekeeping. Try to keep your daily TRF score to less than 30. But if an occasional meal adds another 10 to 15 points to your daily TRF scores, so be it. The goal is long-term consistency, not dietary celibacy.

There are a vast number of compelling and evidence-based data that have clearly shown that long-term dietary and lifestyle modifications can reduce the risk of cardiovascular diseases by over 80%, diabetes by over 90%, cancers of the breast, colon, lung and prostate (the leading causes of cancer deaths) by over 90%. Dietary and lifestyle modifications should always be the first line of defense against a long list of diseases. Preventing disease is even more essential considering the soaring cost of healthcare and the vast number of people who are uninsured or underinsured. The goal is to start today and stay the course! Here is a summary of what Twenty Risk Factor Diet suggestions are...

PRINCIPLES OF THE TWENTY RISK FACTOR DIET

AVOID: Mayonnaise, stick margarine, shortening, cooking fats and foods or snacks made with them, such as cakes, cookies, chocolate (dark chocolate is usually permitted), croissants, donuts, pastries, pies and deep-fried foods, butter, creams, and creamy or buttery sauces such as Alfredo, béarnaise, hollandaise. However, no single meal or a single day of any dietary indiscretion will cause irreparable harm! What counts is the long-term trend and adherence to the principles outlined here.

CUT DOWN: All sweets, including sugar and high fructose corn sweeteners, "honeyed," "sugared" or frosted cereals, high glycemic carbohydrates, and starches such as white bread, pasta, potato and brown or white rice. All sodas, including sugar-free varieties (phosphoric acid in sodas increases calcium loss through the kidneys and contributes to osteoporosis). Limit alcohol to no more than two drinks with dinner.

EAT: Three to five seafood meals per week and five or more servings of fruits (apples, apricot, berries, figs, plums, peaches, nectarines, oranges, red or black grapes, melons) and darker vegetables (celery, lettuce, spinach, watercress, herbs, broccoli, and green, yellow or red peppers, tomato), and various legumes.

Among nuts, choose almond, hazelnut, pistachio, and walnut (all have high concentrations of desirable monounsaturates and low levels of omega-6 polyunsaturates). All lean meats (small portions) are reasonable choices. Chicken and turkey (not deep-fried) are fine but not as a substitute for fish. Instead of breads, buns or rolls for your sandwiches consider romaine or other types of lettuce to make lettuce-wraps. Several cups of tea or coffee per day, without heavy cream and no or little sugar.

USE OLIVE OIL: Olive oil, preferably extra virgin or virgin (1st or 2nd pressing), for all your cooking needs. For high heat cooking, use canola oil (olive oil tends to smoke at high temperatures).

TRF SCORING SYSTEM

Nutrient	Amount	Score
S=Salt	Each 1,000 mg	+1
HGC=High Glygemic Carbohydrates	Each 10 gm	+1
Ch=Cholesterol	Each 100 mg	+1
Omega-6 PUFA	Each 5 gm	+1
TFA=Trans Fatty Acids	Each 1 gm	+1
SFA=Saturated Fatty Acids	Each 1 gm	+2
VF and N=Vegetables, Fruits and Nuts	Each 2 servings	+2
MUFA=Monounsaturated Fatty Acids	Each 2 gm	−1
Omega-3 PUFA (Plant-derived) Polyunsaturated fatty acids	Each 2 gm	−1
Omega-3 PUFA (Marine-derived) Polyunsaturated fatty acids	Each 1 gm	−1

•Dietary carbohydrates and proteins are neutral (score 0) in the TRF system
•VF and N=vegetables, fruits, and nuts; also represents their antioxidants, flavonoids and other cardio-protective ingredients

The TRF score of a food or snack is the sum of art its ingredients. This single score provides an instantaneous understanding of the total nutritional impact of a given food, instead of focus on a single ingredient. The lower the TRF score of a food or snack is, the more coronary-friendly it is. The goal is to keep the total TRF scores of all foods and snacks under +30 points per day, preferably closer to +20.

TRF SCORES OF OILS AND FATS
(Per 2 Tablespoons)

Coconut {A}	+48	Chicken Fat	+14
Palm Kernel {A}	+44	Cottonseed	+15
Vegetable Shortening	+26	Turkey Fat	+14
Butter {A}	+25	Safflower {B}	+8
Palm	+23	Sunflower {B}	+8
Beef Tallow	+22	Corn {B}	+6
Lamb Tallow	+21	Soybean	+6
Stick Margarine	+17	Peanut	+5
Mayonnaise	+18	Sesame	+3
Lard	+17	Olive {C}	−2
Soft Margarine	+15	Canola {C}	−3
Duck Fat	+14	Hazelnut {C}	−5

{A}-Coconut Oil, Palm Kernel Oil, and Butter have highest percentage of saturated fatty acids: 86%, 81%, and 62%, respectively.
{B}-Safflower, Sunflower, and Corn Oil contain the highest percentage of Omega-6 PUFA: 77%, 69%, and 61%, respectively.
{C}-Olive, Canola, and Hazelnut Oil are rich sources of monounsaturated fatty acids and contain 72%, 56%, and 78%, respectively.

TRF SCORES OF MARGARINES
(Per 2-Tablespoon Serving)

All Fat-Free Margarines	0	Land O' Lakes, Stick*	+13
Benecol Spread++	+1	Land O' Lakes, Fresh Buttery*	+12
Blue Bonnet	+13	Land O' Lakes Spread*	+12
Blue Bonnet, Home Style*	+7	Mazola*	+18
Brummel & Brown Spread++	+4	Mazola, Diet 100% Corn Oil Imitation	+5
Canoleo from Canola Oil	+2	Mazola, Unsalted*	+18
Country Crock Churn Style*	+8	Mrs. Filbert's 100% Corn Oil*	+14
Country Crock, Spread*	+8	Mrs. Filbert's Golden*	+17
Country Crock, Stick*	+17	Mrs. Filbert's Soft Golden*	+15
Empress, Soft*	+14	Mrs. Filbert's Whipped Margarine*	+15
Empress Stick*	+18	Mrs. Filbert's Whipped Spread*	+11
Fleischmann's Squeezable*	+6	Parkay Stick*	+15
Fleischmann's, Stick	+11	Parkay Squeezable*	+8
Fleischmann's, Light++	+4	Parkay Calcium Plus	+3
Fleischmann's Move Over Butter*	+15	Parkay Light*	+11
Fleischmann's Premium Blend*++	+7	Parkay Spread*	+8
Fleischmann's Today's Choice*	+6	Promise, Stick*++	+10
I Can't Believe It's Not Butter*	+14	Promise, Buttery Light++	+4
I Can't Believe It's Not Butter, Light*	+8	Promise, Fat-Free	0
I Can't Believe It's Not Butter, Spread++	+4	Promise, Spread*++	+8
I Can't Believe It's Not Butter, Sweet Cream and Calcium	+4	Smart Balance, Soft++	+5
		Smart Beat, Spread++	0
Imperial, Soft*	+12	Take Control, Spread++	+1
Imperial, Stick*	+15	Weight Watchers Extra Light, Stick	+5

*AVOID
++All these products are free of trans fatty acids.

TRF SCORES OF DAIRY AND EGG PRODUCTS
(Per 100 gm or 3.5 oz, Unless Otherwise Noted)

Buttermilk	+1	Cocoa and Chocolate Powder in Nonfat Milk	+3
Buttermilk (1 Cup)	+3	Cocoa and Chocolate Powder with Whole Milk*	+1
Canned Milk, Whole, Evaporated*	+21	Dried, Nonfat Milk Egg Nog*	+7
Canned Milk, Skim, Evaporated	0	Egg Nog (1 Cup)*	+20
Chocolate Milk, 1% Fat (1 Cup)	+2	Egg, Large (1 Whole)	+4
Chocolate Milk, 2% Fat	+2	Egg, Yolk (1 Large)	+4
Chocolate Milk, 2% Fat (1 Cup)*	+6	Egg Whites	0
Chocolate Milk, Regular	+5	Egg, 1 Hard, Soft Cooked, or Poached	+4
Chocolate Milk, Regular (1 Cup)*	+11	Egg, 1 Scrambled with Olive or Canola Oil	+3
Evaporated, Condensed and Sweetened Milk*	+17	Egg, 1 Scrambled with Added Milk and Margarine*	+5
Evaporated, Condensed and Sweetened Milk (1 Cup)*	+43	Egg, 1 Sunny Side Up Cooked with Margarine*	+10
Milk, Skim (No Fat)	0	Egg, 1 Omelette Cooked in Butter or Margarine*	+11
Milk, Low-Fat (2%)	+2		
Milk, Whole (4% Fat)	+4	Egg, 1 Omelette Cooked in Butter or Margarine* with Added Cheese*	+13
Milk, Whole (4% Fat) (1 Cup)*	+9		
Milk, Vanilla Shake (8 Oz)*	+9		

*AVOID

TRF SCORES OF CHEESES AND OTHER DAIRY PRODUCTS
(Cheese 1 Per oz Slice, Other Dairy Products Per 3.5 oz, Unless Otherwise Noted)

American*	+11	Cottage, Creamed	+6
American Spread (2 Tbs)	+7	Cottage, 2%	+3
Blue*	+10	Cottage, 1%	+2
Brie	+9	Cream Cheese (2 Tbs)*	+12
Camembert	+7	Cream Cheese, Light (2 Tbs)	+5
Cheddar*	+12	Cream Cheese, Smoked Salmon (2 Tbs)	+7
Cheddar, Shredded	+23	Cream Cheese, Olive & Pimento (2 Tbs)	+6
Colby*	+11	Cream Cheese, Fat-Free	0

TRF SCORES OF CHEESES AND OTHER DAIRY PRODUCTS (*Continued*)

Cream Cheese, Soft (2 Tbs)	+7	Ricotta, Part Skim (2 Tbs)	+3
Feta (2 Tbs)	+8	Romano*	+10
Gouda*	+10	Roquefort*	+12
Gruyere*	+11	Swiss*	+10
Havarti*	+13	Swiss, Low-Fat	+5
Mozzarella	+8	Ice Cream, Regular*	+13
Mozzarella, Part Skim	+6	Ice Cream, Rich (16% Fat)*	+19
Muenster*	+11	Ice Cream, Soft (3% Fat)	+2
Parmesan, Hard	+9	Sherbet (2% Fat)	+4
Parmesan, Grated (2 Tbs)	+4	Yogurt, Whole Milk	+3
Pimento*	+11	Yogurt, Frozen, Fat-Free	0
Provolone	+8	Yogurt, Frozen, Fat-Free (8 oz. container)	+7
Ricotta (2 Tbs)	+4	Yogurt, Low-Fat Milk, Plain	+2

*AVOID
Although all cheeses with TRF scores of more than +10 should be avoided, an occasional piece of cheese will not have any detrimental impact. Clearly, added slices of processed cheese to an otherwise lean sandwich, or "cheese lovers" pizza, are counterproductive.

PREPACKAGED CHEESES
(Per 1 oz. Serving or as Otherwise Noted)

Kraft

American	+4	Deli Deluxe Provolone*	+10
Cheddar Jack, with Jalapeño (¼ Cup*)	+10	Deli Deluxe Skim Swiss*	+11
Classic Melt, 4 Cheeses (¼ Cup)*	+10	**Kraft Fat-Free**	
Classic Melt, Cheddar and American (¼ Cup)*	+12	Mexican Taco (¼ Cup)*	+10
Classic Melt, Mexican (¼ Cup)*	+10	Mild Cheddar (¼ Cup)*	+12
Deli Deluxe American*	+7	Mozzarella (¼ Cup)*	+7
Deli Deluxe, Hearty Taste*	+11	Mozzarella, 2% Fat	+5
Deli Deluxe, Deli Thin, Aged Swiss	+4	Mozzarella and Parmesan (¼ Cup)*	+8
Deli Deluxe, Deli Thin, Mozzarella*	+8	Parmesan Italian (¼ Cup)*	+2
Deli Deluxe Mild Cheddar*	+15	Sharp Cheddar	+4
Deli Deluxe Old English*	+14	Singles, American*	+7
		Singles, Pepper Jack, 2%	+4

PREPACKAGED CHEESES (*Continued*)

		Sargento	
Singles, Swiss, 2% Fat	+4	**Sargento**	
Velveeta*	+9	Cheddar Jack*	+9
Velveeta, Light	+5	Double Cheddar*	+9
		Fancy Mild Cheddar*	+9
Kraft Cracker Barrel		Fancy Monterey Jack*	+9
Velveeta, Mexican*	+9	Fancy Parmesan	+2
Baby Swiss*	+12	Fancy Sharp Cheddar*	+9
Extra Sharp*	+14	Fancy Swiss*	+8
Extra Sharp, 2% Milk*	+8	Italian 6 Cheese*	+7
New York Aged Sharp*	+14	Italian with Garlic*	+8
Sharp Cheddar*	+12	Light Mexican	+6
Sharp White*	+12	Light Mozzarella	+5
		Mexican 4 Cheese*	+11
Kraft Cubes (per 8 cubes)		Mild Cheddar*	+9
Vermont Sharp White*	+12	Mild Cheddar, Light	+6
Cheddar and Monterey Jack*	+13	Mozzarella	+6
Colby and Monterey Jack*	+13	Mozzarella, Light	+5
Mild Cheddar*	+13	Nacho and Taco*	+9
		Parmesan, Mozzarella and Romano*	+8
Kraft Strips (per 1 strip)		Pepper Jack*	+9
Sharp Cheddar*	+13	Pizza*	+8
Polly-0 String-ums	+7	Stringsters (1 Stick)	+7
Polly-0 Superlong*	+8		
Polly-0 Twist-ums	+5		
Rip-ums*	+8		

*AVOID
Always try to choose among lighter cheeses with Lower TRF scores.

TRF SCORES OF POULTRY
(Per 100 gm or Per Serving)

Chicken, Fried

Breast with Skin	+7
Breast without Skin	+3
Breast without Skin with Batter	+5
Breast without Skin with Flour	+4
Drumsticks with Skin (2)	+7
Drumsticks without Skin (2)	+5
Drumsticks with Skin and Batter (2)*	+10
Drumsticks with Skin and Flour (2)	+9
Drumsticks without Skin with Batter (2)	+8
Drumsticks without Skin with Flour (2)	+7
Leg with Skin (1)*	+10
Leg with Skin with Batter (1)*	+13
Leg with Skin with Flour (1)*	+11
Leg without Skin (1)	+5
Leg without Skin with Batter (1)	+8
Leg without Skin with Flour (1)	+6
Thighs with Skin (2)*	+10
Thighs without Skin (2)	+6

Chicken, Roasted

Breast with Skin	+5
Breast without Skin	+3

*AVOID

Drumsticks with Skin (2)	+5
Drumsticks without Skin (2)	+3
Leg with Skin (1)	+5
Leg without Skin (1)	+3
Thighs with Skin (2)	+8
Thighs without Skin (2)	+5

Other Poultry

Cornish Hen with Skin, Roasted	+6
Duck with Skin, Roasted *	+15
Duck without Skin, Roasted	+6
Pheasant with Skin, Roasted	+5
Pheasant without Skin, Roasted	+2
Turkey, Breast (Sliced)	+2
Dark Meat with Skin	+6
Dark Meat without Skin	+4
White Meat with Skin	+5
White Meat without Skin	+3

TRF SCORES OF BEEF AND ORGAN MEATS
Per 100 gm or 3.5 oz

Boneless Chuck, Trimmed*	+16	Porterhouse Steak, Choice*	+25
Chuck Roast, Choice (without Bone)*	+24	Rib Roast without Bone, Choice*	+28
Chuck Steak, Choice (without Bone)*	+24	Round Steak, Lean	+10
Chuck, Ground, Lean*	+16	Rump Roast, Choice*	+20
Chuck, Rib Roast*	+28	Sirloin Steak, Choice*	+20
Chuck, Ground, Extra Lean	+11	T-bone Steak, Choice*	+25
Chuck Roast, Lean*	+13	Tenderloin, Lean	+6
Chuck Steak, Lean*	+13	Beef Brain*	+22
Chopped Sirloin, Extra Lean	+7	Beef Heart	+5
Corned Beef, Cooked*	+23	Beef Liver	+7
Corned Beef Hash (with potato)*	+10	Beef Tongue*	+14
Ground Beef, Lean (20% Fat)*	+17	Beef Tongue, Lean	+8
Ground Beef, Extra Lean (10% Fat)	+8	Chicken Heart	+5
Ground Round, Lean*	+12	Chicken Liver	+9
Ground Rump, Extra Lean	+8	Chicken Liver Pate (1 oz)	+5
Ground Rump, Regular*	+21	Duck Liver	+8
London Broil, Flank Steak, Choice	+6		

*AVOID

TRF SCORES OF LAMB, PORK, VEAL AND VENISON PRODUCTS
(Per 100 gm, Unless Otherwise Noted)

Lamb		Chop, Loin, Broiled, Grilled, Lean Meat Only, 2 Chops	+6
Chop, Broiled, Grilled	+8	Leg, Roasted	+10
Chop, Broiled, Grilled, Lean Meat Only, 2 Chops	+9	Leg, Roasted, Lean Meat Only	+4
Chop, Loin, Broiled, Grilled	+9	Rib, Roasted*	+20
Chop, Loin, Broiled, Grilled, 2 Average Chops*	+21	Rib, Roasted, Lean Meat Only*	+8

TRF SCORES OF LAMB, PORK, VEAL AND VENISON PRODUCTS (*Continued*)

Shoulder, Roasted*	+14	Pork Chop, Pan Fried, Lean Meat Only	+6
Shoulder, Roasted, Lean Meat Only*	+7	Pork, Ribs, Roasted*	+14
		Pork, Ribs, Roasted, Lean Meat Only*	+8
Pork		Pork Shoulder, Roasted*	+14
Bacon, 3 Slices	+4	Pork Shoulder, Roasted, Lean Meat Only*	+6
Canadian Bacon, 2 Slices	+2	Spare Ribs, Roasted, Broiled*	+19
Ham, Roasted	+5		
Ham, Roasted, Lean Meat Only	+5	**Veal**	
Ham, Canned	+3	Cutlet, Lean	+4
Ham, Leg Roasted	+4	Chop, Broiled, Grilled	+8
Ham, Leg Roasted, Lean Meat Only	+4	Chop, Broiled, Grilled, Lean Meat Only	+4
Ham, Lunch Meat, 2 Slices	+3	Rib, Roasted	+9
Pork Chop, Broiled, Grilled	+9	Rib, Roasted, Lean Meat Only	+4
Pork Chop, Broiled, Grilled, Lean Meat Only	+4	**Venison**	
Pork Chop, Pan Fried*	+14	Steak	+3

*AVOID

TRF SCORES OF SEAFOOD*

(Per 100 gm or 3.5 oz)

Barracuda	−1	Halibut	−1
Bass, Freshwater	−1	Herring	−1
Bass, Sea	0	Mackerel, Atlantic	−5
Bass, Striped	−1	Mackerel, King	0
Bluefish	−2	Mahimahi	−2
Catfish	−2	Monkfish	0
Caviar	+1	Mullet	−2
Cod	0	Ocean Perch	0
Croaker	−2	Orange Roughy	−2
Flounder	0	Perch	0
Grouper	0	Pollock	0
Haddock	0	Pompano	+1

Rockfish	−1		Sturgeon	0
Sablefish	−2		Sardines	−1
Salmon, Atlantic	−1		Swordfish	−1
Salmon, Chinook	−4		Trout, Rainbow (Farm-raised)	−1
Salmon, Coho	−3		Trout, Rainbow (Lake)	−3
Shark	−1		Trout, Sea	+1
Snapper	−1		Tuna, Bluefin	−1
Sole	0		Tuna, Yellowfin	−1
Spot	+1		Whitefish	−1

*TRF scores of some fish such as tuna, salmon or rainbow trout may vary depending on where the fish was caught (or canned). Wild fish have higher concentrations of omega-3 PUFA than farm-raised fish.

TRF SCORES OF OTHER SEAFOOD
(Per 100 gm)

Tuna and Salmon (Canned in Water)

Bumble Bee Solid White	−1
Bumble Bee Chunk White	−1
Bumble Bee Pink Salmon	−2
Bumble Bee Red Salmon	−2
Chicken of the Sea Solid White	−1
Chicken of the Sea Chunk White	−1
Chicken of the Sea Salmon	−2
Starkist Chunk Light	−1
Starkist Solid White	−2

Tuna (Canned in Oil)

Bumble Bee Solid White	−1
Bumble Bee Chunk White	+1
Chicken of the Sea Chunk Light	−1
Starkist Chunk White Lunch	−1

Starkist Lunch Kit	-1
Starkist Solid White	0

Shellfish

Clams	0
Crabs, Alaska King	0
Crabs, Dungeness	0
Crayfish	0
Lobster	+1
Mussels	0
Octopus	0
Oysters	0
Scallops	0
Shrimp	+1
Snail	0
Squid	+2

TRF SCORES OF GRAIN PRODUCTS
(Per Serving as Noted)

Bagel, Plain (1)	+4	Italian Bread	0
Bread Crumbs (1 Cup)	+4	Mixed Grain Bread	0
Bread Stuffing (1 Cup)	+8	Oatmeal Bread	0
Cracked Wheat	+1	Pita Bread	0
Dinner Rolls (2)	+2	Pumpernickel Bread	0
English Muffins (1)	+3	Raisin Bread	0
French or Austrian Bread	+3	Rye Bread	0
Hot Dog or Hamburger Rolls (1)	+3	Wheat Bread	0
Hard Rolls (2)	+1	Whole Wheat Bread	+1
Hoagie/Submarine Rolls (1)	+1	White Bread	+1
		Other European Breads	+1

KELLOGG'S CEREALS AND OTHER PRODUCTS

Cereals (per Bowl)

All-bran, Bran Buds	+2	Honey Crunch Corn Flakes	+2
All-bran, Extra Fiber	+1	Just Right Fruit and Nut	+3
All-bran, Original	+1	Marshamallow Froot Loops	+2
Apple Jacks	+2	Mini-wheats, Frosted Bite-Size	+4
Cinnamon Crunch Crispix	+2	Mini-wheats, Frosted Original	+4
Cocoa Rice Krispies	+2	Mini-wheats, Honey Frosted Bite-Size	+4
Complete Oat Bran Flakes	+1	Mini-wheats, Raisin	+3
Complete Wheat Bran Flakes	+1	Mini-wheats, Strawberry	+3
Corn Flakes	+2	Mueslix	+3
Corn Pops	+2	Pokemon	+2
Cracklin' Oat Bran	+2	Product 19	+2
Crispix	+2	Raisin Bran	+2
Froot Loops	+2	Raisin Bran Crunch	+3
Frosted Flakes	+2	Rice Krispies	+4
		Smacks	+3

KELLOGG'S CEREALS AND OTHER PRODUCTS (*Continued*)

Smart Start	+2	Vanilla Yogurt Bar (1)	+2
Special K	+2	Minis, Apple Cinnamon (1 Pouch)	+3

Cereal Bars (per Bar) | | Minis, Blueberry (1 Pouch) | +3 |

		Minis, Strawberry (1 Pouch)	+3
Apple Cinnamon	+2	Twists, Apple Cobbler (1)	+3
Blueberry	+2	Twists, Cappuccino and Créme (1)	+3
Cherry	+2	Twists, Strawberry Cheesecake (1)	+3
Mixed Berry	+2	Rice Krispies Treats (1) Apple Cinnamon*	+4
Raspberry or Strawberry	+2	Caramel Chocolatey Chunk* (1)	+4
Special K Bars	+3	Chocolatey Peanut Butter* (1)	+5

Nutri-grain Products | | Double Chocolatey Chunk* | +5 |

		Original (1)	+2
Blueberry Yogurt Bar (1)	+2	Single Serve* (1)	+4
Strawberry Yogurt Bar (1)	+2		

*AVOID

QUAKER OATMEALS, CEREALS AND GRITS

Oatmeals (per Serving)

		Nutrition for Women, Golden Brown Sugar (1 Packet)	+3
Baked Apple (1 Packet-instant)	+2	Oat Bran Hot Cereal (½ Cup)	+2
Banana Bread (1 Packet)	+2	Sun Country Iron-fortified (½ Cup)	+3
Brown Sugar (1 Packet)	+2		
Cinnamon Roll (1 Packet-instant)	+2	**Cereals**	
Crystal Wedding Oats (½ Cup)	+3	Cap'n Crunch	+2
Dinosaur Eggs (1 Packet)*	+7	Life	+1
Express Instant Oatmeal (1 Packet)	+2	Quaker Oatmeal Cereal	+1
French Vanilla (1 Packet)	+3	Quaker Squares, Brown Sugar	+2
Honey Nut (1 Packet)	+3	Quaker Squares, Cinnamon	+2
Instant Oatmeal, Maple and Brown Sugar	+3	Quisp	+2
Instant Oatmeal, Raisin Cinnamon Swirl (1 Packet)	+4		
Instant Oatmeal, Regular (1 Packet)	+1	**Instant Grits (per Serving or Packet)**	
Instant Oatmeal, Strawberries and Cream (1 Packet)	+3	American Cheese	+2
Multigrain Oatmeal (½ Cup)	+2	Cheddar Cheese Blend	+3
		Country Bacon	+2

QUAKER OATMEALS, CEREALS AND GRITS (*Continued*)

Ham N' Cheese	+3	Real Cheddar Cheese	+1
Original	+1	Red Eye Gravy and Country Ham	+2
Real Butter	+2	3 Cheeses	+1

*AVOID

GENERAL MILLS CEREALS
(Per Bowl)

Apple Cinnamon Cheerios	+1	Multi Bran Chex	+3
Basic 4	+1	Multi Grain Cheerios	0
Boo Berry	+1	Nature Valley Low-Fat Fruit Granola	+3
Cheerios	0	Nesquik	+2
Cinnamon Grahams	+1	Oatmeal Crisp, Almond	+4
Cinnamon Toast Crunch	+2	Oatmeal Crisp, Apple Cinnamon	+3
Cocoa Puffs	+1	Oatmeal Crisp, Raisin	+3
Cookie Crisp	+1	Para Su Familia Cinnamon Stars	+2
Corn or Rice Chex	+2	Para Su Familia Frutis	+2
Count Chocula	+2	Para Su Familia Raisin Bran	+3
Country Corn Flakes	+2	Raisin Nut Bran	+2
Fiber One	+1	Reese's Peanut Butter Puffs	+3
Franken Berry	+1	Total Brown Sugar and Oats	+2
French Toast Crunch	+2	Total Corn Flakes	+2
Frosted Cheerios	+1	Total Raisin Bran	+2
Golden Grahams	+2	Total Whole Grain	+2
Gold Medal Raisin Bran	+2	Trix	+2
Harmony	+3	Wheat Chex	+2
Honey Nut Cheerios	+1		
Honey Nut Chex	+2	**Wheaties**	
Honey Nut Clusters	+3	Breakfast of Champions	+1
Kaboom	+2	Frosted Wheaties	+2
Kix and Berry Berry Kix	+2	Wheaties Energy Crunch	+3
Lucky Charms	+2	Wheaties Raisin Bran	+3

TRF SCORES OF NUTS, VEGETABLES AND FRUITS

Nuts (Per 1 oz Serving)

Almonds, Dried or Dry Roasted	−1
Almonds, Oil Roasted	−1
Beechnuts, Dried or Roasted	+1
Brazil nuts, Dried or Roasted	+7
Butternuts, Dried or Roasted	+2
Cashew Nuts, Dried or Roasted	+2
Chestnuts, Dried or Roasted	0
Coconut, Dry Meat*	+17
Coconut, Dried, Shredded*	+17
Coconut, Raw Meat, 2"x2" Piece*	+26
Filberts, Dried or Roasted	−4
Ginkgo Nuts, Dried	0
Hickory Nuts, Dried	+1
Macadamia Nuts, Dried or Roasted	−3

*AVOID

Mixed Nuts, Dried or Roasted	+1
Peanuts, Dried or Roasted	+2
Peanut Butter (2 Tbs)	+4
Pecans, Dried or Roasted	−2
Pine Nuts, Dried or Roasted	+3
Pistachio Nuts, Dried or Roasted	−1
Pumpkin Kernels	+4
Sesame Seeds, Roasted or Toasted	+2
Sunflower Kernels	+4
Walnuts, Dried or Roasted	+2

Fruits and Vegetables (Per 2 Servings)

All Fruits	+−1
Most Vegetables**	−1

**The TRF Scores for Olives and Avocados is −2.

TRF SCORES OF FROZEN ENTREES

Budget Gourmet

Beef Cantonese	+6
Cheese Manicotti with Meat Sauce*	+22
Chicken Marsala	+9
Chinese Style Vegetables and Chicken	+4
Fettucine Alfredo with Four Cheeses*	+26
Glazed Turkey	+4
Italian Sausage Lasagna*	+18
Italian Style Vegetables and Chicken	+4

Linguini with Tomato Sauce and Italian Sausage*	+12
Macaroni and Cheese*	+10
Mandarin Chicken	+3
Oriental Beef*	+10
Orange Glazed Chicken Breast	+3
Penne Pasta with Chunky Tomatoes*	+10
Pepper Steak	+6
Rigatoni in Cream Sauce with Broccoli and Chicken	+7
Scalloped Noodles and Turkey*	+21

TRF SCORES OF FROZEN ENTREES (*Continued*)

Sirloin Tips with Country Style Vegetables*	+11	Beef Sirloin Salisbury Steak	+5
Spaghetti with Chunky Tomato and Meat Sauce	+7	Herbed Chicken Breast with Fettucine	+7
Spicy Szechuan Style Vegetables and Chicken	+5	Roast Chicken Breast with Herb Gravy	+4
Swedish Meatballs*	+32	Shrimp Mariner	+5
Three Cheese Lasagna*	+21	Special Recipe Sirloin Beef	+6
Wide Ribbon Pasta with Ricotta and Chunky Tomatoes*	+15	Stuffed Turkey Breast	+5
		Yankee Pot Roast	+4

*AVOID

TRF SCORES OF CANNED BEANS AND PASTA ENTREES
(*Per 100 gm*)

Campbell's

Baked Barbecue Beans	0	Lasagna*	+8
Baked Beans, Brown Sugar, Bacon-flavored	+3	Meat Tortellini	+4
Baked Beans, New England Style	+2	Mini Ravioli in Tomato and Meat Sauce	+7
Pork N' Beans	+2	Pasta with Mini Meatballs	+7

Chef Boyardee

		Spaghetti and Meatballs*	+7
Beefaroni	+7	Teenage Mutant Ninja Turtles	+7
Beef Ravioli	+7	Tic Tac Toe with Meatballs*	+7
Cheese Ravioli	+4		
Cheese Tortellini	+4	**Franco-American**	
Chomps-a-lot Bite-Size Lasagna	+4	Spaghettios in Cheese Sauce	+5
Chomps-a-lot Bite-Size Beef Ravioli	+4	Spaghettios with Meatballs*	+9
Dinosaurs	+4	Spaghettios in Cheese Sauce Teddyos	+5
Fettucine in Meat Sauce	+7	Spaghettios with Sliced Franks*	+10
		Garfield Ravioli in Meat Sauce*	+9

*AVOID

TRF SCORES OF BOXED PASTA ENTREES
(Per Serving)

Rice-a-Roni

Angel Hair Pasta with Parmesan Cheese	+5
Corkscrew Pasta with Four Cheeses	+6
Fettucine	+5
Fettucine with Alfredo Sauce	+6
Fettucine with Romanoff Sauce	+7
Linguini with Chicken and Broccoli Sauce	+5
Penne Pasta, Herb and Butter	+4
Rigatoni with White Cheddar and Broccoli	+6

Hamburger Helper

Beef Noodle	+2
Cheeseburger Macaroni	+5
Italian Rigatoni	+4
Lasagna	+4
Pizza Pasta	+4
Stroganoff	+4
Tuna Helper, Cheesy Noodles	+4
Zesty Italian	+2

Lipton Noodles N' Sauce

Alfredo*	+11
Beef	+6

Chicken	+5
Creamy Chicken*	+7
Mild Cheddar Bacon	+5
Parmesan*	+9
Romanoff	+6
Stroganoff	+5

Lipton Pasta & Sauce

Cheddar Broccoli	+4
Creamy Garlic	+4
Tini Primavera	+5

Lipton Golden Sauté

Angel Hair with Chicken N' Broccoli	+3
Penne Pasta, Herb with Garlic	+5
Rice and Vermicelli with Chicken Flavor	+5

Kraft Macaroni & Cheese

Dinomac	+4
Original	+5
Super Mario	+6

*AVOID

TRF SCORES OF PROCESSED FOODS
(Per Slice)

Butterball

Roasted Chicken	+1
Roasted Turkey	+1
Roasted Turkey Breast	+1

Healthy Choice

Baked Cooked Ham	+1
Bologna, Turkey	+1
Smoked Turkey Breast	+1
Turkey	+1

Hebrew National

Beef Bologna*	+6
Beef Salami*	+6

Louis Rich

Bologna*	+6
Cooked Turkey Salami	+2
Roasted Turkey Breast	+1
Salami	+4
Smoked Turkey	+1
Turkey Bologna	+5
Turkey Pastrami	+1
White Turkey	+1

*AVOID

Oscar Mayer

Beef Bologna*	+8
Bologna*	+8
Bologna (Thin Sliced)	+4
Corned Beef (Thin Sliced)	+1
Hard Salami	+2
Healthy Favorites	+4
Light Beef Bologna	+1
Oven Roasted Chicken	+1
Oven Roasted Turkey	+1
Pastrami	+2

Oscar Mayer Lunchables (Per Package)

Bologna with American Cheese*	+28
Chicken with American Cheese*	+20
Lean Chicken with Monterey Jack*	+20
Lean Ham with American Cheese*	+20
Lean Ham with Swiss Cheese without Dessert*	+18
Lean Turkey with Cheddar Cheese and Reese's Cup*	+20
Lean Turkey with Cheddar Cheese and Trail Mix*	+26

CAMPBELL'S CONDENSED SOUPS
(Per Cup [Prepared])

Healthy Request

Bean with Ham and Bacon	+3
Chicken and Rice	+3
Chicken Noodle	+3
Chicken Vegetable	+2
Cream of Broccoli	+3
Cream of Celery	+3
Cream of Chicken	+3
Cream of Chicken and Broccoli	+3
Cream of Mushroom	+3
Hearty Pasta and Vegetables	+1
Minestrone	+1
Tomato	+2
Vegetable	+1
Vegetable Beef	+2

Regular

Bean with Bacon	+4
Beef Noodle	+3
Beef with Vegetable and Barley	+3
Beefy Mushroom	+3
Black Bean	+1
California Style Vegetables	+1
Cheddar Cheese*	+9
Chicken Alphabet with Vegetable	+3
Chicken and Dumplings	+3
Chicken and Stars	+2
Chicken Gumbo	+2*
Chicken Noodle	+2
Chicken Noodle O's	+3

Chicken with Rice	+2
Chicken with Vegetables	+2
Chicken with Wild Rice	+2
Cream of Asparagus*	+5
Cream of Broccoli*	+5
Cream of Broccoli and Cheese*	+5
Cream of Celery*	+5
Cream of Chicken*	+5
Cream of Chicken and Broccoli*	+6
Cream of Chicken Dijon*	+6
Cream of Chicken Mushroom*	+6
Cream of Chicken with Herbs	+4
Cream of Mushroom*	+5
Cream of Mushroom with Garlic	+3
Cream of Onion*	+5
Cream of Potato	+4
Cream of Potato with Shrimp*	+5
Creamy Chicken Noodle*	+5
Curly Chicken Noodle	+3
Double Noodle in Chicken Broth	+3
Fiesta Chili Beef with Beans*	+5
Fiesta Nacho Cheese*	+8
French Onion	+2
Fun Shapes Pasta with Chicken	+1
Golden Mushroom	+2
Green Pea	+3
Hearty Vegetable with Pasta	+1
Homestyle Chicken Noodle	+3
Italian Tomato with Basil and Oregano	+1

CAMPBELL'S CONDENSED SOUPS (*Continued*)

Manhattan Clam Chowder	+1	Split Pea with Ham*	+5
Mega Noodle in Chicken Broth	+2	Tomato	+1
Minestrone	+2	Tomato Bisque	+3
New England Clam Chowder	+2	Tomato Noodle	+1
Noodle and Ground Beef*	+5	Tomato with Garlic and Herbs	+1
Old-Fashioned Tomato Rice	+2	Turkey Noodle	+3
Old-Fashioned Vegetable	+2	Turkey Vegetable	+2
Oyster Stew*	+8	Vegetable	+1
Pepper Pot	+4	Vegetable Beef	+1
Scotch Broth	+3	Won Ton	+1
Southwestern Chicken Vegetable	+1		

*AVOID

CAMPBELL'S READY-TO-SERVE SOUPS
(*Per 1 Can or as Noted*)

Healthy Request

Chicken Noodle	+2	Chicken with Rice	+2
Chicken Vegetable	+1	Creamy Tomato*	+5
Creamy Potato with Garlic	+2	Minestrone	+2
Hearty Chicken with White and Wild Rice	+1	Tomato	+2
Hearty Country Vegetable	+1	Vegetable with Beef Stock	+2
Hearty Vegetable	+1		

Select

Hearty Vegetable Beef	+2	Bean and Ham	+3
New England Clam Chowder	+1	Chicken and Potato with Garlic	+2
Split Pea with Ham	+2	Chicken and Rice	+1
Tomato Ravioli with Vegetables	+3	Chicken Vegetable	+2
		Chicken with Egg Noodles	+3

Classic

		Country Mushroom Rice	+2
Bean and Bacon	+4	Country Vegetables	+2
Chicken Noodle	+3	Creamy Potato with Roasted Garlic*	+6

CAMPBELL'S CONDENSED SOUPS (*Continued*)

Fiesta Vegetable	+2
Grilled Chicken with Sundried Tomatoes	+2
Italian Style Chicken with Vegetables	+3
New England Clam Chowder*	+12
Old World Minestrone	+3
Oriental Noodles with Vegetables	+2
Roasted Chicken with White and Wild Rice	+2
Savory Lentil	+1
Split Pea with Ham	+3
Tomato Garden	+2
Tuscany Style Minestrone	+4
Vegetable Beef	+2

Soup At Hand

Blended Vegetable Medley*	+5
Classic Tomato	+3
Cream of Broccoli*	+5
Creamy Chicken*	+6

Simply Home

Chicken Vegetable Pasta	+2
Chicken Noodle	+2
Chicken with White and Wild Rice	+4
Country Vegetable	+2
Minestrone	+2
Vegetable Garden	+3
98% Fat-Free Cream of Broccoli	+3
98% Fat-Free Cream of Celery	+3
98% Fat-Free Cream of Mushroom	+3

Chunky Soups (Per ½ Can)

Baked Potato with Steak and Cheese*	+9
Baked Potato with Bacon and Chives*	+5
Baked Potato with Bacon and Cheese*	+7
Beef with Country Vegetables*	+4
Beef with White and Wild Rice*	+5
Cheese Tortellini with Chicken and Vegetables	+3
Chicken Broccoli Cheese and Potato*	+9
Chicken Corn Chowder*	+11
Chicken and Dumplings*	+5
Clam Chowder, Manhattan-Style	+3
Classic Chicken Noodle	+3
Grilled Chicken with Vegetables and Pasta	+2
Grilled Sirloin with Hearty Vegetables	+3
Hearty Chicken with Vegetables	+3
Herb Roasted Chicken with Potato	+3
Honey Roasted Ham with Potato*	+4
Old Fashioned Potato Ham Chowder*	+11
Old Fashioned Vegetable Beef*	+4
Pepper Steak	+3
Salisbury Steak with Mushrooms*	+7
Savory Chicken with White and Wild Rice	+2
Seasoned Beef with Potatoes and Herbs	+3
Sirloin Burger with Country Vegetable*	+9
Slow Roasted Beef with Mushrooms	+3
Split Pea 'N' Ham	+3
Steak 'N Potato	+2
Tomato Cheese Ravioli with Vegetable	+5
Vegetable	+3

*AVOID

PROGRESSO SOUPS
(Per 1 Cup)

Beef and Baked Potato	+3	Homestyle Chicken with Vegetables and Pearl Onion	+1
Beef and Mushroom Portobello	+3	Lentil	+1
Beef and Vegetable*	+4	Manhattan Clam Chowder	+1
Chicken and Wild Rice	+1	Minestrone	+1
Chicken Barley	+1	New England Clam Chowder*	+11
Chicken Noodle	+1	Potato Chowder with Broccoli and Cheese*	+5
Creamy Mushroom*	+13	Roasted Chicken Rotini	+1
French Onion	+2	Roasted Chicken with Garden Herbs	+1
Grilled Chicken Italiano with Vegetables and Penne	+2	Southwestern Style Corn Chowder	+1
Grilled Steak with Vegetables and Penne	+3	Tomato Rotini	+2
Hearty Tomato	+2		

*AVOID

TRF SCORES FOR SAUCES
(Per ½ Cup = 120 ml)

Classico

Four Cheese	+3	Garlic and Herbs	+1
Mushroom and Ripe Olives	+2	Traditional	+1
Onion and Garlic	+2	Zesty Italian	+1
Spicy Red Pepper	+2		
Sweet Peppers and Onions	+2	**Newman's Own**	
Tomato and Basil	+3	Sockarooni	+1
		Venetian with Mushroom	+1

Healthy Choice

Chunky Garlic and Onions	+1	**Prego**	
Chunky Mushroom	+1	Diced Onion and Garlic	+2
Extra Chunky Mushroom	+1	Flavored with Meat	+3
Flavored with Meat	+1	Fresh Mushroom	+3
		Garden Combination	+2

TRF SCORES FOR SAUCES (*Continued*)

Low Sodium	+2	Chunky Garden Super Mushroom	+2
Mushroom and Diced Onion	+3	Chunky Mushrooms and Green Peppers	+3
Mushroom and Diced Tomato	+2	Chunky Super Vegetable Primavera	+2
Diced Onion and Garlic	+2	Homestyle Flavored with Meat	+3
Flavored with Meat	+3	Homestyle with Mushroom	+2
Fresh Mushroom	+3	Homestyle Tomato and Herb	+2
Garden Combination	+2	Light Garden Harvest	+1
Low Sodium	+2	Light Tomato and Herb	+1
Mushroom and Diced Onion	+3	Old World Style Traditional	+2
Mushroom and Diced Tomato	+2	Old World Style with Meat	+3
Diced Onion and Garlic	+2	Thick and Hearty Mushroom	+2
Flavored with Meat	+3	Thick and Hearty with Meat	+2
Fresh Mushroom	+3	Thick and Hearty Tomato and Herb	+2
Tomato and Basil	+2		
Tomato, Onion and Garlic	+3	**Other Sauces**	
Traditional	+4	Béarnaise*	+8
Zesty Basil	+4	Hollandaise	+3
Zesty Garlic and Cheese	+4	Marinara (Tomato Based)	0
Zesty Mushroom with Cheese	+3	Spaghetti with Meat	+1
		Spaghetti with Meatballs	+1
Ragu		Tartar	+4
Chunky Gardenstyle	+2		

*AVOID

TRF SCORES OF SALAD DRESSINGS
(Per 2 Tablespoons)

Kraft		Caesar Ranch	+4
Bacon and Tomato*	+5	Classic Caesar*	+5
Blue Cheese*	+6	Coleslaw	+4
Catalina	+4	Creamy Italian*	+6

TRF SCORES OF SALAD DRESSINGS (*Continued*)

Creamy Parmesan Romano	+5	**Newman's Own**		
Creamy Roasted Garlic	+4	Balsamic Vinaigrette	+2
Cucumber Ranch*	+5	Caesar	+3
Deliciously Right Italian	+2	Creamy Caesar*	+6
Deliciously Right Ranch	+4	Light Italian	+3
Deliciously Right Thousand Island	+2	Olive Oil and Vinegar	+3
Deliciously Right Catalina	+2	Parisienne Dijon Lime	+1
French	+4	Parmesan	+1
Greek Vinaigrette	+3	Parmesiano Italiano	+3
Honey Dijon*	+5	Ranch	+3
Italian, Olive Oil	+4		
Peppercorn Ranch*	+5	**Hidden Valley**		
Ranch*	+5	Bacon*	+4
Ranch Sour Cream and Onion*	+5	Blue Cheese	+3
Salsa Zesty Garden	+2	Honey Dijon	+3
Tangy Tomato Bacon	+3	Ranch Italian	+3
Thousand Island	+4	All Reduced-Calorie Varieties	+2
Zesty Italian	+4	All Low-Fat/Reduced-Calorie	0

Ken's

Wishbone

Caesar Lite	+2	Chunky Blue Cheese*	+5
Creamy Parmesan Lite	+3	Classic Caesar	+5
Raspberry Walnut Vinaigrette	+2	Italian	+2
Red Wine Vinegar and Olive Oil	−1	Ranch*	+5
Steak House Blue Cheese*	+16	Red Wine Vinaigrette	+1
Steak House Basil Vinaigrette	+4	Robusto Italian	+2
Steak House Sweet Vidalia Onion	+3	Russian	+3
Thousand Island*	+5	All Fat-Free Varieties	0

*AVOID

TRF SCORES OF CAKES
(Per One Slice or 1/16 of Cake)

Angel Food	+3	Gingerbread (Butter)*		+9
Caramel, No Icing (Vegetable Shortening)*	+5	Marble Cake		+6
Caramel, No Icing (Butter)*	+8	Plain (Vegetable Shortening)		+11
Caramel, with Icing (Vegetable Shortening)*	+8	Plain (Butter)*		+11
Caramel, with Icing (Butter)*	+11	Plain, with Chocolate Icing (Vegetable Shortening)*		+10
Carrot, with Cream Cheese Frosting*	+9	Plain, with Chocolate Icing (Butter)*		+11
Cheesecake*	+20	Pound Cake (Vegetable Shortening)*		+7
Chocolate, No Icing (Vegetable Shortening)*	+9	Pound Cake (Butter)*		+8
Chocolate, No Icing (Butter)*	+10	Sponge Cake		+5
Chocolate with Icing (Vegetable Shortening)*	+21	Caramel Icing (2 Tbs)		+3
Chocolate with Icing (Butter)*	+22	Chocolate Icing (2 Tbs)		+6
Coffeecake, No Icing (Vegetable Shortening)	+6	Coconut Icing (2 Tbs)		+6
Coffeecake, with Icing	+8	Chocolate Fudge Icing (2 Tbs)		+6
Fruitcake (Vegetable Shortening)	+1	Chocolate Syrup*		+14
Fruitcake (Butter)	+5	Chocolate Syrup (Fat-Free)		+2
Gingerbread (Vegetable Shortening)*	+8			

*AVOID

TRF SCORES OF HERSHEY'S CHOCOLATE PRODUCTS

Butterscotch	+3	Chocolate, Milk, with Peanuts*	+7
Caramel, Plain	+4	Chocolate Coated Almonds	+5
Caramel with Chocolate	+5	Chocolate Covered Raisins	+6
Caramel with Nuts	+3	Chocolate Fudge	+5
Chocolate, Bittersweet*	+12	Chocolate Fudge with Nuts	+5
Chocolate, Semisweet*	+8	Chocolate Fudge with Walnuts	+4
Chocolate, Milk, Plain*	+8	Peanut Bar	+5
Chocolate, Milk, with Almonds*	+7	Peanut Brittle	+4

TRF SCORES OF HERSHEY'S CHOCOLATE PRODUCTS (*Continued*)

Yogurt Covered Nuts	+1		**Hershey's Bites**	
Yogurt Covered Raisins	+2		Almond Joy (8)*	+7
Other Candies without Milk, Fat, or Chocolate	+2		Cookies 'n' Creme (8)*	+6
5th Avenue (1)	+4		Milk Chocolate Eggs (4)*	
Almond Joy, Small Size (1)*	+5		Milk Chocolate with Almonds (7)*	+7
Almond Joy, Regular Size (1)*	+8		York Peppermint Pattie (9)	+4
Caramello (1)*	+5			
Heath Bar (1)	+3		**Hershey's Miniatures (1 Piece)**	
Kisses (4)*	+8		Krackel	+3
Kisses with Almond (4)*	+7		Milk Chocolate	+3
Kit Kat Wafer Bar (1)	+3		Mr. Goodbar	+3
Krackel Chocolate Bar (1)*	+6		Special Dark	+3
Milk Chocolate Bar (1)*	+7		Cookies 'n' Creme	+3
Milk Duds (7 Pieces)	+3		Dark Chocolate with Almonds	+3
Mounds (1)*	+9		Milk Chocolate	+4
Mr. Goodbar (1)	+4		Milk Chocolate with Almonds	+3
Reese's Cups (1)	+2		Milk Chocolate with Almonds and Toffee	+3
Reese's Eggs (1)	+4		Milk Chocolate with Raisins and Almonds	+3
Reese's Nutrageous (1)	+4			
Rolo Caramels in Milk Chocolate (1)	+4		**Hershey's Sweet Escapes (1 Bar)**	
Sixlets (3 8-ball Tubes)*	+7		Caramel and Peanut Butter	+3
Symphony Chocolate Bar (1)*	+7		Crispy Caramel Fudge Bar	+3
Whatchamacallit (1)*	+7		Crunchy Peanut Butter	+3
Whoppers (9 Pieces)*	+7		Triple Chocolate Wafer Bar	+4
York Peppermint Pattie (1)	+4			
Zagnut, Snack Size (1)*	+7			

*AVOID

TRF SCORES OF HERSHEY'S OTHER PRODUCTS
(Per Serving as Listed)

Classic Caramels, Creme (3)*	+5
Classic Caramels, Soft and Chewy (3)	+4
Crispy Rice Snacks, Peanut Butter (1)	+2
Good and Plenty (1 Box)	+1
Good 'n Fruity	+1

Hershey's Tastetations Candies

Butterscotch (3)	+3
Caramel (3)	+3
Jolly Rancher Candies (3)	+1
Jolly Rancher Lollipop (1)	+1
Payday (1 Bar)	+1
Rainblo Bubblegum Balls (2)	0
Reese's Pieces (2)	+1

Robin Eggs

Mini (10 Pieces)*	+5
Medium (4 Pieces)*	+5
Large (2 Pieces)	+4

Twizzlers

Cherry Candy (1)	+1
Chocolate Candy (1)	+1
Licorice Candy (1)	+1
Nibs Cherry or Licorice (9)	+1
Pull 'n' Peel (1)	+1
Strawberry (1)	+1
Zero Candy Bar	+1

Hershey's Grocery Products

Candy Coated Sprinkles (1 Tbs)*	+5
Caramel Sundae Syrup (1 Tbs)	+2
Chocolate Fudge (1 Tbs)*	+5
Chocolate Syrup (2 Tbs)	+2
Chocolate Syrup, Lite (2 Tbs)	+1
Cocoa (1 Tbs)	+2
Double Chocolate (1 Tbs)	+2
European Style Cocoa (1 Tbs)	+2
Fat-Free Chocolate Syrup (1 Tbs)	+2
Hot Fudge Syrup (1 Tbs)	+3
Reese's and Milk Chocolate (1 Tbs)*	+5
Strawberry Syrup (2 Tbs)	+2
Whoppers Malt Syrup	+2

Hershey's Bake Shoppe

Butterscotch Chips (1 Tbs)*	+5
Milk Chocolate Chips (1 Tbs)*	+6
Mini Chocolate Chips (1 Tbs)*	+6
Mini Kisses (1 Tbs)*	+7
Premier White Milk Chocolate Chips (1 Tbs)*	+7
Raspberry Chips (1 Tbs)*	+6
Reese's Peanut Butter Chips (1 Tbs)*	+5
Semisweet Chocolate Chips (1 Tbs)*	+6
Semisweet Mini Chips (1 Tbs)*	+6
Skor, English Toffee Bits (1 Tbs)*	+6

*AVOID

TRF SCORES OF MARS PRODUCTS

M&M's Snacks (Per Serving)

Milk Chocolate, Large Bar (1.7 Oz)*	+15
Milk Chocolate, Fun Size*	+6
Peanut, Large*	+12
Peanut, Fun Size	+5
Peanut Butter, Large*	+20
Almond (1.3 Oz)*	+9
Crispy, Large Pack (1.5 Oz)*	+13
Crispy, Fun Size (3 Packs)*	+13
Mini (1-oz Tube)*	+13
Dove Dark Chocolate (1 Piece) (6 G)	+3
Dove Milk Chocolate Caramel 1 Piece	+2
Dove Milk Chocolate, 1 Piece	+3

3 Musketeers

Chewlicious Candy, 1 Bar	+3
Fun Size, 2 Bars*	+7
Large Bar, 1 Bar*	+13
Miniatures, 7 Pieces*	+9

*AVOID

Milky Way

Fun Size, 2 Bars*	+9
Large Bar, 1 Bar*	+13
Miniatures, 5 Pieces*	+9
Midnight, 1 Bar*	+12

Snickers

Large (1 Bar)*	+13
Fun Size (2 Bars)*	+9
Miniatures (4 Pieces)*	+9
Cruncher, Fun Size (3 Pieces)*	+11

Other Candy Bars

Almond Joy, Large Bar*	+20
Baby Ruth, Large Bar*	+21
Butterfinger, Large Bar*	+15
Kit Kat, Big Kat*	+23
Mounds, Large Bar*	+22

Starburst

Fruit Chews, 1 Pack (2 Oz)	+4
Fruit Chew Pop, 1 Lollipop	+1
Hard Candy (1)	+1

TRF SCORES OF PIES
(Per One Regular Slice or 1/8 of Pie)

Apple*	+10	Cherry*	+10
Banana Custard	+8	Chocolate Chiffon*	+11
Blackberry*	+10	Chocolate Meringue*	+12
Blueberry*	+5	Coconut Custard*	+12

TRF SCORES OF PIES (*Continued*)

Custard*	+7	Sweet Potato*	+9
Lemon Chiffon	+3	Walnut	+5
Lemon Meringue	+9	Apple Pie Filling	+2
Peach	+8	Cherry Pie Filling (½ Cup)	0
Pecan	+8	Applesauce Pie Filling (½ Cup)	0
Pineapple	+9	Cranberry (½ Cup)	0
Pumpkin*	+10	Mincemeat (½ Cup)	0
Raisin	+8	Libby Pumpkin Pie Filling (½ Cup)	0
Strawberry	+8		

*AVOID

TRF SCORES OF COOKIES

Archway Cookies (Per Cookie)

Apple 'n Raisin*	+5	Coconut, Chips Deluxe (10)*	+6
Chocolate Chip and Toffee*	+6	Country Style Oatmeal and Raisins (2)	+3
Date-filled Oatmeal*	+7	Frosted Animals Cookies (1 Pack)*	+20
Dutch Cocoa*	+8	Fudge Shoppe Clusters, Double Fudge 'n Caramel (2)*	+8
Frosty Lemon*	+6	Fudge Shoppe Clusters, Peanut (1)*	+6
Fat-Free Oatmeal Raisin*	+5	Fudge Shoppe Deluxe Grahams (3)*	+10
Fat-Free Fruit Bar	+3	Fudge Shoppe Fudge Stripes (3)*	+10
Fat-Free Granola	+3	Fudge Shoppe Fudge Stripes, Reduced Fat (3)*	+7
Golden Oatmeal	+3	Fudge Shoppe Grasshopper (4)*	+9
Oatmeal	+3	Fudge Shoppe Fudge Sticks (3)*	+9
Old-Fashioned Molasses*	+6	Mini Fudge Shoppe Stripes (4)	+3
Rocky Road*	+6	Mini Fudge, Chips Deluxe (4)*	+7

Keebler

		Peanut Butter Fudge Sticks (3)*	+3
Chocolate Chip, Original (1)	+3	Peanut Butter, Chips Deluxe (1)	+4
Chocolate Lovers, Chips Deluxe (1)*	+6	Rainbow, Chips Deluxe (1)	+4
Club Mini Sandwiches (1 Package)*	+7	Sandies Chocolate Chip & Pecan (1)	+2

TRF SCORES OF COOKIES (*Continued*)

Sandies Mini Pecan Shortbread (4)*	+5
Sandies Pecan Shortbread (1)	+1
Sandies Simply Shortbread (1)	+4
Soft 'n Chewy, Chips Deluxe (1)	+2
Vienna Fingers (4)*	+8

Mrs. Fields (Per Cookie)

Macadamia*	+9
Milk Chocolate*	+10
Semisweet Chocolate	+10
Oatmeal with Nuts and Raisins	+7

Nabisco

Chips Ahoy! (3)*	+3
Chips Ahoy! Candy Blast (1)	+2
Chips Ahoy! Chocolate Chewy (3)*	+6
Chips Ahoy! Chunky (1)	+4
Chips Ahoy! Cremewiches (2)*	+6
Chips Ahoy! Peanut Butter (1)	+3
Chips Ahoy! Reduced Fat (1)	+4
Ginger Snaps (4)	+2
Grahams, All Varieties (28)	+3
Grahams, Dora Explorer (8)	+3
Mini Oreo, Bite-Size (9)	+3
Mini Oreo, Chocolate Creme (9)	+3
Newtons, Apple, Fig, or Berries (2)	+1
Nutter Butter (1 Package)*	+5
Oreo (3)	+4
Oreo Cookie Bar (1)*	+15
Oreo Double Delight (2)	+4
Oreo Double Stuf (4)*	+7

Oreo Fudge (1)	+3
Oreo Fudge Mint (1)	+3
Pinwheels, Pure Chocolate (1)*	+6

Nabisco Snackwell's

Chocolate Chip Bite-Size (6)	+2
Chocolate Sandwich (2)	+2
Creme Sandwich (2)	+2
Devil's Food, Fat-Free (1)	+1
Ginger Snaps (4)	+2
Mint Creme (2)	+3
Sugar-Free Chocolate Chip (3)	+2
Sugar-Free Chocolate Sandwich (3)	+3
Sugar-Free Lemon Creme (3)	+2
Sugar-Free Oatmeal (1)	+1

Nabisco, Other Snacks

Treasures, Chocolate Creme (3 Pieces)*	+14
Treasures, Peanut Butter (3 Pieces)*	+13
Treasures, Toasted Coconut (3 Pieces)*	+18

Pepperidge Farm

Bordeaux (4)*	+6
Brussels (3)*	+7
Chantilly (2)	+3
Chessmen (3)*	+7
Crème Magnifique (2)*	+6
Decadent Chocolate (2)*	+8
Delectables (3)*	+8
Dessert Bliss (3)*	+7
Geneva (3)*	+8

TRF SCORES OF COOKIES (*Continued*)

Ginger Man (4)	+3		Nantucket*	+7
Golden Orchard (5)*	+5		Nantucket Dark Chocolate*	+6
Lemon Nut (3)*	+5		Nantucket Double Chocolate*	+7
Lido (2)*	+6		Santa Cruz	+3
Milano (3)*	+8		Sausalito*	+7
Milano, Endless Chocolate (3)*	+11		Sausalito Milk Chocolate Macademia*	+6
Milano, Milk Chocolate (3)*	+8		Sedona*	+5
Pirouettes (2)*	+8		Tahoe*	+7
Salzburg, Chocolate Mocha (2)*	+5			
Shortbread (2)*	+5			

Others

Spritzers (5)	+4
St. Tropez (2)*	+6
Verona (3)*	+5

Pepperidge Farm Soft Chocolate Chunks (1)

Caramel*	+5
Chesapeake*	+6
Chesapeake Dark Chocolate*	+6
Laredo*	+5

Chocolate Chip Cookies with Butter* (1)	+9
Chocolate Chip Cookies with Shortening*	+8
Fig Bars (1)	+2
Gingersnaps (3)	+3
Oatmeal Cookies with Raisins (3)	+4
Raisin Cookies (3)	+3
Sugar Wafers (3)	+3

*AVOID

TRF SCORES OF DUNKIN' DONUTS

(Per 1 Donut)

Apple Crumb*	+7		Blueberry Crumb*	+8
Apple Fritter*	+7		Boston Kreme*	+5
Apple N' Spice	+4		Bow Tie Donut Ring*	+11
Banana Kreme*	+5		Chocolate Coconut Cake*	+8
Bismark Chocolate Iced*	+10		Chocolate Frosted Coffee Roll*	+5
Black Raspberry*	+5		Chocolate Glazed Cake*	+8
Blueberry Cake*	+8		Chocolate Kreme Filled*	+8

TRF SCORES OF DUNKIN' DONUTS (*Continued*)

Cinnamon Bun*	+12	**Munchkins (Per 3)**	
Cinnamon Cake*	+7	Chocolate Glazed*	+5
Coconut Cake*	+11	Butter Nut*	+7
Coffee Roll*	+7	Cinnamon*	+7
Double Chocolate Cake*	+9	Coconut*	+8
Dunkin' Donut*	+7	Glazed*	+5
Eclair*	+7	Plain*	+7
Glazed Cake*	+7	Powdered*	+7
Glazed Chocolate Cruller*	+8	Sugar Raised*	+7
Glazed Cruller*	+8	Toasted Coconut*	+7
Glazed Donut	+4	Yeast, Glazed*	+5
Glazed Fritter*	+7	Yeast, Jelly Filled*	+6
Jelly Filled	+4	Yeast, Lemon Filled	+4
Jelly Stick*	+7	Yeast, Sugar Raised*	+6
Lemon Donut*	+5		
Maple Frosted Coffee Roll*	+7	**Muffins, Danish and Scones**	
Maple Frosted Donut*	+5	Apple Danish*	+7
Marble Frosted Donut*	+5	Banana Nut Muffin*	+16
Old Fashioned Cake Donut*	+7	Blueberry Muffin*	+16
Plain Cruller*	+7	Blueberry Scone*	+12
Powdered Cruller*	+7	Cheese Danish*	+10
Powdered Cake Donut*	+7	Chocolate Chip Muffin*	+25
Strawberry Filled Donut	+4	Coffee Cake Muffin*	+24
Strawberry Frosted Donut*	+5	Corn Muffin*	+12
Sugar Cruller*	+7	Cranberry Orange Muffin*	+14
Sugar Raised Donut*	+7	Honey Bran Raisin Muffin*	+12
Toasted Coconut*	+12	Maple Walnut Scone*	+13
Vanilla Frosted Coffee Roll*	+7	Raspberry White Chocolate Scone*	+17
Vanilla Frosted Donut*	+8	Reduced Fat Blueberry Muffin*	+20
Whole Wheat Glazed Donut*	+9	Strawberry Cheese Danish*	+8

TRF SCORES OF DUNKIN' DONUTS (*Continued*)

Chocolate Chunk*	+16	Oatmeal Raisin Pecan*	+12
Chocolate Chunk with Walnut*	+14	White Chocolate Chunk*	+16

*AVOID

TRF SCORES OF KRISPY KREME DONUTS
(Per 1 Donut)

Apple Cinnamon Sugar*	+7	Glazed Yeast*	+7
Blueberry Powdered Sugar*	+9	Honey Bun*	+14
Cake Glazed Cruller*	+8	Old Fashioned Honey and Oat*	+7
Chocolate Enrobed*	+17	Old Fashioned Sour Cream*	+7
Chocolate Enrobed Mini Cake*	+20	Plain Mini Cake*	+9
Chocolate Iced, Creme Filled*	+12	Powdered Raspberry Filled*	+10
Chocolate Iced, Custard Filled*	+10	Powdered Strawberry Filled*	+9
Chocolate Iced, Glazed*	+8	Powdered Sugar Cake*	+7
Cinnamon Bun*	+9	Powdered Sugar Mini Cake*	+7
Cinnamon Twist*	+7	Sugar Donut*	+7
Cranapple Crunch Filled*	+11	Traditional Cake Donut*	+7
Glazed Blueberry*	+9	Traditional Chocolate Iced*	+8
Glazed Cherry*	+10	Vanilla Iced Cake with Sprinkles*	+8
Glazed Cinnamon*	+7	Vanilla Iced, Custard Filled*	+9
Glazed Creme Filled*	+12	Vanilla Iced, Creme Filled*	+12
Glazed Custard Filled*	+9	Yeast, Chocolate Iced with Sprinkles*	+8
Glazed Devil's Food*	+12		
Glazed Donut*	+7	**Pies (One)**	
Glazed Lemon Filled*	+10	Apple*	+15
Glazed Mini Cruller*	+8	Cherry*	+15
Glazed Pumpkin Spice*	+14	Coconut Creme*	+15
Glazed Raspberry Filled*	+10	Peach*	+18
Glazed Twist*	+7		

*AVOID

TRF SCORES OF KELLOGG'S POP-TARTS AND EGGOS

Pop-tarts Pastry Swirls (Per 1)

Apple Cinnamon*	+9
Cheese*	+8
Cheese and Cherry*	+8
Cinnamon and Creme*	+9
Strawberry*	+9

Pop-tarts Snak-stix (Per 1)

Frosted Caramel Chocolate*	+5
Frosted Cookies and Creme*	+6
Frosted Double Chocolate*	+6
Frosted Strawberry*	+5

Pop-tarts (Per 1)

Apple Cinnamon	+3
Blueberry	+3
Chocolate Chip*	+5
Frosted Blueberry*	+5
Frosted Brown Sugar Cinnamon	+3
Frosted Cherry*	+4
Frosted Chocolate Vanilla Creme*	+4
Frosted Grape*	+4

*AVOID

Frosted Raspberry	+3
Frosted S'mores*	+4
Frosted Strawberry*	+4
Frosted Wild Berry*	+4
Frosted Wild Magiburst*	+4
Frosted Low-Fat Brown Sugar Cinnamon	+3
Frosted Low-Fat Chocolate Fudge	+3
Frosted Low-Fat Strawberry	+3

Eggo Waffles (Per 2) and Pancakes (Per 3)

Apple Cinnamon, Banana Bread, Blueberry, and Waf-fulls Waffles	+4
Buttermilk, Chocolate Chip, Homestyle, Minis, and Strawberry Waffles*	+5
Cinnamon Toast Waffles*	+7
Special K Waffles	+2
Buttermilk Pancakes*	+5

TRF SCORES OF SWEET SNACKS

Hostess	Serving Size	
Fruit Pie, Apple	1*	+22
Fruit Pie, Blueberry	1*	+23
Fruit Pie, Cherry	1*	+24
Fruit Pie, Lemon	1*	+26
Ho Hos	3 Pieces*	+26
Mini-muffins, Banana	3 Pieces*	+5
Mini-muffins, Blueberry	3 Pieces*	+5
Mini-muffins, Brownie	3 Pieces*	+8
Mini-muffins, Cinnamon Apple	3 Pieces*	+6
Mini-muffins, Chocolate Chip	3 Pieces*	+7
Twinkies	1 Piece	+4
Twinkies, Chocolate Cake	1 Cake*	+5
Twinkies, Ding Dongs	2 Cakes*	+22
Twinkies, Low-Fat	1 Cake	+2
Twinkies, Sponge-Cake	1 Cake	+2

Tastykake	Serving Size	
Butterscotch Krimpets	3 Cakes*	+6
Cherry Pie	1 Pie*	+9
Chocolate Cupcakes	3 Cakes*	+7
Chocolate Iced Tasty Klair	1 Pie*	+16
Chocolate Kandykakes	2 Pieces*	+10
French Apple Pie	1 Piece*	+6
Frosted Mini-donuts	2 Pieces*	+9
Ghostly Goodies	2 Pieces*	+16
Jelly Krimpets	2 Pieces*	+1
Koffee Kakes	2 Cakes*	+7
Koffee Kakes, Low-Fat	2 Cakes	+2
Kreepy Kakes	2 Cakes*	+5
Lemon Pie	1 Pie*	+7

TRF SCORES OF SWEET SNACKS (*Continued*)

Snak Bar Chocolate Chip	1 Bar*	+10
Iced Fudge	1 Bar*	+7
Oatmeal Raisin	1 Bar*	+17
Witchy Goodies	2 Pieces*	+16

Quaker Chewy Granola

Caramel Apple Bar	1	+5
Chocolate Chip Granola Bar	1	+5
Peanut Butter Bar	1*	+6
Trail Mix Granola Bar	1*	+5

Others

Brownies with Butter*	1.5*	+8
Brownies with Nuts*	1.5*	+7
Coconut Bar*	3 Pieces	+8
Danish, Small Plain*	1	+8
Danish, Small with Fruit*	1	+7
Donut, Chocolate Covered*	1	+11
Donut, with Custard Inside*	1	+12

*AVOID

TRF SCORES OF CHIPS & PRETZELS
(*Per Serving Size or Pieces*)

Doritos

Baked Nacho Cheese (15)	+3
Cool Ranch (14)*	+7
Four Cheese (14)*	+7
Nacho Cheese (12)*	+7
Spicier Nacho (11)*	+7
3 D Jalapeno (27)*	+6
3 D Nacho Cheese (27)*	+6
3 D Maximum Cheddar (27)*	+7

Lays

Baked Masterpiece (11)	+2
Baked Original (11)	+2
Bistro Gourmet/Applewood (12)*	+8
Bistro Gourmet/Garlic (15)*	+8

TRF SCORES OF CHIPS & PRETZELS (Continued)

California Cool Dill (17)*	+10	**UTZ (Per 20 Pieces)**	
Classic (20)*	+10	Bar-b-q*	+8
Classic Russets (20)*	+7	Crisp, All Natural*	+7
Hickory BBQ (13)*	+8	Ripples*	+8
Masterpiece (15)*	+9	Sour Cream & Onion*	+9
Original (11)*	+10	Wavy Crisp*	+7
Sour Cream & Onion (17)*	+10	Wavy Honey Bar-b-q	+8

Robert's Amer. Gourmet

Rolled Gold Pretzels

Original Flyers (1½ Oz Bag)	+2	Classic Thins (9)	+3
Original Veggie Chips (1½ Oz)	+2	Hard Sourdough (1)	+2
Pirate's Booty Chips (1½ Oz)	+3	Honey Mustard (13)	+2
Smart Puffs with Cheddar (1½ Oz)	+3	Sticks (40)	+2
		Tiny Twists (17)	+3

Terra

		Twist, Braided (8)	+2
Blues (15)*	+4		
Red Bliss (12)*	+6	**Snyder's**	
Red Bliss Olive Oil/Garlic (13)	+2		
Stix (50)*	+7	Jalapeno, or Cheese (½ Cup)*	+4
Sweet Potato (17)*	+8	Mini (20)	+2
Vegetable Chips (10)*	+7	Nibblers (16)	+2
Yukon Gold (8)*	+6	Old Thyme (30)	+2
		Rods (3)	+2

Tostitos

		Sourdough Hard (1)	+2
Bite-Size (24)*	+6	Sourdough Specials (6)	+2
Crispy Rounds (13)*	+7	Snaps (24)	+2
Scoops (13)*	+6	Sticks (28)	+2
White Corn (13)*	+5	Thin (11)	+2
White Lime (13)*	+5		

*AVOID

TRF SCORES OF CRACKERS

Pepperidge Farm Goldfish

Baby Goldfish (90) 5 Pieces	+3
Cheddar (5 Pieces or 1 Oz)	+3
Cheese Trio (58)	+3
Pizza (14)	+3
Pretzel (41)	+2
Snack Mix (½ Cup)	+4
Snack Sticks (5)	+4

Nabisco Crackers

Better Cheddar (22)	+4
Better Cheddar, Reduced-Fat (25)	+3
Ritz Jalapeño Cheddar (33)	+3
Ritz Mini Cheddar or Original (33)	+3
Ritz, Reduced-Fat (5)	+2
Ritz, Regular or Low-Sodium (5)	+2
Sociables (5)	+1
Teddy Grahams Bearwiches (Pack)	+3
Triscuit (7)	+2
Triscuit, Reduced-Fat (7)	+1
Triscuit, Deli-Style Rye (7)	+2
Triscuit Garden Herb (6)	+2
Triscuit Thin Crisps (14)	+2
Wheat Thins, Crispy Thins, Ranch (10)	+1
Wheat Thins, Multigrain (7)	+2
Wheat Thins, Reduced-Fat (16)	+2
Whole Wheat, Reduced-Fat (5)	+0

Sunshine Crackers

Big Baked Snack Crackers (13)	+3
Cheddar Jack (26)	+3
Cheese It, Baked Crackers (14)	+4
Cheese It, Club Mini Sandwiches (14)*	+5
Cheese It, Mini Sandwiches (14)*	+5
Cheese It, Reduced-Fat (29)	+2
Cheese It, White Cheddar (26)	+3
Original Krispy Mild Cheddars (5)	+1
Original Krispy Saltine (5)	0
Parmesan & Garlic (26)	+3

Keebler Crackers

Cinnamon Crisp Grahams (8)	+3
Chocolate Grahams (8)	+3
Club, Mini Sandwiches (1 Package)*	+7
Club, Reduced-Fat (5)	+0
Harvest Bakery Crackers (2)	+1
Honey Grahams (8)	+3
Honey Grahams, Low-Fat (9)	+1
Town House (5)	+1
Wheatables, 7 Grain (17)*	+5
Wheatables, Honey Or Low-Fat (17)	+2
Wheatables, Original (15)	+3

Stella D'oro

Breadsticks (1)	+3
Fat-Free Breadstick (1)	+1
Sesame Breadstick (1)	+3

*AVOID

TRF SCORES OF BURGER KING

Breakfast

Biscuit*	+8
Biscuit with Egg*	+12
Biscuit with Sausage*	+20
Biscuit with Sausage, Egg and Cheese*	+30
Cini-minis, without Icing*	+12
Croissan'wich with Sausage and Cheese*	+26
Croissan'wich with Sausage, Egg and Cheese*	+33
French Toast Sticks (5)*	+25
Hash Browns, Small*	+19
Hash Browns, Large*	+35

Sandwiches/Side Orders

BK Broiler Chicken*	+14
BK Broiler Chicken without Mayo*	+11
BK Big Fish*	+34
Chicken Whopper*	+11
Chicken Whopper without Mayo*	+7
Chicken Tenders (4)*	+7
Chicken Tenders (5)*	+9
Chicken Tenders (8)*	+15
Big Veggie Burger	+4
French Fries, Small*	+12
French Fries, Medium*	+18
French Fries, King*	+26
Onion Rings, Medium*	+15
Onion Rings, Large*	+22
Onion Rings, King*	+25

Burgers

Bacon Cheeseburger*	+20
Bacon Double Cheeseburger*	+35
Big King*	+36
Cheeseburger*	+18
Double Cheeseburger*	+33
Double Whopper*	+45
Double Whopper, without Mayo*	+42
Double Whopper with Cheese*	+53
Double Whopper with Cheese, without Mayo*	+54
Hamburger*	+13
Whopper*	+28
Whopper without Mayo*	+25
Whopper with Cheese*	+37
Whopper with Cheese, without Mayo	+34
Whopper Jr.*	+20
Whopper Jr., without Mayo*	+17
Whopper Jr., with Cheese*	+23
Whopper Jr., with Cheese without Mayo*	+21

Desserts/Drinks

Dutch Apple Pie*	+13
Chocolate Shake, Small*	+9
Chocolate Shake, Medium*	+12
Strawberry Shake, Small*	+9
Strawberry Shake, Medium*	+11
Vanilla Shake, Small*	+9
Vanilla Shake, Medium*	+11

*AVOID

TRF SCORES OF KENTUCKY FRIED CHICKEN

Crispy Strips (3 Strips)

Colonel's Strips*	+14
Spicy, Honey BBQ, or Blazin' Strips*	+12

Extra Crispy

Breast*	+20
Drumstick*	+8
Thigh*	+18
Whole Wing*	+10

Hot & Spicy Chicken

Breast*	+20
Drumstick*	+6
Thigh*	+20
Whole Wing*	+8

Original Recipe Chicken

Breast*	+16
Chicken Pot Pie*	+28
Drumstick	+7
Thigh*	+18
Whole Wing*	+8

Popcorn Chicken & Wings

Individual Popcorn Chicken*	+18
Kid's Popcorn Chicken*	+10
Large Popcorn Chicken*	+27
Honey BBQ Wings*	+22
Hot Wings*	+22

*AVOID

Sandwiches

Original Roast with Sauce*	+14
Original Roast without Sauce*	+10
Tender Roast with Sauce*	+8
Tender Roast without Sauce	+5

Other Sandwiches

Twister*	+31
Honey BBQ Flavored	+4
Triple Crunch without Sauce*	+18
Triple Crunch Zinger without Sauce*	+16

Sides

Biscuit (1)*	+5
Cole Slaw	+4
Corn on the Cob (without Butter)	0
Mashed Potatoes*	+5
Mean Greens	+3
Potato Salad*	+7
Potato Wedges*	+10

Desserts

Double Chocolate Chip Cake*	+10
Parfait, Fudge Brownie*	+9
Parfait, Lemon Creme*	+17
Pecan Pie*	+10

TRF SCORES OF MCDONALD'S

Breakfast

Bacon, Egg and Cheese Biscuit*	+28
Biscuit*	+6
Breakfast Burrito*	+20
Egg McMuffin*	+13
English Muffin	+3
Hash Browns*	+6
Hotcakes*	+11
Hotcakes with Margarine and Syrup*	+22
Sausage*	+9
Sausage Biscuit*	+17
Sausage Biscuit with Egg*	+27
Sausage McMuffin*	+22
Sausage McMuffin with Egg*	+25
Scrambled Eggs*	+14

Chicken McNuggets

Chicken McNuggets (4)*	+8
Chicken McNuggets (6)*	+11
Chicken McNuggets (9)*	+18
Chicken McGrill*	+9
Chicken McGrill without Mayo	+6
Crispy Chicken*	+12

French Fries

Small*	+17
Large*	+20
Super Size*	+26

*AVOID

Burgers/Sandwiches

Big Mac*	+19
Big N' Tasty*	+27
Big N' Tasty with Cheese*	+31
Cheeseburger*	+12
Crispy Chicken Deluxe*	+14
Fish Filet Deluxe*	+14
Grilled Chicken Deluxe*	+10
Hamburger	+7
Quarter Pounder*	+17
Quarter Pounder with Cheese*	+25

Salads & Dressings

Caesar Salad with Grilled Chicken	+3
Chef Salad*	+8
Garden Salad	+4
Caesar Dressing (1 Package)	+4
Ranch Dressing (1 Package)	+4
Red French Dressing (1 Package)	+2

Desserts

Baked Apple Pie*	+10
Butterfinger Mcflurry*	+35
Chocolate Chip Cookie (1)*	+18
Hot Caramel Sundae*	+15
Hot Fudge Sundae*	+17
Strawberry Triple Thick Shake*	+32
Vanilla Triple Thick Shake*	+32

TRF SCORES OF PIZZA HUT
(Pizzas per 2 Slices)

Beef Topping

Hand Tossed*	+31
Pan*	+28
Stuffed Crust*	+32
Thin N' Crispy*	+20

Cheese

Hand Tossed*	+21
Pan*	+25
Stuffed Crust*	+32
Thin N' Crispy*	+18

Ham

Hand Tossed*	+14
Pan*	+15
Stuffed Crust*	+22
Thin N' Crispy*	+13

Italian Sausage

Hand Tossed*	+22
Pan*	+24
Stuffed Crust*	+31
Thin N' Crispy*	+25

Meat Lovers

Hand Tossed*	+24
Pan*	+23
Stuffed Crust*	+44
Thin N' Crispy*	+29

Pepperoni

Hand Tossed*	+17
Pan*	+17
Stuffed Crust*	+29
Thin N' Crispy*	+16

Personal Pan (Per Pizza)

Cheese*	+21
Pepperoni Lovers*	+24
Supreme*	+26

Pork

Hand Tossed*	+21
Pan*	+21
Stuffed Crust*	+29
Thin N' Crispy*	+25

Supreme

Hand Tossed*	+21
Pan*	+20
Stuffed Crust*	+32
Thin N' Crispy*	+20

Super Supreme

Hand Tossed*	+19
Pan*	+21
Stuffed Crust*	+34
Thin N' Crispy*	+21

Veggie Lovers

Hand Tossed*	+12
Pan*	+15

TRF SCORES OF PIZZA HUT (*Continued*)

Stuffed Crust*	+25
Thin N' Crispy*	+9

Pepperoni Lovers

Hand Tossed*	+25
Pan*	+30
Stuffed Crust*	+37
Thin N' Crispy*	+25

Spaghetti

Spaghetti with Marinara	+2
Spaghetti with Meatballs*	+20
Spaghetti with Meat sauce	+10

Other

Apple Dessert	+4
Bread Stick (1)	+2
Bread Stick Sauce	0
Cavatini Pasta*	+12
Cavatini Supreme*	+15
Cherry Dessert	+2
Garlic Bread	+2
Ham and Cheese Sandwich*	+15
Hot Buffalo Wings (4)	+6
Mild Buffalo Wings (5)	+8

*AVOID

TRF SCORES OF SUBWAY

Classic Sandwiches

BLT	+8
Cold Cut Trio*	+14
Italian BMT*	+17
Seafood, Light Mayo*	+9
Seafood, Regular Mayo*	+15
Tuna, Light Mayo*	+9
Tuna, Regular Mayo*	+21

6 Grams Fat Or Less (6")

Ham	+4
Roast Beef	+5
Roast Chicken Breast	+5
Subway Club	+5
Turkey Breast	+4
Turkey Breast and Ham	+4
Veggie Delite	+3

6" Select

Chipotle Southwest Steak and Cheese*	+15
Chipotle Southwest Turkey and Bacon*	+11
Dijon Horseradish Melt*	+17
Honey Mustard Ham	+4
Red Wine Vinaigrette Club	+8
Sweet Onion Chicken Teriyaki	+4

Extreme Sandwiches

Dijon Horseradish Melt*	+18
Southwestern Onion Chicken Teriyaki	+7
Southwestern Turkey and Ham*	+13
Vinaigrette Club*	+9

TRF SCORES OF SUBWAY (*Continued*)

Double Meat Sandwiches

Chicken Breast	+8
Cold Cut Trio*	+28
Ham	+7
Italian BMT*	+31
Meatballs*	+35
Roast Beef	+8
Seafood and Crab*	+15
Steak and Cheese*	+16
Subway Club*	+9

*Avoid

Subway Melt*	+21
Tuna*	+19
Turkey Breast	+7
Turkey and Ham	+7

Salads

BLT*	+8
Chicken Taco*	+14
Italian BMT*	+13
Veggie Delite	0

TRF SCORES OF TACO BELL

Border Wraps

Chicken Fajita*	+12
Chicken Fajita Supreme*	+16
Steak Fajita*	+12
Steak Fajita Supreme*	+16
Veggie Fajita*	+9
Veggie Fajita Supreme*	+12

Breakfast

Burrito*	+22
Fiesta Burrito*	+12
Gordita*	+17
Quesadilla*	+19
Quesadilla, Bacon*	+24
Quesadilla, Cheese*	+20
Quesadilla, Sausage*	+22

Quesadilla, Steak*	+20

Burritos

Bean	+8
Chili Cheese*	+18
Fiesta, Beef*	+12
Fiesta, Chicken	+8
Fiesta, Steak	+8
Grilled Stuft, Beef*	+21
Grilled Stuft, Chicken*	+16
Grilled Stuft, Steak*	+17
Supreme, Chicken or Steak*	+12

Nachos and Sides

3 Cheese Sauce (Serving)	+4
Nachos*	+16
Nachos Bellgrande*	+22

TRF SCORES OF TACO BELL (*Continued*)

Nachos Pintos 'n Cheese*	+8
Nachos Supreme*	+17
Mexican Rice*	+8

Gorditas & Quesadillas

Gordita Baja Beef*	+12
Gordita Baja Chicken*	+9
Gordita Baja Steak*	+9
Gordita Nacho Cheese, Beef*	+9
Gordita Nacho Cheese, Chicken*	+9
Gordita Nacho Cheese, Steak	+7
Gordita Supreme, Beef*	+13
Gordita Supreme, Chicken*	10
Gordita Supreme, Steak*	+11
Quesadilla, Cheese*	+25
Quesadilla, Cheese Extreme*	+24
Quesadilla, Chicken*	+24
Quesadilla, Steak*	+25

Chalupas

Baja Beef*	+14
Baja Chicken*	+13
Baja Steak*	+14
Nacho, Beef or Steak*	+13
Nacho Chicken*	+10
Supreme Beef*	+17
Supreme Chicken or Steak*	+14

Tacos

Enchirito, Beef*	+19
Enchirito, Chicken	+15
Enchirito, Steak*	+16
Mexican Melt*	+15
Mexican Pizza*	+22
Southwest Steak Bowl*	+22
Taco Salad with Salsa*	+30
Taco Salad with Salsa, without Shell*	+22
Tostada*	+9
Zesty Chicken Border Bowl without Dressing*	+21

*AVOID

TRF SCORES WENDY'S

Fresh Stuffed Pitas

Chicken Caesar*	+10
Classic Greek*	+15
Garden Ranch Chicken*	+8
Garden Veggie	+6

Pita Dressings

Caesar Vinaigrette	+3
Garden Ranch Sauce	+3

Potatoes

Blue Cheese*	+13

TRF SCORES WENDY'S (*Continued*)

Baked Potato, Plain	+7	Oriental Sesame*	+7
Potato with Bacon and Cheese*	+20	Spring Mix with Cheese*	+12
Potato with Broccoli and Cheese*	+15	Taco Supremo Salad*	+21
Potato with Cheese*	+15		

Salad Dressings/Garnish

Potato with Chili and Cheese*	+18
Potato with Sour Cream and Chives*	+15
Potato with Whipped Margarine*	+11

Creamy Ranch or Honey Mustard*	+9
Creamy Ranch, Reduced Fat	+4
French	+3
Honey Roasted Almonds or Pecans	+1
House Vinaigrette*	+7
Sour Cream*	+7

Nuggets, Chili and Fries

Chicken Nuggets (4)	+6
Chicken Nuggets (5)	+7
Chili, Small	+6
Chili, Large*	+9
Chili with Shredded Cheddar	+7
French Fries, Medium*	+13
French Fries, Biggie*	+15

Sandwiches

Big Bacon Classic*	+27
Breaded Chicken Fillet*	+9
Cheeseburger, Kids' Meal	+11
Chicken Club*	+10
Grilled Chicken	+5
Hamburger, Kids' Meal	+7
Jr. Bacon Cheeseburger*	+16
Jr. Cheeseburger*	+11
Jr. Cheeseburger Deluxe*	+14
Jr. Hamburger	+7
Plain Hamburger*	+11
Hamburger with Everything*	+16
Spicy Chicken	+8

Desserts

Chocolate Chip Cookie*	+12
Frosty, Junior (6 Oz)*	+6
Frosty, Small (12 Oz)*	+12
Frosty, Medium (16 Oz)*	+17

Salads

Caesar with One Packet Dressing*	+7
Honey Mustard Dressing*	+9
Mandarin Chicken	+4

*AVOID

5

HOW TO ESTIMATE YOUR OWN RISK OF A HEART ATTACK

More than half of American adults die of cardiovascular diseases. Most of these deaths and cardiovascular disease-related disabilities occur in people in their 40s, 50s, or 60s. Why would anyone in his or her prime want to suffer a disabling or fatal heart attack, stroke or aortic aneurysm?

Unlike strep throat, pneumonia or appendicitis, random events like heart attacks are not really "sudden." A heart attack is the culmination of long-term exposure to multiple risk factors. Eliminate or greatly modify these risk factors as early as you can, and you may prevent practically *every* heart attack.

Coronary artery disease is multifaceted. Each person's risk profile depends on the number and strength of each risk factor. To forecast someone's long-term heart attack risk accurately, every risk factor should be considered.

For the past two decades, many cardiovascular organizations, including the American Heart Association, have stubbornly relied on the Framingham (Massachusetts) Heart Study's "Risk Scores" for their recommendations for prevention or treatment of coronary heart disease. The Framingham Risk Scores were first proposed in 1991 and revised in 1998. To estimate the 10-year probability of a coronary event, Framingham scores are based on the traditional risk factors including age, LDL-cholesterol, HDL-cholesterol, blood pressure, smoking and diabetes. On the basis of these limited data, the 10-year probability of a cardiovascular event is estimated as low (5%), moderate (under 10%), moderately high (10% to 20%), and very high (over 20%).

Unfortunately, someone with a strong family history of premature cardiovascular disease, high homocysteine, sleep apnea, rheumatoid arthritis, abdominal obesity, terrible eating habits, and a sedentary lifestyle would be placed in the low-risk category using the Framingham Risk scores. Recent data have shown that, collectively, low-risk individuals account for two-thirds of cardiovascular risk in the entire population. For 30% of these "low-risk" individuals, the first manifestation of a cardiovascular disease is a fatal or nonfatal heart attack.

Moreover, low risk or moderately low risk does not mean "No" risk. Low-risk individuals are classified as such because many of the major

SCORES FOR MAJOR CORONARY RISK FACTORS

Risk factor	Score
1- Diabetes	+5
2- Abdominal obesity	+3
3- Sedentary lifestyle	+3
Light exercise	−1
Regular, vigorous exercise	−3
4- Atherogenic, "Western" diet	+3
Twenty Risk Factor diet	−3
5- HDL level in mg/dl:	
Under 40	+3
40–45 for men	+1
40–55 for women	+1
Over 45 for men, Over 55 for women	−3
6- LDL-Cholesterol over 100 mg/dl*	+3
7- Triglycerides over 130 mg/dl	+3
8- Age: Men over 45, women over 55**	+3
9- Smoking	+3
10- Chronic kidney disease	+3
11- Chronic inflammation	+3
12- Blood pressure over 120/80	+3
13- Lipoprotein(a) over 30 mg/dl	+3
14- Family history of CAD	+3
15- Homocysteine over 9 mmol/l	+2
16- Negative affect	+2
17- Hematocrit over 48%	+2
18- Platelets over 300,000/ml	+2
19- Obstructive sleep apnea or chronic lung disease	+2
20- Birth weight under 6 lb (under 2.7 kg)	+2

*LDL-cholesterol should be under 70 mg/dl in diabetes, and those with metabolic syndrome, multiple coronary risk factors or pre-existing cardiovascular or chronic kidney disease.

**Score for age over 65 in men or over 70 in women is 10.

To estimate your risk of a cardiovascular event, add up the scores of all your known risk factors and compare with the table.

---

risk factors (outside the six traditional ones) are ignored, but including some of these risk factors, many low-risk individuals are actually silently at high risk.

If my car has decent brakes, new tires, and I haven't had any alcohol, and I am not speeding, my probability of a traffic accident would be very low, based on these limited risk factors. Right? However, what if it is dark and raining, my headlights are out, my windshield wipers smear my windshield and I am driving on a winding mountain road? Is my risk of an accident still very low? You see my point? You can't rely on a risk assessment system that is flawed. Yet, in its 2007 update, the AHA still relies on Framingham risk scores in its guidelines for cardiovascular disease prevention.

I have looked at all the 20 major coronary risk factors and include all of these in my risk estimates. Instead of describing levels of risk as low, moderate, or high, I calculate the percentage risk from under 5% to more than 90%, providing readers with a personalized report card. I believe this personal risk estimate is not only far more inclusive and therefore more reliable, it also avoids

ESTIMATED 10-YEAR RISK OF A CARDIOVASCULAR EVENT

Total score	% risk of an event
1–5	less than 5
6–10	10
11–15	15
16–20	20
21–25	35
26–30	45
31–35	60
36-40	75
more than 41	more than 90

the misclassifications that are so common using the Framingham risk scores.

Of the 20 major risk factors for coronary artery disease, 10 can be determined on the initial visit to a healthcare provider interested in the prevention and management of coronary artery disease. These 10 major risk factors are a personal or family history of cardiovascular disease or diabetes, abdominal obesity, sedentary lifestyle, diet, blood pressure, smoking status, age, negative affect, obstructive sleep apnea or chronic lung disease, and low birthweight.

The other major risk factors may all be determined (or confirmed) with blood tests that are readily available at nearly all laboratories (or sent out by local laboratories to a "reference lab" elsewhere). These include tests for diabetes, HDL, LDL, triglycerides, lipoprotein(a), tests to confirm suspected chronic inflammatory diseases such as rheumatoid arthritis or systemic lupus or AIDS, if warranted, kidney function tests, homocysteine and a complete blood count to measure red blood cells, white blood cells and platelets. Additional tests for relevant minor risk factors such as fibrinogen or thyroid function can be done at the same time. So, a comprehensive cardiovascular risk profile will be available for your next visit to the healthcare provider.

The table provides a comprehensive risk assessment tool that can be used at home or by healthcare providers to accurately estimate an individual's probability of a coronary event within a ten-year time frame. To improve the accuracy of risk estimates, data from numerous long-term studies of coronary risk factors have been pooled and incorporated into these tables.

The risk-estimate charts represent the most thorough and accurate tool *ever* developed. Rather than relying on a few traditional risk factors and ignoring all others, as is currently done with both Framingham and Reynolds risk scores. Although precision is improved by including all major risk factors, flexibility is built into these estimates for an accurate assessment of the 10-year probability of a coronary event even if some risk factors have not been included.

Ideally, the 10-year risk estimate of a coronary event for men and women under 60 should be close to zero. But since at least one-half of men past 40 years of age (and one-third of women) have some degree of coronary artery disease, the average risk is much higher, ranging from 10% to 20%. When the 10-year risk of a coronary event is 10% or higher, vigorous intervention is essential. Do not accept a doctor's assurance that, "Your risk is no higher than the average," or, "Let's wait and see what happens." What you need to do is to take my risk assessment charts to your healthcare provider and jointly agree on a proactive course. As your risk level changes by correcting various risk factors, you can calculate your own progress on your PDA, computer or on paper.

Ideally you should address all risk factors. Obviously, we can't change our birth weight, family history or age. However, the impact of these seemingly fixed factors can be dramatically reduced by diligently controlling or correcting other risk factors, most of which have some genetic roots. We can't cure diabetes, chronic kidney disease or rheumatoid arthritis, but we can effectively treat or control them, which will help significantly lower your risk of a cardiovascular event. The table provides a practical tool with which you and your healthcare provider can determine your risk level and how best to reduce it. ❧

6

CARDIAC TESTING: WHAT DOES IT TELL US?

The purpose of cardio-vascular testing is to determine the presence of heart and vascular disease or damage, cardiovascular risk factors, and response to treatment. This information can be used to assess the prognosis and plan a course of action to improve cardiovascular health and reduce the risk of angina, heart attack, heart failure, stroke, peripheral vascular complications and cardiovascular disabilities or deaths.

Electrocardiogram (ECG)

The standard ECG captures minute electrical activity of the heart muscle, by placing electrodes on the chest wall. When coronary artery disease is well advanced to the point that the lumen of a particular branch is narrowed by more than 60% to 70%, the blood flow may still be adequate when the heart is beating 60 to 80 times a minute. But when the heart has to beat a lot faster, at times even more than 140 beats a minute during recreational exercise, specially in those who lack cardiovascular fitness, or during the "stress" exercise test, the blood flow through the narrow artery is not sufficient to provide that section of the heart muscle with nutrients and adequate

oxygen. It is this ischemia (reduced blood flow) or hypoxia (reduced oxygen supply) to the heart muscle that alters its electrical activities, which will be picked up on the ECG. It is also precisely this absence of ischemia/hypoxia that results in "your ECG is great!"—a hollow assurance.

The standard ECG has a high positive predictive value, but a poor negative predictive value. A "positive" ECG means that either it has detected damage that has already been done, or changes that suggest ischemia. In other words, the test will detect damaged heart muscle or impaired blood flow to a portion of the heart, either from severe clogging or spasm of the artery.

It's very important to note that a "negative" ECG does not mean that arteries are normal. There may be multiple plaques in the artery wall, and narrowed lumen (by as much as 50%). As long as the blood flow to the heart muscle is adequate in a resting state, the muscle is not deprived of oxygen and nutrients. Thus the electrical signature the heart muscle will appear normal and the ECG will be "negative.' As you can see, a negative ECG does not mean normal coronary arteries; it means that coronary artery *may* be normal, or there may be multiple plaques that are not severe enough yet to impede blood flow to the heart muscle. The standard ECG does not have the ability to predict a coronary event. This explains why someone with a normal ECG one day may have a heart attack the next day or the next week.

Exercise Stress ECG

Exercise increases the heart rate and heart workload and is a good means of determining the adequacy of blood flow to the heart muscle. Although the bicycle is quieter and allows better ECG recordings, the treadmill is more widely used in the US.

In addition to continuous ECG recording, many other cardiovascular responses are monitored during and shortly after the exercise test. For example, the blood pressure behavior is an important clue to cardiovascular fitness. During the exercise, systolic blood pressure may range from 160 to 200 mmHg. A more pronounced or sustained hypertensive response may be a sign of significant cardiovascular disease. Failure to raise the blood pressure during exercise is also abnormal and may reflect significant heart muscle damage, low blood volume due to dehydration, or anemia and the use of antihypertension drugs. Within two minutes after exercise, the blood pressure should go back to prestress levels. Sustained post-exercise hypertension also indicates preexisting cardiovascular disease.

Heart rate response to exercise is also an important clue to cardiovascular health. For people with no significant cardiac disease, an exercise-induced rapid heart rate normally slows down—back to its pre-exercise level—within a few minutes. A significant rise in heart rate after low-intensity testing, or a continued rapid heart rate for more than a few minutes after the test is a reason for concern, and may be a sign of...

- Poor cardiovascular fitness

- Poor conditioning

- Low blood volume

- Coronary artery disease

Certain drugs, such as beta blockers, may prevent the heart rate from increasing during exercise. However, for well-conditioned athletes or regular runners, a slower heart rate is due to their cardiovascular fitness, and not a heart disease.

Nuclear Stress Tests

Many people may not be able to complete a maximal or adequate bicycle or treadmill stress test for a variety of reasons. They include cardiovascular diseases, age, physical limitations, such as poor conditioning, fatigue, shortness of breath and chronic lung disease, leg cramps, a severe hypertensive response, chest pain, preexisting joint diseases or obesity. In these cases, the stress test is either terminated or performed with much less intense exercise (under 85% of capacity).

Unfortunately, submaximal tests are inadequate to determine the cardiovascular health. One alternative or addition to exercise test is nuclear imaging of the heart muscle function.

For this test, a person is given an intravenous injection of adenosine or dipyridamole, drugs that temporarily increase blood flow to the heart muscle. Note that different drugs may be used for some people, especially asthmatics. That's because these drugs may cause a bronchial spasm or provoke an asthma attack. Other people may already be taking dipyridamole as an anticlotting agent. In these cases, another drug, dobutamine, is used.

One of these drugs will be administered intravenously, and then a small amount of a medical-grade radioactive agent (a "tracer") is also injected intravenously. Images of blood flow (perfusion) in different parts of the heart muscle are then captured in color by a special scanner called a Single Photon Emission Computed Tomography or SPECT.

The tracer most often used for nuclear studies of the heart is Thallium-201, which behaves very much like potassium. Potassium is a major mineral in muscle cells and most other human cells, but it is virtually absent in scar tissues. Since thallium cannot penetrate into any scar within the heart muscle, it is a very suitable tracer for differentiating between live or dead (and scarred) heart muscle tissue.

Thallium nuclear tests can be combined with a modified exercise test. One advantage of thallium is that if a defect in the heart muscle is seen initially, additional scans can be obtained three or four or even 24 hours later. If the defect disappears, it indicates a reversible problem with blood perfusion of that segment that is still viable.

This kind of reversible "thallium defect" is often due to significant occlusive disease of the artery supplying that segment. Thus revascularization, either by placement of stents in the narrowed segment or through bypass surgery can save the heart muscle from permanent damage. On the other hand, a persistent defect on delayed scans, even after reinjecting a small amount of thallium-201 at rest, indicates the presence of scarred tissue.

One disadvantage of thallium-201 is that it has a long half-life (73 hours). So some harmless residual radioactivity may be present for a week or two. Even this minimal radioactivity can be picked up by most airport security. If you plan to travel by air within 20 days of the test, ask your doctor for a written statement or documentation as to the date of your nuclear stress test. This will help expedite your security clearance at the airport. Some centers also use another tracer, Technetium-99, alone or combined with thallium (referred to as double isotope test), especially in very obese persons.

As with standard ECG, exercise or nuclear (SPECT) stress testing has an excellent positive predictive value. A positive test usually indicates the presence of significant coronary artery disease, or preexisting heart muscle damage. However, a person could have multiple plaques in the thickened wall of one or more branches of coronary artery without protruding into the lumen to cause a serious blockage and still have a "negative" stress test.

Importantly, in some cases collateral branches grow out near the narrowed part of an artery, and compensate for reduced blood flow through the narrowed section. As long as during the few minutes of stress testing the lumen of the artery is still open enough to allow adequate blood flow to the heart muscle, regardless of how many coronary plaques there are, the stress test will give us a "false negative" result. Thus a negative stress test does not exclude the presence of significant, nonocclusive coronary artery disease.

Nearly 80% of heart attacks are caused by rupture of one or more nonocclusive plaques, resulting in the formation of rapidly expanding clots that clog the lumen of the artery within an hour or two.

Echocardiography

Echocardiography is based on the principle of transmitting ultrasonic waves through the chest wall, directed at the heart muscle or heart valves. The returned sound waves (or echoes) are received by a transducer that directs the information to a computer, which converts that information into an image called an echocardiogram.

Echocardiography can check on the function or any abnormalities of the heart's four valves. It is also used to image the wall motion of different chambers of the heart to see if the heart muscle functions properly. Certain structures in the back portion of the heart, including the left upper chamber (left atrium) and aorta after it leaves the heart are difficult to image by directing the ultrasound waves through the front. The spinal column in the back creates additional barrier to penetration of ultrasound waves to and from the heart. In these situations, a miniaturized transducer is attached to a small instrument that can be inserted through the mouth into the esophagus, a procedure called *trans-esophageal echocardiogram* (or TEE).

TEE is done under moderate intravenous sedation and a topical anesthetic to numb the throat, minimizing any gagging or other discomfort. Since a portion of the esophagus is adjacent to the heart, it provides an excellent advantage to visualize the hidden or blind spots of the heart.

Intravascular Ultrasound vs. Coronary Angiography

For over three decades catheterization of coronary arteries by injecting a contrast material into the artery and taking X-rays of coronary artery branches (*coronary angiography*), has been considered the "gold standard" for diagnosing coronary artery disease. In my view, two major problems with coronary angiography have often been ignored.

- First, coronary angiography is based on X-ray pictures of the lumen, not the wall of the arteries. Think of coronary artery disease as a bagel; the problem is not in the hole, but in the thickened wall!

- Second, many studies have defined coronary artery disease as a greater than 50% occlusion of the lumen, and other studies define it as occlusion of a segment of the artery by more than 70%! So a vast majority of people with coronary artery disease are given the proverbial "clean bill of health" when, in fact, they may well have significant coronary artery disease. This hollow assurance that "your coronary artery is wide open," which I hear in my office quite frequently, gives people a false sense of security, and may make them complacent about dealing with their major coronary risk factors.

More recently, ultra-miniaturized ultrasound transducers have been developed. They can be inserted inside a small catheter and advanced through femoral artery (in the groin) into the coronary artery, similar to how it is done for coronary angiography. *Intravascular ultrasound imaging* (IVUS) technique provides high resolution views of the heart structures, and both the lumen and the wall of coronary artery. Now we can at last see and focus on the wall and not just the lumen!

Given the invasive nature and inherent pitfalls, cardiac catheterization should be reserved for urgent interventions to place stents in occluding or occluded arteries, or to provide a road map for the surgeon to determine which branches of coronary artery need bypass surgery. Thus for diagnosis of coronary artery disease or determination of plaque burden, people should no longer be subjected to cardiac catheterization without IVUS.

Doppler Echocardiogram and Vascular Imaging

Doppler ultrasound technique is another excellent noninvasive way to *assess the presence of any significant plaques in the wall of the arteries and of any abnormalities in blood flow through various large arteries or veins*. It is especially applicable to carotid arteries of the neck to detect occluding plaques, which may cause stroke; kidney arteries to detect narrowing of kidney arteries as a cause of hypertension; and the legs to detect any peripheral vascular disease. However, Doppler is unsuitable for assessment of coronary arteries, especially because of motion artifacts created by heart beats.

Magnetic Resonance Imaging (MRI)

Cardiovascular MRI is often referred to as *Cardiovascular Magnetic Resonance* or CMR. As a noninvasive procedure, CMR has added significant precision to cardiac testing. It provides excellent images of the heart structures, and the perfusion of the heart muscle when combined with dobutamine-induced stress. CMR is not yet suitable for assessment of coronary arteries due to small size of coronary artery branches, their twists and turns within the heart muscle, and the artifacts produced by the heart and respiratory motions.

Most of these limitations are being addressed so that within the next few years CMR may become a more accurate alternative to nuclear and radiographic imaging. At this time imaging larger arteries such as those of the kidneys, carotid or the brain, provides excellent information on the lumen and the wall of these arteries.

Electron-Beam Computed Tomography for Coronary Calcium (EBCT)

As you've read here, the coronary and cerebral artery plaques have many ingredients. They contain oxidized LDL-cholesterol debris, white blood cells, smooth muscle cells, and collagen (scar) fibers. Some plaques may randomly contain iron or calcium deposits.

Several years ago, some researchers thought measuring calcium content of coronary arteries by a modified CAT scanner (EBCT) might have a prognostic value. They believed that calcium deposits reflect the presence of advanced coronary artery disease, and that this might provide additional information about the course of coronary artery disease. So the entrepreneurial forces took over, proclaiming EBCT as the next best hope for prevention of a heart attack!

EBCT offers virtually no useful information to help prevent or treat coronary artery disease...

1. The vulnerability of atherosclerotic plaques to crack or rupture (responsible for about 80% of all heart attacks) does not depend on its calcium content. It depends on the fat content, inflammatory process, and oxidative turmoil within the plaque.

2. High calcium scores or content merely suggests the presence of coronary artery plaques, hence it suggests the obvious—people with coronary artery disease have a higher risk of a heart attack. Statin therapy (to lower cholesterol level) along with other risk factor modifications dramatically reduce the risk of a heart attack, at times by over 90%. Yet, the calcium score (content) may continue to rise and not reflect the stabilization or improvement in plaque structure.

3. Some people argue that detecting calcium deposits in the coronary artery proves that there is coronary disease and that people may become more active in fighting the disease. Unfortunately, many smokers with chronic lung disease, alcoholics with liver disease or cirrhosis, and people with severe obesity and multiple coronary risk factors, are aware of their self-destructive behaviors and do not take the necessary steps to help themselves. A negative or low coronary calcium score may create a false sense of security just as a negative ECG or exercise stress test might. This may also increase resistance to reasonable interventions to correct existing coronary risk factors, allowing the disease to progress unchecked.

4. EBCT costs about $500 to $600, and it is not reimbursable by most insurance carriers. Many commercial outfits with free-standing CAT scanners are also quite aggressive with

a bait-and-switch program of pushing a lung scan and abdominal scan for another $400 to $500 out-of-pocket.

Computed Tomographic (CT) Angiography

Imaging the coronary artery with a new generation of CAT scanner is a reliable and noninvasive technique for detection of significant coronary occlusion. After an intravenous injection of a contrast solution, rapid CAT scan of the heart and coronary heart branches is obtained.

This technique has been immensely helpful in emergency room settings where patients are brought in with chest pain and the suspicion of a heart attack. Immediate 64-slice CT of the heart and coronary artery can accurately exclude significant narrowing or thrombosis (blood clot) in the lumen of the artery.

More than two-thirds of such patients (whose coronary artery narrowing is under 25%) can be discharged rather than waiting in the ER for 24 hours for the results of repeated blood tests and ECGs. Patients with coronary narrowing of over 70 (about 10% of cases) may be sent for coronary catheterization and placement of stents or for bypass surgery. The remainder (about 25% of cases) with coronary artery narrowing between 25% to 70% will require a stress nuclear imaging, which can help doctors decide on the best treatment. One major drawback of super fast CT angiography is that it does not provide meaningful information about the wall of coronary artery or the extent of any plaques therein. It is more suitable for use as a tool to exclude a significant occlusive disease.

What About "Other" Blood Tests?

C-reactive protein (CRP): CRP is a protein compound produced by the liver in response to any inflammation or infection in the body, whether acute or chronic, bacterial or viral. In the absence of apparent inflammation or infection, a raised blood level of CRP is a surrogate for inflammation within the vascular tree, including coronary artery. Thus CRP is not risk factor for coronary artery disease; instead it is a risk marker, telling us there is active inflammatory turmoil somewhere within the vascular tree.

Does this information help us? Perhaps not! Recent studies have shown that CRP provides no further prognostic information beyond the 20 risk factors. Still, when CRP is greater than 3 mg/l, it may suggest a more active vascular turmoil, and is associated with a higher risk of stroke and unstable angina. Thus periodic testing for CRP might help in ruling out an active inflammatory vascular process, or perhaps encourage the healthcare provider to be more aggressive in treating various risk factors.

Minor risk factors such as elevated fibrinogen (a potent clotting factor), gout and persistently elevated white blood cells may play a small part in aggravating preexisting cardiovascular diseases. An overactive thyroid may contribute to atrial fibrillation even in young people, but not coronary artery disease. An underactive thyroid can significantly raise the LDL-cholesterol and triglycerides, making a bad situation worse. Blood tests are needed to rule out other potential co-conspirators for these reasons.

So What Is the Single Best Test to Let Me Know if I Have Coronary Artery Disease?

In a disease with 20 major risk factors and a slow destructive course that smolders for many years, no single noninvasive test can detect the ongoing inflammatory process or nonocclusive plaques within the wall of the arteries. Thus you should use tables fff and ggg to provide you with a reliable estimate of your risk for a future cardiovascular event.

For an urgent diagnosis, CT angiography is a quick, noninvasive, and accurate test to exclude obstructive plaques or a significant occlusion of the lumen of an artery by a recent blood clot (thrombosis).

For non-urgent cases or to find out if you have moderate to advanced coronary plaques, MRI angiography, once some technical problems are solved, should be a reasonable noninvasive test.

The gold standard for the invasive diagnosis of coronary artery disease at any stage is intravascular ultrasound (IVUS). ❦

GLOSSARY

Angiography—Injecting a dye into an artery and taking X-ray pictures to check for narrowing or clogging of the arteries.

Angioplasty—Removing debris from the clogging and plaques in the arterial wall to open or at least widen the lumen of an artery. This is usually done through special catheters inserted into the arteries. At times, tiny balloons are passed through these catheters and placed within the narrow segments of the vessels. By gently dilating the balloons repeatedly, some narrow segments can be dilated to allow an adequate blood flow. This is called "balloon angioplasty."

Apoproteins—Also called apolipoproteins (or apo). These important proteins are the "managers" or the "drivers" of lipoprotein-cholesterol molecules. They direct where the good or bad cholesterol particles go, and what they do. The important apoproteins are: apo A-1, which is carried by HDL-cholesterol and is cardio-protective, and apo B-100, which is carried by LDL-cholesterol and is damaging to the inner wall of the arteries.

Arteriosclerosis—Hardening (= sclerosis), thickening, and loss of elasticity of the arteries, due to degenerative changes.

Atherogenic—Having the potential to cause atheroma formation (see **atheroma**).

Atheroma—An area of the arterial wall that is bulging with a collection or deposits of various substances. Atheroma is commonly made up of blood platelets, white blood cells that have gobbled up and are engorged with oxidized-cholesterol (foam cells), dysfunctional smooth muscle cells, and deposits of collagen fibers and various minerals, such as iron, calcium, copper, etc. Rupture of an atheroma is the principal cause of heart attack.

Atherosclerosis—When there are numerous atheromas along the arterial tree, especially in coronary arteries or brain arteries, the condition is referred to as atherosclerosis.

Cis and trans fatty acids—The molecules of fatty acids are arranged like bracelets or chains made up of carbon atoms. Hydrogen atoms dangle from these carbon atoms like charms on a bracelet. When hydrogen atoms are on one side (up or down) of unsaturated carbons in a polyunsaturated fat, it is called a cis form. Cis fatty acids are usually liquid at room temperature. When the hydrogen atoms are on both sides (up and down) of the chain, it is called a trans fatty acid (Figure 13-B). Trans fatty acids are produced during the hydrogenation process of vegetable oils, and are usually solid or semisolid at room temperature.

243

Cholesterol—One of many fatty substances in blood and tissues of all animals. No plant contains cholesterol.

Cholesterol look-alikes—These are plant versions of cholesterol that are called phytosterols (phyto=plant). Phytosterols are usually not absorbed by the human intestine. They also reduce or block the absorption of dietary cholesterol.

Coronary Artery Disease (CAD)—When any segment or branch of the heart's artery (= coronary artery) is distorted or clogged (either partially or more extensively), the condition is referred to as coronary artery disease or atherosclerosis of the coronary artery.

Coronary Heart Disease (CHD) (or ischemic heart disease)—When CAD has progressed and caused certain coronary events such as angina (chest pain), heart failure, or heart attack, it is called CHD. Since in CHD the damage to heart muscle is the result of poor circulation (ischemia), Europeans often refer to it as "ischemic heart disease."

Down-regulating—Slowing down, suppressing, inhibiting.

Endogenous—Produced within the human body.

Endothelium—The thin inner lining of arteries made up of a single layer of cells. Injury to, or dysfunction of, the endothelium is the first and the most important step in the development of coronary artery disease.

Enzyme—Important substance within the human body that facilitates a variety of functions, without which the body cannot function.

Essential—When used in the context of the human body, it implies that it must be provided through dietary intake, since the body cannot produce it. Some amino acids and fatty acids are "essential" for the body's function, but carbohydrates or most fats are not.

Exogenous—Provided from outside the body, such as through diet or in the form of medications or supplements (the opposite of endogenous).

Fatty Acids—These are the smaller by-products of the breakdown or digestion of various fats. There are several kinds of fatty acids. When one molecule of fatty acids is joined to one molecule of glycerol, it is called "monoglyceride." When two or three fatty acids are attached to one molecule of glycerol, they form "diglycerides" and "triglycerides." If the carbon molecules in fatty acids are fully occupied with hydrogen atoms, they are called saturated, otherwise they are unsaturated.

Foam cells—These white blood cells, called "monocytes," reside inside the wall of the arteries and gobble up large amounts of LDL-cholesterol. When viewed under a microscope, the cholesterol-laden monocytes look foamy or bubbly, hence the name.

Free Radicals, also Oxygen Free Radicals, Superoxides, and Hydroxyl Radicals—Each living cell, especially in humans and higher animals, is a nonstop microscopic factory where hundreds of biochemical reactions are constantly taking place. During these activities, certain unstable and toxic by-products are produced which are referred to as "free radicals." Some free radicals have very unstable oxygen atoms, hence oxygen free radicals. Normally, almost all of these unstable by-products are immediately neutralized within the cells by other chemicals, enzymes, and reactions. Excessive production or inadequate neutralization of these free radicals may have important roles in certain cancers, damage to the heart muscle, liver, lungs, and many other organs (see **Oxidize**).

Hydrogenation—A processing technique in which hydrogen atoms are added to unsaturated fatty acids. This is done to convert a liquid fat (oil) into a solid fat which improves its stability and shelf life. During partial hydrogenation of natural oils, a number of trans fatty acids are produced which are actually harmful. Recent advances in food technology have enabled margarine manufacturers to produce some spreads with very little or no trans fatty acids (see **Cis and trans fatty acids**).

Lipids—Various fatty substances, including those in blood circulation, such as cholesterol, lipoproteins, etc.

Lipoproteins—These are tiny pellets that contain various fats (lipids) and proteins (hence, lipoproteins). Lipoproteins are nature's "limousines" for cholesterol to ride on and be transported throughout the body. The more protein they have, the denser they are. Conversely, higher concentrations of various fats make them less dense, very much like lean versus fatty meats. Based on their density, they are classified as very low density lipoproteins (VLDL) with the highest fat, to intermediate density lipoproteins (IDL), low density lipoproteins (LDL), and high density lipoproteins (HDL) with the lowest amount of fat and highest concentration of protein (Figure 1).

Macrophages—see **Monocytes**.

Monocytes—These are specialized human white blood cells which often play the role of scavengers in various tissues. Larger monocytes are called macrophages and act like a biological "pac-man," clearing debris, oxidized cholesterol, etc. from various sites in the human body.

Morbidity—Complications and disabilities of a disease.

Mortality—Death rate from a given disease. Mortality can be expressed per 100, 1,000, or 10,000 cases, depending on how common the death rate is for a given disease.

N-3 and N-6 polyunsaturated fatty acids (PUFA)—also called omega-3 and omega-6 PUFA (Figure 13). If the first double bond (unsaturated carbon) of a PUFA is three carbons away from the left end of the chain, it is called an n-3, or omega-3 PUFA. If the first double bond is six carbons away, it forms an n-6 PUFA. The position of this first double bond confers profoundly different biological functions to PUFA (Chapter 3, "Omega-6 Polyunsaturated Fat" through "Omega-3 Polyunsaturated Fat").

Omega-3 and Omega-6 polyunsaturates—see above.

Oxidants (or Oxidizing Agents)—Any compound that gives up oxygen, or attracts hydrogen or electrons from another compound. Antioxidants inhibit or reduce these reactions.

Oxidize—To combine with oxygen, or to give up hydrogen or electrons. A compound is oxidized when it is combined with oxygen, or coerced to give up hydrogen or electrons. Oxidation should not be confused with oxygenation. The browning of an apple after a bite or rusting of a nail are examples of oxidation.

Oxygenation—The process of delivering oxygen to various tissues. Since oxygen is carried by red blood cells, uninterrupted blood circulation is essential for tissue oxygenation.

Polymerization—Most fats, especially polyunsaturated fatty acids, form larger molecules or polymers when exposed to relatively high temperatures. Polymerization reduces the bioavailability of polyunsaturated fatty acids, making them less absorbable.

Psyllium (pronounced silly-om)—A water soluble fiber from the husk of a plant. Psyllium is used as a supplement (or is in some cereals) to provide additional fiber to the diet.

Receptor Activity and Receptor Sites—To work properly in the human body, many chemical and biochemical substances must enter various cells through specific receiving docks or entrances. These entrances are called "receptors" or "receptor sites." If an adequate number of receptors are not available, or have already been occupied ("competitively") by other substances, then the receptor activity is low. For example, a low receptor activity for LDL-cholesterol will prevent LDL particles from entering the liver and other tissues for disposal. Under these circumstances, LDL-cholesterol particles have no place to "dock," so they return to blood circulation and raise the blood cholesterol level. In some cases, there are plenty of LDL receptors, but because they are defective, or "mutants," they cannot allow LDL particles to enter liver cells. So far, over 350 mutant or abnormal types of LDL receptors have been identified.

Responder and Nonresponder—In medicine, these terms are used to identify individuals who will or will not respond to a particular form of treatment or intervention. For example, many people are salt nonresponders, meaning that no matter how much salt they eat, it will not affect their blood pressure. Similarly, about 70% of the population are cholesterol nonresponders whose blood cholesterol levels will not rise appreciably with cholesterol feeding.

Sterols—The basic skeleton of certain chemicals made in animal or plant tissues. Cholesterol is a sterol that is produced in animal tissues only.

The plant version of sterol or its cholesterol look-alike is called phytosterol (phyto = plant).

Superoxides—Potent oxidants that are generated within human tissues, usually under metabolic stress (see **Oxidants**).

T-lymphocytes or T-cells—Special white blood cells which are enormously important in defending against various bacterial and viral infections. When the number of T-cells is abnormally low, immune defenses are broken down, making an individual very susceptible to infections and certain cancers.

Thrombogenic—Having the potential to cause a thrombosis, or clotting of the blood inside the arteries or veins.

Thrombosis—Clotting of blood inside an artery or a vein. Thrombosis of a coronary artery chokes off the circulation, causing a heart attack. The same process in a cerebral artery results in a stroke, whereas a thrombosis in a vein results in phlebitis.

TPA Tissue Plasminogen Activator—One of the most potent clot-busting anti-coagulants. TPA is the drug used in emergency departments as soon as someone with a heart attack (or coronary thrombosis) arrives. The goal is to dissolve the clot and open up the artery's lumen before severe, irreversible damage to the heart muscle occurs.

Trans fatty acids—see **Cis** and **trans fatty acids**.

INDEX